Schriftenreihe Neurologie
Neurology Series 21

M. Oehmichen

Mononuclear Phagocytes in the Central Nervous System

Origin, Mode of Distribution, and Function of Progressive Microglia, Perivascular Cells of Intracerebral Vessels, Free Subarachnoidal Cells, and Epiplexus Cells

Translated by Margaret M. Clarkson

With 38 Figures

Springer-Verlag
Berlin Heidelberg New York 1978

Privatdozent Dr. Manfred Oehmichen
Institut für Gerichtliche Medizin
Postfach 1749, D-7400 Tübingen

ISBN-13: 978-3-642-46387-7 e-ISBN-13: 978-3-642-46385-3
DOI: 10.1007/978-3-642-46385-3

Library of Congress Cataloging in Publication Data. Oehmichen, Manfred. Mononuclear phagocytes in the central nervous system. (Neurology series; 21) Bibliography: p. Includes index. 1. Central nervous system. 2. Monocytes. 3. Microglia. I. Title. II. Series: Schriftenreihe neurologie; 21. [DNLM: 1. Central nervous system—Cytology. 2. Central nervous system—Physiology. 3. Phagocytes—Cytology. 4. Phagocytes—Physiology. 5. Neuroglia. Wa SC344 Bd. 21/WL300.3 028m] QP370.02713 599'.01'88 78-15718

Softcover reprint of the hardcover 1st edition 1978

Offsetprinting and Binding: Brühlsche Universitätsdruckerei, Lahn-Gießen 2123/3130-543210

Preface

A number of years ago Prof. J. Peiffer (Tübingen/FRG) asked whether cerebrospinal fluid cells originate in blood cells. With this question, the first seeds were sown for the research which resulted in this book. The original question was eventually expanded to whether extravascular hematogenous cells are present in the nervous system. In the course of my research this question became more and more concentrated on the demonstration of monocyte derivatives (i.e., mononuclear phagocytes) within the nervous system.

While these questions are certainly not new, they regularly crop up when microglia are to be classified, particularly progressive microglia. Three extensive surveys were published during the past few years, all of which arrived at different conclusions (Cammermeyer, 1970b; Vaughn and Skoff, 1972; Fujita and Kitamura, 1976). In addition to progressive microglia, other active phagocytes were observed which I refer to as "perivascular cells," "free subarachnoidal cells," and "epiplexus cells." These cells were seldom described in the literature, and then predominantly in another context. A presentation based on the hypothesis that the cell types of the central nervous system have potentially identical kinetics and functional potency has not been published.

My study was purposely constructed to exclude some possible misinterpretations made by other authors resulting from unavoidable errors that might have occurred in the various methods. I also tried to obtain additional information by using other methods. The experiments, some of which were extremely elaborate, were carried out during my seven-year association with the Institute for Brain Research, University of Tübingen (Tübingen/FRG) and were supported in part by the Deutsche Forschungsgemeinschaft. During the course of the years the methods, and therefore also the experimental models, were necessarily altered.

Various observations presented in the literature as well as my own findings associated with the problem of whether there is evidence for the presence of mononuclear phagocytes within the nervous system are summarized in this book. My research tends to indicate that such evidence exists. As the author, I am fully aware that these conclusions are just as dependent on the methods used as were the conclusions of the other authors cited. This book therefore should not be considered a definitive work on the subject, but rather a *starting point* and a *work paper* for discussion of many problems which I feel are extremely important for all immunologic questions involving the specific or nonspecific inflammatory reactions in the context of pathogen and tumor defense and the development of autoimmune diseases. A compilation of individual findings, some of which have already been published elsewhere, seemed justified since this made a comprehensive survey of the problem of mononuclear phagocytes in the nervous system possible.

These experiments were made possible with the support and help of the following people: Mr. Helmut Grüninger, demonstrator at the Institute for Brain Research, Uni-

Mrs. Mira Gencic, medical technologist at the Institute for Brain Research, University of Tübingen, who provided both practical assistance and emotional support; Dr. M. E. Greaves (London/England), Prof. H. Huber (Innsbruck/Austria), Dr. Y. Narita, university instructor (Tokyo/Japan), Drs. R. Saebisch, G. Schütze, W. Treff, H. Wiethölter (Tübingen/FRG), and Prof. A. Torvik (Oslo/Norway), all of whom worked with me on various experiments; Prof. J. Peiffer, Director of the Institute for Brain Research, University of Tübingen, who offered both encouragement and constructive criticism; Prof. W. Schlote, Director of the Department for Submicroscopic Pathology and Neuropathology at the Institute of Pathology, University of Tübingen, who continuously offered sound and practical advice. I would also like to express my gratitude to all those colleagues and assistants at the Institute for Brain Research, who, either directly or indirectly, were responsible for the technical execution of these experiments. I am especially grateful to Ms. Margaret Clarkson for translating the manuscript into English. This book could not have been published without the financial support of the Schaper and Brümmer Pharmaceutical Company (Salzgitter/FRG). Therefore I am particularly indebted to Prof. M. Földi, Director of the research department of Schaper and Brümmer. I would also like to express my gratitude to Dr. H. Selzer (Private Clinic for Multiple Sclerosis, Schönmünzach/FRG) for his generosity. Most of all, I would like to thank my wife Bri and my children Holger and Kim for their patience and understanding during the long years of research.

Tübingen, Summer 1978 MANFRED OEHMICHEN

Contents

Abbreviations

ADPase: adenosine diphosphatase
AGG: aggregated gamma globulin
AHGG: anti-human gamma globulin from goats
AHGR: anti-human gamma globulin from rabbits
AMGG: anti-mouse gamma globulin from goats
ANA-esterase: α-naphthyl acetate esterase
APase: acid phosphatase
ARGG: anti-rabbit gamma globulin from goats
ATPase: adenosine triphosphatase
C: complement
CNS: central nervous system
Cr: chromium
CSF: cerbrospinal fluid
DPNase: diphosphopyridine nucleotide diaphorase
E: washed sheep erythrocytes
EA: sheep erythrocytes sensitized by sheep erythrocyte antibodies produced in rabbits
EA-IgG: sheep erythrocytes sensitized by the immunoglobulin G fraction of sheep erythrocyte antibodies produced in rabbits
EA-IgM: sheep erythrocytes sensitized by the immunoglobulin M fraction of sheep erythrocyte antibodies produced in rabbits
EN: sheep erythrocytes sensitized with neuraminidase
^{3}H-DFP: diisopropyl fluorophosphate labeled with tritium
^{3}H-TdR: thymidine labeled with tritium
IgG: immunoglobulin G
M: median
MP: mononuclear phagocyte
MPS: mononuclear phagocyte system
NASA-esterase. naphthol AS acetate esterase
NAS-DCA-esterase: naphthol AS-D chloroacetate esterase
PAS: periodic acid Schiffs reaction
PBS: phosphate buffered saline
RES: reticuloendothelial system
SRBC: sheep red blood cells
Succ.ase: succinic dehydrogenase
SD: standard deviation
TPNase: triphosphopyridine nucleotide diaphorase
UDPase: uridine diphosphatase
VBS: veronal buffered saline
VD: variability coefficient

Introduction

The central nervous system is isolated from the rest of the body by virtue of its location (enclosed in the skull and surrounded by dura mater) and its functional characteristics (barrier mechanisms such as the blood-brain barrier). These factors could provide a partial explanation for the varied reactions of the central nervous system to different noxae. Moreover, the general nervous system (i.e., central and peripheral nervous systems) is characterized by highly differentiated cell types and cell functions typical for this system. A comparison is not always possible especially between these specific cell reactions and reactions of other cells. Such specific cell reactions include the mode of removal of endogenous waste products (e.g., siderin in a cerebral hemorrhage) and exogenous corpuscles or antigens (e.g., viral). In other words, there are typical reactions for this particular system during the course of nonspecific and specific inflammatory processes.

In addition to these characteristic reactions of the nervous system, criteria are present under inflammatory conditions that permit a comparison between these reactions and reactions in other areas of the body. Extravascular erythrocytes, therefore, are considered endogenous in the central nervous system, but waste products outside the vessels since they must be removed. Migrated bacteria, however, are considered foreign protein because they stimulate the formation of antibodies and an antigen-typic cell reaction.

It is important that organ-specific reactions be distinguished from general reaction patterns to facilitate the theoretical treatment of the question and to deal with the relevant therapeutic consequences and procedures. Cytologically, the classification of the various cell types appearing during the course of inflammatory processes according to cell reactions raises the questions of where certain cells in a cell reaction originate and of the appearance of these cell types.

For the most part, it has been accepted that granulocytes, lymphocytes, and monocytes are the typical cell components involved in a general inflammatory reaction. Granulocytes and lymphocytes can usually be definitely recognized by their morphology. However, monocytes and macrophages, recently classified under the term "mononuclear phagocytes," are often difficult to identify because of their highly varied polymorphism. The location of the cell as well as developmental and functional conditions, for example, influence polymorphism. The appearance of monocytes within nerve tissue has been discussed, but their demonstration in damaged and undamaged nerve tissue has usually been disputed or not dealt with.

The purpose of this study is to clarify whether cells are present in normal or damaged nerve tissue that, in terms of their kinetics and function, could be derived from monocytes and/or macrophages. A detailed presentation is made of the problem itself together with the results of current research. A description of the author's own investigations then follows this background information. Finally, the author's investigations are discussed in the light of findings published by other researchers.

A. Formulation of the Problem and Relevant Literature

As mentioned above, the question has recently been raised as to whether or not extravascularly located, so-called mononuclear phagocytes (MP) are present in the central nervous system (CNS) and/or the peripheral nervous system (PNS). In order to approach the problem, the *current situation* in which the question has developed is discussed; the *morphologic studies conducted in the past* which interpreted the problem similarly are summarized. Finally, on the basis of the available literature a *synopsis* of the classification of a series of highly active phagocytic cells in the CNS is presented. Unfortunately, a certain amount of repetition could not be avoided in working through the relevant literature under these various aspects.

I. "Mononuclear Phagocyte System"

On the basis of recent electron-microscopic, enzyme-histochemical, cell kinetic, and immunologic findings, a group of authors associated with Van Furth have suggested the term "mononuclear phagocyte system" (MPS) (Langevoort et al., 1970). In spite of all qualifying criticism, most authors after 1970 tended to accept this term (e.g., Van Furth et al., 1972, 1975; Page et al., 1974; Warr and Sljivic, 1974; Jzumi et al., 1975; Widmann and Fahimi, 1975; Volkman, 1976; Meuret, 1977). Some of the cells included in this system had been previously classified under other terms or in the "reticuloendothelial system" (RES) of Aschoff (1924).

Mononuclear cells of the MPS are cells with similar morphology, kinetics, and function which possess pronounced phagocytic activity, even if they came from different locations or were previously classified under a different nomenclature. The following three developmental and functional conditions were differentiated according to origin and location: promonocyte (bone marrow) → monocyte (peripheral blood) → macrophage (tissue). The so-called macrophages (Metschnikoff, 1891) are found in almost all tissues and organs. The descriptive terms given to them vary considerably, e.g., histiocyte (connective tissue); Kupffer's cell (liver); osteoclast (bone); alveolar and peritoneal macrophages; free and fixed macrophages in the spleen, lymph nodes, bone marrow, and mesangial cells (renal glomerulus, see Camazine et al., 1976). Under pathologic conditions epitheloid cells and polynuclear giant cells could originate from monocytes and/or macrophages (Goldstein, 1959; Papadimitriou et al., 1973; Mariano and Spector, 1974). For some of the above-mentioned cell types, only a few isolated findings tend to indicate that these cells belong to the monocyte-macrophage series. Reticular cells, dendritic cells in the follicles of the spleen and the lymph nodes, endothelial cells, and fibroblasts can definitely be *excluded* from this series because of their different functions, kinetics, and morphology.

Even though this term has been extensively applied to a cell series and, therefore, has more or less found acceptance, an exact definition of a mononuclear phagocyte is difficult to formulate (see also Gesner and Howard, 1967). *Morphologic findings* are of almost no help whatsoever. The difference in location and the developmental and functional conditions are responsible, in part, for the wide range of variations. It is precisely the difficulty of recognizing common morphologic criteria which calls the uniformity of such a cell system into question. Some authors considered argyrophilia (Marshall,

1956) and ruffling of the plasma membrane demonstrated by phase contrast or electron microscopy (Hirsch and Fedorko, 1970; Deams and Bredereoo, 1970) to be relatively specific morphologic characteristics.

Kinetic findings, however, are constant and, together with the functional observations, formed the rationale for coining this classification. As mentioned above, transformation stages of blood monocytes that originate from bone marrow (Volkman and Gowans, 1965a, b; Van Furth and Cohn, 1968; Van Furth, 1976) are found in all cell types included in the mononuclear phagocyte system. After differentiation, these cells showed only a slight tendency toward proliferation in the tissue or in the peripheral blood. The ability to divide locally, however, can be stimulated under certain circumstances (Forbes, 1966; North, 1969; Spector, 1970; More et al., 1973). Apparently, macrophages survive for a relatively long period of time in the tissue and, under certain pathologic conditions, can recirculate via the blood stream or the lymphatic system (Roser, 1965, 1968, 1970a, b).

The uniform *functional characteristic* is the ability for phagocytosis and pinocytosis. Observation of phagocytosis stimulated by incubating cells with colloidal solutions (Gosselin, 1956) and the lysosomal enzyme content (Cohn, 1970) proved to be relatively specific. The tendency to adhere to glass (Bennett and Cohn, 1966) and the presence of surface receptors for IgG subfractions 1 and 3 as well as for the third component of the complement (Huber et al., 1970; Shevach et al., 1973; Huber and Holm, 1975) are also characteristic of mononuclear phagocytes. A series of typical reactions have also been observed for mononuclear phagocytes following administration of sera or drugs (for survey, see Leder, 1967; Nelson, 1969; Van Furth, 1970c, 1975; Roos, 1970; Carr, 1973).

The authors associated with Van Furth (1970c) questioned if cells are present in the nervous system (particularly microglia cells) which could be included in the "mononuclear phagocyte system." This question is particularly important for the neuropathologist since more and more highly differentiated functions concerning defensive immune responses to infection and tumors are being attributed to monocytes and macrophages (for survey, see Laskin and Lechevalier, 1972; Van Furth, 1975; Nelson, 1976; Fink, 1976; Mathé et al., 1976).

Conclusion

Variously located cells with the same origin and function are included under the term "mononuclear phagocyte system." The question arises if cells that morphologically, kinetically, and functionally resemble monocytes and macrophages from other areas of the body are also present in the nervous system. The relevant literature is so voluminous that only the important findings can be surveyed in the context of this study.

II. Literature Dealing with Mononuclear Phagocytes in the Central Nervous System

The evolution of the terminology and the understanding of the morphology, classification, and possible identical cytogenetics of phagocytes in the CNS from various locations is not only an important part of the history of neurocytology, neurohistology, and neuropathology, but also of the history of the development of special methods. The problem dealt with here is the same question that arose in the middle of the last century: Are phagocytic cells present in the CNS? If so, what do they look like and into which cell system should they be classified?

Phagocytic ability has been assumed for almost every cell type in the CNS: *nerve cells* in the fetal period (Matsuyama et al., 1975), *astrocytes* (Schwalbe, 1881; Friedmann, 1890; Nissl, 1899; Spielmeyer, 1922; Andrew, 1941; Niessing, 1954; Field, 1957; Blinzinger, 1968; Raisman, 1969; Robain, 1970; Davidoff, 1973), *oligodendrocytes* (Pruijs, 1927; Ferraro and Davidoff, 1928; Takano, 1964; Maxwell and Kruger, 1966; Schlote, 1970; Cook and Wisniewski, 1973; Davidoff, 1973), *ependymal cells* (Wüllenweber, 1924; Arnvig, 1948), *choroidal cells* (Van Rijssel, 1946; Kappers, 1953), and *endothelial cells* (Blinzinger, 1968a; Cancilla et al., 1972; Stenwig, 1972). Most of the relevant methods of demonstration tend to indicate that, after a given time, basically extracellular material can also be found intracellularly in the above-mentioned cell types. Whether this is an active process such as phagocytosis or passive diffusion is open to discussion.

The main problem, however, appears to be that of quantity. In the literature, a series of cells within the nerve tissue have been described which, in contrast to the above-mentioned elements, ingest and assimilate extracellular material much more quickly (in minutes or hours, instead of days and weeks) and in much larger quantities. These cells from various locations were referred to as "progressive microglia," "perivascular cells from intracerebral vessels," "free subarachnoidal cells," and "epiplexus cells."

1. Progressive Microglia

Gluge (1841) first described the mesodermal origin of phagocytic cells inside damaged brain tissue. He referred to these cells as "inflammatory corpuscles" *(Entzündungskugeln)* and suggested that they were derived from leukocytes. Later these cells were sometimes called "Gluge's corpuscles" (*Gluges-Kugeln,* see Ribbert, 1882). In 1846, Virchow also noted that mesenchymal cells participated in the glial reaction. In 1867, he used the term "foam cells" *(Schaumzelle)* for such cells; the term is still used today. In 1854, Virchow distinguished neurologia from nerve cells in general and referred to them as an independent cell type. In 1889, His suggested that nerve cells and neurologlia originated from different cell populations.

The discussion regarding the appearance of mesenchymal cells in the CNS began in 1881 when Schwalbe stated that glial cells could originate from mesoderm as well as from neuroectoderm (see also Friedmann, 1890). Stroebe (1894, see also Schmaus and Sacki, 1901) supported this hypothesis after he observed two cell types that appeared at different times following traumatic brain damage. Shortly after the trauma, he observed segmented leukocytes containing cell components. Later he found cells that he designated phagocytizing "granule cells" *(Körnchenzellen)* or "granule corpuscles" *(Körnchenkugeln)*. After observing the glial reaction following brain damage, Nissl (1899) suggested that glial cells take over that function in brain tissue which would normally be carried out by macrophages in other areas of the body. He coined the term "rod cells" *(Stäbchenzelle)*. At about the same time, Robertson (1900a) postulated that local glial cells lose their prolongations after traumatic damage and then develop into granule cells. Within the same year (1900b), he was able to identify prolongations on "adendritic" cells in the CNS. He referred to these cells as "mesoglia" and suggested that they were precursors of the granule cells. Later Cajal (1920) also used the term mesoglia.

Capobianco (1901) established that large quantities of mesodermal elements appeared in the leptomeninges during the early postnatal period. Apparently the elements grew into the CNS with the invading vessels. According to Capobianco, these mesodermal elements, which had partially retained the ability for phagocytosis, transformed into neuroglial cells. Nissl (1903) reached a similar conclusion in his investigations. He suggested that phagocytes in the CNS originated from the adventitial connective tissue of the intracerebral vessels. He referred to these cells as "compound granular corpuscles" *(Gitterzelle)* (1904) and suggested that they, together with Langhans' giant cells and foreign-body giant cells, originated from the mesoderm. Since, for Nissl, an invasion through the intact limiting membrane (basement membrane) of the glia was highly improbable, he did not assume that compound granular corpuscles were derived from blood cells. Many authors after Nissl, however, have accepted the adventitial origin of these cells. Other authors (Minor, 1904; Devaux, 1908; Farrar, 1908) assumed that blood cells also participated to some extent in the early stages of the traumatic reaction. Even these authors, however, attributed most of the compound granular corpuscles to a local proliferation of adventitial connective tissue cells. A few authors (Kaufmann, 1904; Borst, 1904; Schmaus, 1904) did, however, consider leukocytes basically precursors of phagocytes in the CNS. Pick (1904) suggested that phagocytes were derived from blood, adventitial connective tissue, and local glial cells. Other authors (Forster, 1908; Marchand, 1909) followed Nissl (1899) and Robertson (1900a) and concluded that phagocytes originated from neuroglial cells. Merzbacher, who coined the term "scavenger cell" *(Abräumzelle)* in 1910, must also be included in this group.

These considerations were based almost entirely on observations of phagocytic ability, location, frequency of mitosis, and morphology of cells in the CNS under normal and pathologic conditions as demonstrated by nonspecific stains. Selective staining of astrocytes with gold mercuric chloride solutions was first made possible by Cajal's technique (1913a, b). Cajal demonstrated a third cell type in addition to nerve cells and glial cells in the sense of astrocytes. For lack of a better term, he referred to these cells as the "third element of the CNS" and suggested that they originated in the mesoderm.

With his silver carbonate staining method, Rio Hortega (1917) obtained a selective demonstration of two cell types in addition to nerve cells and astroglial cells (macroglial). He referred to these two cells types as "microglia" (1919a, b) and "oligodendroglia" (1921a). Whereas he identified oligodendroglia as neuroectodermal cells, he thought "microglia" originated in the mesoderm. As Capobianco in 1901, Rio Hortega also observed an accumulation of microglial cells in the leptomeninges of the tela choroidea superior and the pedunculus cerebri during the embryonic period. In the early stages of embryonic development, the cells migrated from these "fountains" or "sources" into the CNS along the blood vessels (see also Beletzky, 1932; Andersen and Matthiessen, 1966). A few microglial cells also invaded the brain tissue from the leptomeninges at other locations. According to Rio Hortega, these (basically resting) cells proliferate under pathologic conditions and became phagocytes of the CNS, so-called progressive microglia. To a lesser extent, these activated cells were also derived from adventitial cells of intracerebral vessels and from invading leptomeningeal cells (for survey, see Rio Hortega, 1921b, 1930a, b, 1932).

The precursor cells in the leptomeninges and/or in the adventitial connective tissue were cells with a nucleus similar to that of a lymphocyte. These cells were observed wherever large quantities of microglia were demonstrated. Rio Hortega (1939) referred to these cells, which were also capable of changing into macrophages, as "polyblasts" or "histiocytes" of the connective tissue. After Rio Hortega and Penfield (1927) had published a description of transformations from resting microglia to progressive microglia (compound granule corpuscles) many authors were willing to accept the idea that phagocytes in the CNS originated primarily from resting microglia (Asua, 1927; Bolsi, 1928; Cone, 1928) and only secondarily from adventitial cells and blood monocytes (Testa, 1928; Gozzano, 1931).

Independent of this classification of cells, almost all authors now tend to agree that resting microglial cells represent a uniform cell population identifiable via light microscopy (Niessing, 1952; Glees, 1955; Scheibel and Scheibel, 1958; Naoumenko and Feigin, 1963; Tsujiyam, 1963; Kreutzberg, 1966; Sjöstrand, 1966a, b; Cammermeyer, 1966; Hommes and Leblond, 1967; Ibrahim et al., 1968; Lewis, 1968; Feigin, 1969). After selective demonstration with Hortega method, resting microglia (Fig. 1A) can be recognized with light microscopy in nondamaged brain tissue as pleomorphic, elongated, or triangular cell bodies (perikaryon). These cell bodies possess a feltwork of fine, intertwining branches of cytoplasm which vary in size and number. The nucleus is oval or round. This cell can be observed in all species, although considerable species-specific variations can be found (Field, 1955; Cammermeyer, 1966, 1970b). Since microglial cells are also found in animals raised under sterile conditions (Cammermeyer, 1970b), they do not signify a pathologic condition. This cell type can be demonstrated in almost all regions of the CNS, except for those regions in which some researchearchers could not observe them with electron microscopy (e.g., facial nucleus: Toryik and Skjörten, 1971b; hypoglossal nucleus: Davidoff, 1973). This cell type is usually located perineuronally (Fig. 1B) and perivascularly (Rio Hortega, 1932; Cammermeyer, 1970b) in the gray matter (Figs. 1D and 2D). Approximately 5–10% of all nonneuronal cell nuclei in the neuropil can be identified as so-called microglial cells (cerebral cortex: Brownson, 1956; Pope, 1958; corpus callosum: Mori and Leblond, 1969; optic nerve: Vaughn and Peters, 1968; Stensaas, 1977; for survey, see Cammermeyer, 1970b).

In addition to the resting microglial cells of normal brain tissue, so-called progressive or activated microglia were described. These cells are actively phagocytic and, under pathologic conditions, may vary considerably in morphology. The cells usually possess an indented, darkly staining nucleus within a swollen body of cytoplasm (Fig. 1C). The processes may be fine or coarse and may vary in number depending on the thickness of the surrounding neuropil (Figs. 1D and 13A). Frequently, they can only be demonstrat-

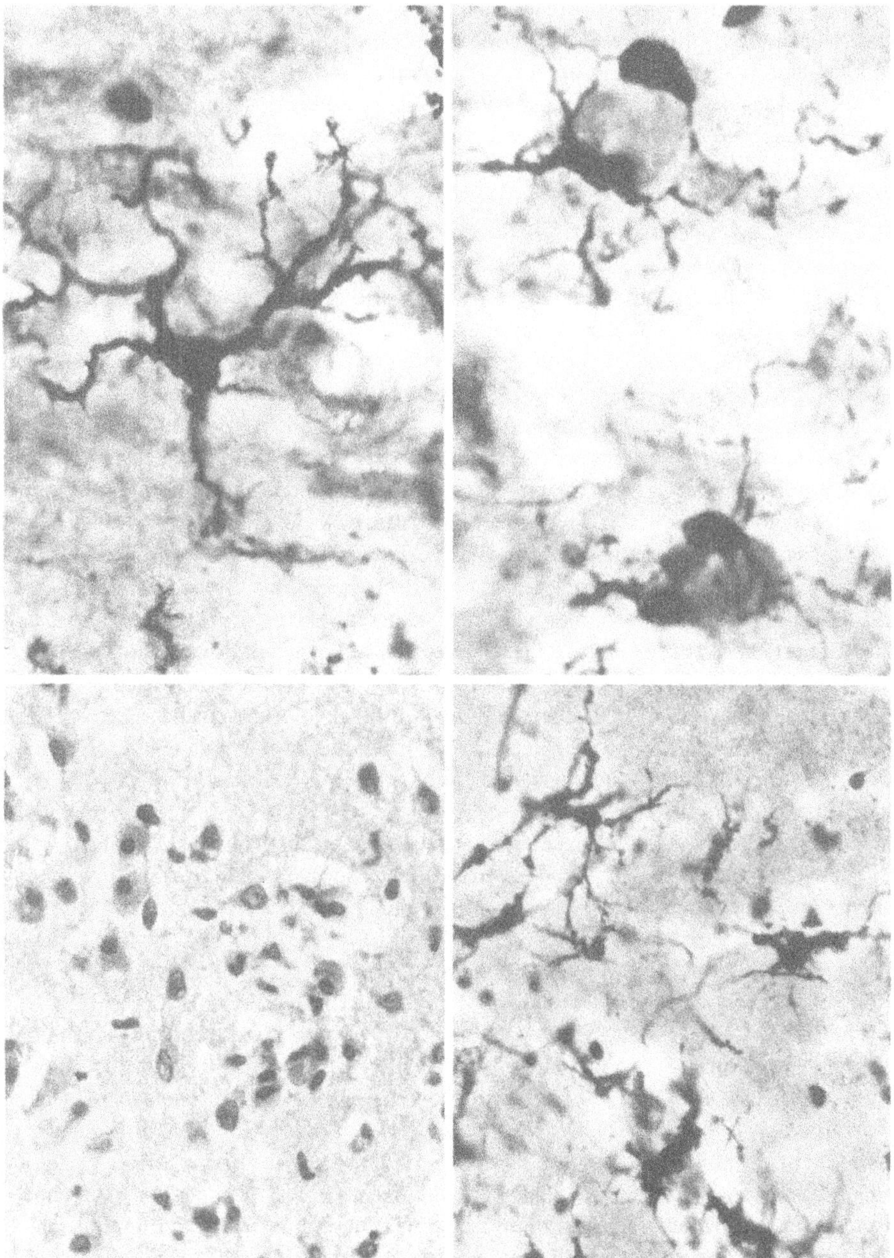

A B C D

Fig. 1 A–D. Microglia. (A) Resting microglia in cerebral white matter of rabbit. (B) Resting microglia in cortical region of rabbit (so-called perineuronal microglia). (C) Progressive microglia in viral encephalitis in man; note the morphologic similarity in the HE stain between microglia and macrophages. (D) Progressive microglia in rabbit following stab wound; note perivascular localization and irregular structure. [(A, B, D) author's modification of Weil and Davenport stain; (C) HE stain; magnification: (A and B) x 1200; (C and D) x 500] ed as pseudopodialike processes. These cells often contain phagocytized material composed in part of erythrocytes, iron, and fat.

These light-microscopic findings were questioned to some extent after the electron microscope was developed. Microglial cells could not be identified primarily with electron microscopy. After having classified astrocytes, oligodendrocytes, and nerve cells, several authors suggested that microglial cells were as yet unclassified small elements with high electron density (Farquhar and Hartmann, 1956; Luse, 1956; Schultz et al., 1957; Palay, 1958; Peters, 1960; De Robertis and Gerschenfeld, 1961; Gray, 1961, 1964; Bunge et al., 1962; Bodian, 1964; Coulter, 1964; Herndon, 1964; Mugnaini and Walberg, 1964). As a result, distinctly different cell types were described as microglial cells (see also the extensive discussion by Mori and Leblond, 1969). Mugnaini and Walberg (1965), Mori and Leblond (1969), and Peters and co-workers (1970) suggested that the darkly staining elements were fixation artifacts. Kruger and Maxwell (1966), however, suggested that the subtile differentiation of oligodendroglia and microglial cells could be demonstrated neither with electron microscopy nor with Hortega's impregnation method. They referred to the phagocytes observed under pathologie conditions as "reactive oligodendrocytes" (see also Caley and Maxwell, 1968).

Two groups of authors were able to make a clear-cut identification of microglia via electron microscopy. By preparing a series of ultrathin sections, Stensaas and Stensaas (1968) distinguished between microglial and oligodendroglial cells (see also Stensaas and Reichert, 1971; Ling et al., 1973). Using the silver impregnation method, Vogel and Kemper (1962) as well as Mori and Leblond (1969) identified these cells primarily as microglial cells via light microscopy. These authors then observed the same cells with the electron microscope. The descriptions of identical cells made by both groups of authors corresponded to previous descriptions from other authors (see below). Since other histologists, however, have been unable to observe this cell type, they concluded that no microglial cells were present in undamaged brain tissue (Malmfors, 1963, Eager and Eager, 1966; Wendell-Smith et al., 1966a, b; King, 1968; Sotelo and Palay, 1968; Caley and Maxwell, 1968; Kruger and Maxwell, 1969; King and Schwyn, 1970).

Based primarily on electron-microscopic observations, Vaughn and his co-workers (Vaughn and Peters, 1968; Vaughn, 1969; Peters et al., 1970; Vaughn et al., 1970; Vaughn and Pease, 1970; Skoff and Vaughn, 1971; Vaughn and Skoff, 1972) proposed a "third" ectodermal multipotential "glial cell type." This glial cell type was identical to the microglial cell described by other authors. After examining normal and degenerating optic nerves in rats, Vaughn and his co-workers suggested that the "third neuroglial element of the CNS" was a glioblast that could develop into an astrocyte or an oligodendrocyte in immature tissue. This cell type was also present in mature tissue, but to a lesser extent. Here it assumed the phagocytic function normally attributed to microglia. The description of this cell type also indicated that it was the same element that other authors had referred to as the microglial cell (see also Vaughn et al., 1970). During embryonic development, these "glioblasts" were usually found around the developing vessels and along the subpial border (Vaughn, 1969; Vaughn and Peters, 1971). Arguing on the basis of Fujita's (1965) autoradiographic investigations of the developing spinal cord in chicks, Vaughn and co-workers rejected a mesodermal origin. Fujita had concluded that cells inside the embryonic pia mater must be differentiated from subpial glioblasts and that no cells could migrate into the neuropil from the pia mater. Recently Fujita and Kitamura (for review, see 1976) found indications of two different cell types: resting microglia of unknown (mesenchymal?) origin and progressive microglia of monocytic origin. On the basis of other experiments, Das and Pfaffenroth (1976) also differentiated two cell types; both types (hematogenous and endogenous macrophages) were characterized by their excessive phagocytic activity under pathologic conditions.

The problems involved in making a clear-cut identification via electron microscopy motivated some authors to select other terms for the above-mentioned cell type, e.g., pericytial macrophage (Maxwell and Kruger, 1965), unidentifiable phagocyte (Mugnaini et al., 1967a, b; Westman, 1969), phagocytic glia (Wong-Riley, 1972), "M" cell (Matthews and Kruger, 1973b; Matthews, 1974), and multipotential glia (Vaughn and Peters, 1968; Kerns and Kinsman, 1973a).

With descriptions based on electron-microscopic observations from teams and individual authors (Blinzinger and Hager, 1962, 1964; Mugnaini et al., 1967b; Blakemore, 1969, 1972, 1975; Conradi, 1969; Privat and Leblond, 1972; Baron and Gallego, 1972; Wong-Riley, 1972; Ling et al., 1973; Phillips, 1973), a special cell type was identified as microglia of undamaged brain tissue. These resting microglial cells usually have a relatively small elongated or irregularly shaped nucleus with dense chromatin near the nuclear membrane. The perikaryon is unusually slender. The passage of the individual processes can rarely be demonstrated. The cytoplasm here is relatively dense compared with that of other cells in the CNS. It contains only a few endoplasmatic reticula, ribosomes and mitochondria, a well-developed Golgi apparatus, and several "dense bodies."

The so-called progressive microglia present under pathologic conditions were, for the most part, also consistently identified with electron microscopy (Blinzinger and Hager, 1962, 1964; Mugnaini et al., 1967a; Kirkpatrick, 1968; Blinzinger and Kreutzberg, 1968; Hager, 1968, 1975; Holländer et al., 1969; Fernando, 1971, 1973a; Torvik and Skjörten, 1971b; Stensaas and Gilson, 1972; Torvik, 1972; Torvik and Söreide, 1972; Bignami and Ralston, 1969). These cells usually possess an elongated, irregularly shaped nucleus and a slender perikaryon with short cytoplasmic processes. The cytoplasm are unusually dense and contain small round or oval mitochondria, Golgi membranes, and ribosomes. The endoplasmatic reticulum is characterized by long, twisted cisternae; lysosomes and a few cell inclusions of various sizes can be identified.

2. Perivascular Cells of Intracerebral Vessels

In 1871, Eberth first described perivascular cells and referred to them as "adventitia capillaries" or "vascular perithelium." Two years later, Rouget (1873, 1874, 1879) carefully investigated this cell type. He suggested that perivascular cells located in proximity to the capillaries assumed a contractile function for these vessels, which do not have muscle fibers. After this point, the cell was also called the "Rouget cell" (Vimtrup, 1922, 1923). Marchand (1898, 1924a, b) used the term "adventitial cell" for the same cell type. He also established its phagocytic ability and in 1924, therefore, he suggested that most macrophages were derived from perivascular cells. For this reason, he referred to all macrophages in general as "adventitial cells" (see also Mandelstamm and

Krylow, 1928). Aschoff (1924) included this cell type in his reticuloendothelial system because of its clear-cut phagocytic ability. He called such cells "histiocytes" (Aschoff and Kiyono, 1913, see also Cappel, 1929). For the same reasons, he referred to Maximow's cells (1927, 1928) as "resting wandering cells" or "primitive mesenchymal cells." Other authors used terms such as "pyrrole cell" (because of the affinity for pyrrole blue, Goldmann, 1913), "lipoid cell" (Ciaccio), "macrophage" (Nutschnikoff), "granule cell" (Tschaschin, 1914), "endothelial phagocyte" (Foot, 1925), and clasmocyte" (Kubie, 1927).

In 1922, Vimtrup accepted Rouget's theory regarding the contractile ability of this cell type (cf. Le Beaux and Willemot, 1978). Relying on experiments with vital stains developed in the meantime, the group of researchers with Vimtrup (Bensley and Vimtrup, 1928; Krogh and Vimtrup, 1932) tried to demonstrate the similarity between this cell type and muscle cells. Schaly (1926) also thought he observed transformation forms between these cells and smooth muscle tissue. On the basis of histochemical investigations, Landers and his co-workers (1962) concluded that pericytes could be considered the muscle cells of the capillaries.

Zimmermann (1923) convincingly questioned this hypothesis when he successfully obtained a selective demonstration of the cell type ("pericyte") with silver dichromate (for similar stains, see Aguirre, 1971; Stensaas, 1975). After the in vivo experiments conducted by Clark and Clark (1925, see also Ohno, 1924), another idea was suggested. These researchers noticed that a few of the temporarily migrating cells in the transparent tail of the tadpole adhered to the outer wall of the capillaries. When these cells rounded off and anchored their processes on the vessel, they were transformed into "Rouget cells." Clark and Clark identified these temporarily migrating cells as "fibroblasts." According to Benninghoff (1930), theories concerning the fibroblastlike nature of these cells were found as early as 1872 (Ranvier). Benninghoff (1926) observed that the cytoplasm of these perivascular cells in mammals was identical with that of the fibroblasts. He also noted that, with certain stimuli, the same cells could react like histiocytes and were able to incorporate vital stains. Using electron microscopy, the Han and Avery (1963) investigations tended to indicate that this cell type ought to be capable of fibrillogenesis. It was, therefore, assumed that such cells were most probably fibroblasts (see also Cliff, 1963).

The results of the investigations mentioned thus far have been almost exclusively obtained in vessels located outside the CNS. Plenk (1929; cf. Tschaschin, 1914) first referred *expressis verbis* to similar elements in the neighborhood of the intracerebral vessels. Compared with vessels in other parts of the body, special conditions were present that were characterized functionally by the blood-brain barrier and morphologically by the appearance of so-called perivascular spaces between the nerve tissue and the vascular wall. Pestalozzi (1849), Virchow (1851), and then Robin (1859) first described the perivascular space. This space has since been demonstrated repeatedly by staining experiments. Key and Retzius (1875) established the following information: The capillaries were composed of an endothelial duct surrounded externally by a fine, monostratified adventitial tube (see also Nissl, 1904; Held, 1909; who referred to the membrana limitans piae and limitans gliae). Quincke (1872), Binswanger and Berger (1898), as well as Lewandowsky

(1910) conducted similar experiments. Trying to maintain physiologic pressure conditions, Weed (1914a, b, 1923, 1938) instilled potassium ferrocyanide and ferric ammonium citrate into the subarachnoid spaces. He found iron in the pericapillary spaces only when the animal was permitted to bleed profusely during the injection. Other authors also questioned if the spaces were physiologic fissures (Schaltenbrand and Bailey, 1928). Later similar experiments employing the subarachnoid injection of a tracer (see Kubie, 1927; Mandelstamm and Krylow, 1928; Patek, 1944; Woollam and Millen, 1954, 1955; Lee and Olszewski, 1960) indicated that the inner surface of the space surrounding the vessels was probably an "inner reticular sheath" resting on the adventitia and was derived from the arachnoidea. The outer border zone was thought to be an "outer reticular sheath" derived from the pia mater; it extended to the marginal border glia. It was assumed that the two reticular sheaths anastomosed in the area of certain vascular sections, but these areas could not be localized. The question as to whether or not this space had a physiologic function could not be answered (Klatzo et al., 1965; Davson, 1967).

Electron-microscopic investigations contributed new insights regarding the presence of the perivascular space in brain tissue. Most authors (Nelson et al., 1962b; Hager, 1961; Frederickson and Low, 1969) described fissures along the walls of the small arteries and veins limited by basement membranes. One membrane was composed of astrocytes; the other, of endothelials (Maynard et al., 1957). These membranes are irregularly formed at birth (Donahue and Pappas, 1962; Caley and Maxwell, 1968; Hauw et al., 1975), and the barrier mechanisms are not yet fully developed at this time (Wenzel and Felgenhauer, 1976). Perivascular cells and their prolongations are localized between the limiting membranes. With the electron microscope, a communication was observed between the subarachnoid space and this perivascular space (Wagner et al., 1974). Apparently, the perivascular space tends to develop only where vessels containing adventitia formed by mesenchymal elements are present. If this adventitia is absent, both basement membranes degenerate and the perivascular space obliterates along the whole length of the vessel. Cerebral capillaries and the smallest veins do not have pericapillary spaces (Nelson et al., 1926b; Shimoda, 1961; Wolff, 1963; Hager, 1964). Wagner and co-workers (1974) noted that the basement-membrane duplication played an important role in the exchange of substances between the cerebrospinal fluid and the extracellular spaces in the brain as well as the intravascular fluid (see also Cancilla et al., 1972). Since the tracer used by these authors spread more rapidly along the capillaries than it did inside the neuropil, they suggested that an open space was present instead of the "obliterated" basement membranes of capillaries as had been assumed previously.

The actual space produced in the brain tissue by the formation of two basement membranes usually contained various quantities of cells. Their location tended to determine the cytomorphology (Fig. 2). Various attempts to classify and to summarize the contradictory morphologic (granular and agranular types: Cammermeyer, 1970b) and histochemical (see Landers et al., 1962; Ibrahim, 1974a, b; Cammermeyer, 1970b) observations made by some authors tend to indicate that elements from *two* cytogenetically different cell types were described and called pericytes, adventitial

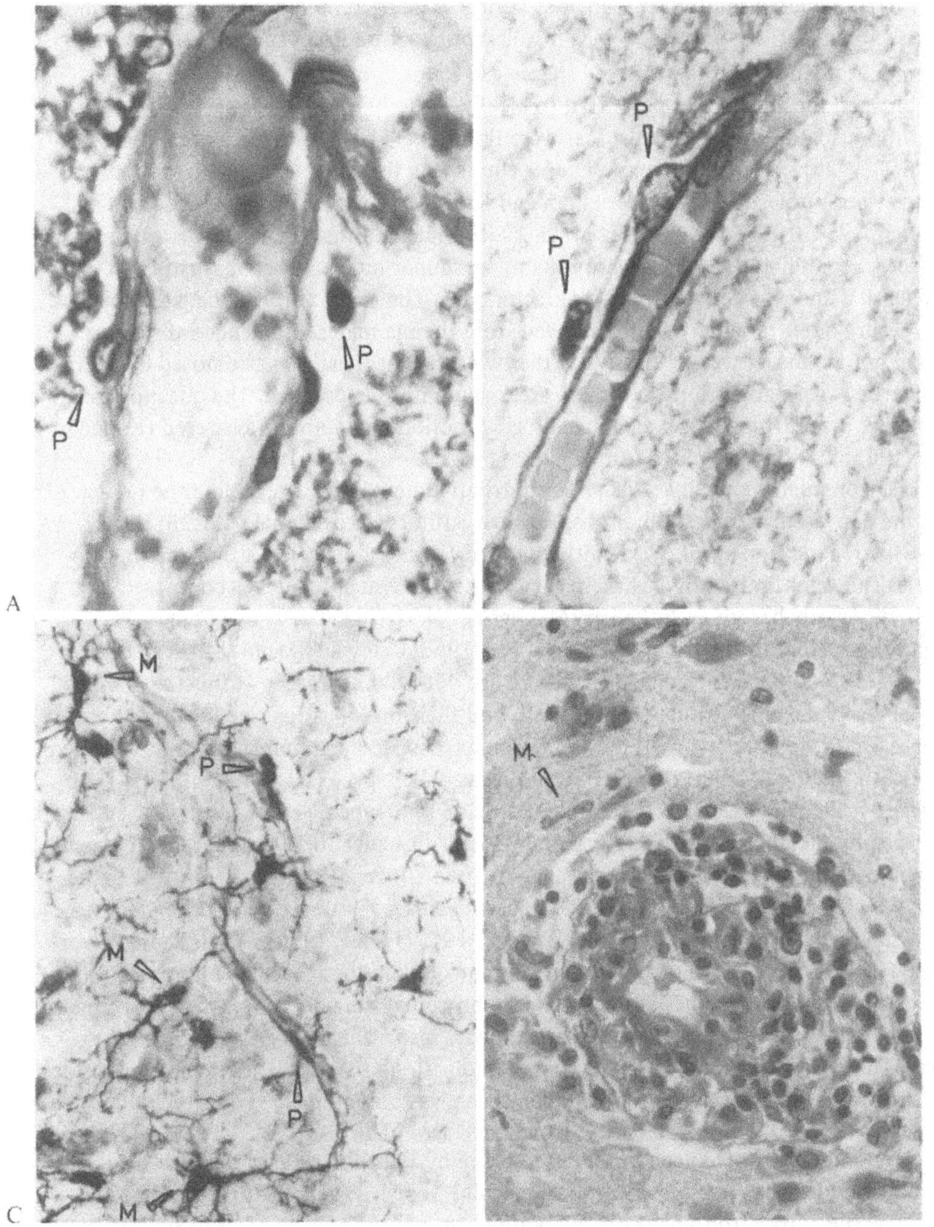

Fig. 2 A–D. Perivascular cells in intracerebral vessels around vein (A), around capillary (B), after demonstration of microglia (C), and under pathologic conditions of meningovascular syphilis (D). Note the different relationship of two perivascular cells (*P*) to the basement membrane in (A and B). In (C) the relationship of resting microglial cells (*M*) to the capillaries can be seen following silver impregnation; the perivascular cells (*P*) are also demonstrated. In (D) the number of perivascular cells is increased and the cells are activated; the number of perivascular microglia is also increased (*M*). Monocytelike cells can be seen in the outer areas of the perivascular space, where cytomorphologic transitions into progressive microglia are present in the neuropil [(A, B, D) HE stain; (C) author's modification of silver impregnation technique for microglia; magnification: (A and B) x 1200; (C and D) x 500]

cells, and/or perivascular cells. Their localization between the basement membranes is the only uniform characteristic of these cells (cf. Figs. 2A and B).

On the one hand, these cells were described as true "pericytes" (Zimmermann, 1923). This cell types is found only next to capillaries. Light-microscopic observations indicated that these cells contain two or more processes that are wound around the capillary surfaces. In contrast to the endothelial cells, the perinuclear zone of these cells penetrates the surrounding brain tissue rather than the vascular lumina. The nucleus contains more chromatin than the nucleus of endothelial cells (Maxwell and Kruger, 1965; Stensaas, 1975; Type I pericyte). Electron-microscopic observations indicate that a round or oval nucleus with uniformly distributed chromatin is characteristic of these cells. They usually have only a scanty margin of slightly staining cytoplasm. The cytoplasm itself contains some organelles, e.g., a few mitochondria, one or two bits of rough or smooth endoplasmatic reticula, a few dispersed filaments and ribosomes, a small Golgi apparatus, as well as a few vacuoles and dense bodies (Han and Avery, 1963; Wong-Riley, 1972; Lafarga and Palacios, 1975). When observed with the light or electron microscope, this cell type is not similar to resting or progressive microglia (Wong-Riley, 1972; Stensaas, 1975). This cell type exhibited no remarkable phagocytic activity.

In addition to the pericytic cell forms, a second cell type was described that is primarily found within the perivascular spaces of venules. For this cell type the ability to incorporate dyes via phagocytosis is particularly characteristic. The cell type is similar in certain respects to progressive microglia (McDonald, 1962; Wong-Riley, 1972; Wagner et al., 1974; Stensaas, 1975), even though it can be observed under normal conditions when no damage is present. Wagner and co-workers (1974) investigated the varied phagocytic behavior of cell types inside the basement membranes. They reported findings similar to those illustrated by the photographs from Cancilla and coworkers (1970, 1972) and Baker and co-workers (1971).

Even though a clear-cut differentiation of this second cell type cannot be made at present with the light microscope [granular type: Cammermeyer (1970b)?; acid phosphatase-positive cell: Barka and Anderson (1962)?; autofluorescent cell: Fleischhauer (1964)?; PAS-positive cell: Fleischhauer (1964); Ashton (1966)?; lipid-containing cell: Cerletti (1910); Dunning and Furth (1935); or Törö (1942)?], certain criteria can be established with electron microscopy. The chromatin is more dense around the nuclear membrane, and the cytoplasm contains more organelles (i.e., rough and smooth endoplasmatic reticula, mitochondria, free ribosomes, dense bodies, varying amounts of vesicles). This cell type was also described as resembling free subarachnoidal cells (Pease and Schultz, 1958; Cancilla et al., 1972). Apparently, the cells proliferate under pathologic conditions. The electron-microscopic photographs from Matthews and Kruger (1973a, b) confirm that, at least under pathologic conditions, mononuclear blood cells pass through the endothelial and glial basement membranes.

It should be noted that, under normal conditions, additional cell types can be demonstrated between the basement membranes, e.g., mast cells (Ibrahim, 1974a, b) or lymphocytes (Kubie, 1927).

3. Free Subarachnoidal Cells

The subarachnoid space should be understood as an extension of the intracerebral perivascular space (Janzen, 1961; Abadia-Fenoll, 1969a, b; Cserr and Ostrach, 1974). Superficially, it is set off from the brain tissue and the peripheral nerve root by monostratified pial cells and by the glial basement membrane. Adventitial cells and endothelial basement membranes limit it from the vascular walls; a superficial layer of arachnoid cover cells connected by an extensive and continuous system of tight junctions (without a continuous basement membrane) limit it from the outlying arachnoidea (Nabeshima et al., 1975). The intervening space is filled with cerebrospinal fluid, collagen fibers, and vessels–large blood vessels as well as capillaries (Hirano et al., 1976). The subarachnoid space, therefore, merges continuously into the perivascular space of intracerebral vessels and terminates around the (obliterated?) glial and endothelial basement membranes (Frederickson and Low, 1969).

The outer layer of the sheath of emerging peripheral nerves within the subarachnoid space is composed of pial cells (Waggener and Beggs, 1967); the inner layer of the sheath of (peripheral) nerves extracerebrally as well as within the subarachnoid space is composed of perineurium (Haller and Low, 1971). Recently several investigations have confirmed that this inner layer of the peripheral nerve sheath terminates as an open-ended tube near the junction of the peripheral nerve and the central nervous tissue. In this way, continuity between endoneural and pial connective tissue spaces is established (Waggener and Beggs, 1967; McCabe and Low, 1969; Haller et al., 1972). Since the pial surface layer is not totally covered and is, therefore, interrupted (Morse and Low, 1971, 1972a, b; Cloyd and Low, 1974; Lopes and Mair, 1974a; Allen and Low, 1975), openings or so-called fenestrae occur. As a result, a continuous space system is present between the subarachnoid and endoneural spaces. The endoneural space also extends extracerebrally. The possibility that labeled proteins flow as a tracer along the endoneural space has already been established (Mellick and Cavanagh, 1968).

Based on experiments with dyes, Weed (1932, 1938) assumed that tissue spaces of intracerebral vessels and periencephalic sheaths were uniform. Later similar experiments by Woollam and Millen (1954, 1955) as well as Rosen and co-workers (1967) substantiated Weed's findings. Final confirmation was possible with electron-microscopic investigations (see among others Maynard et al., 1957; Pease and Schultz, 1958). The tissue lining the subarachnoid space together with an enclosed reticular network and invading vessels was referred to as the leptomeninges. The leptomeninges were considered to be connective tissue that, according to most authors, originated in the mesoderm (His, 1865; Koelliker, 1879; Van Gelderen, 1926; Kershman, 1939; Watanabe, 1950; Schaltenbrand, 1955; Waggener and Beggs, 1967; Frederickson and Low, 1969; Morse and Low, 1972a). Harvey and Burr (1926) as well as Harvey and co-workers (1933) questioned this hypothesis. In their transplantation experiments, they noted that the meninges developed only when parts of neighboring ganglion cell crests were transplanted with the neural tube. Even though Flexner (1929) was unable to confirm these findings with his own experiments, their hypothesis was later used not only to support the ectodermal origin of microglial cells (Rydberg, 1932) and pial cells (Hörstadius, 1950; Millen and Woollam, 1961), but also to refute the ectodermic-layer theory itself (Starck, 1955).

Key and Retzius (1875) first described the cytologic structure forming the basis of the cavity system. They observed cobblestonelike elements lining the arachnoidea and pia which resembled mesothelial cells lining the abdominal cavity (Weed, 1932, 1938; Shabo and Maxwell, 1968a, b; Anderson, 1969). This similarity was not entirely consistent after the cells were observed with the electron microscope (Thomas, 1966; Waggener and Beggs, 1967). Frederickson and Low (1969) found neither a basement membrane consisting of border cells limiting the subarachnoid space [see to the contrary Lopes and Mair (1974b) who observed a discontinuous basement membrane in the human arachnoidea] nor "tight junctions," which might be considered characteristic of epithelial tissue. The demonstrated cell connections for the pia-arachnoid cells seemed to be desmosomal (Frederickson and Low, 1969; Lopes and Mair, 1974b). Since border cells and cells from neighboring vessels, for example, seem to have a similar appearance, Tilney and Riley (1938) suggested that these border cells were endothelial cells. On the basis of electron-microscopic investigations, Pease and Schultz (1958) (see also Nelson et al., 1962c; Iida, 1966) described the cells as fibroblastlike elements. Other researchers, however, observed that the cytoplasm contained only a few mitochondria and endoplasmatic reticula (Morse and Low, 1972a). According to Morse and Low, the cells most closely resembled fibrocytes, i.e., a less active type of collagenous fiber-forming cell (see also Thomas, 1966; Cloyd and Low, 1974). Morse and Low (1972a) also noted that other cells could frequently be observed below the pial cell layer (i.e., between the pial cells and the glial basement membrane) which were best described morphologically as macrophages.

Essick's typical observations (1920) should also be mentioned. After injecting foreign matter into the subarachnoid space, he found that border cells transformed into phagocytes, detached from the pial and arachnoidal cell layer, and became "free cells" in the subarachnoid space. This finding was substantiated by experiments with dyes (Ayer, 1920; Weed, 1920; Woollard, 1924) and by injecting erythrocytes into the subarachnoid space (Bagley, 1928). Since until this time only the phagocytic ability of arachnoid cover cells had been questioned, Wislocki (1928) suggested that this cell type was less active than pial cells. Cushing (1925) also included all phagocytizing cells in the subarachnoid space under the term "meningocytes." Only Kubie and Schultz (1925) distinguished between border cells and phagocytizing free cells of other origins.

Such confirmation of Essick's findings (1920) correlated well with the results acquired later with electron-microscopic investigations concerning experimental *coli* meningitis by Nelson and co-workers (1962a, b, c; see also Shuttleworth and Allen, 1966; Shabo and Maxwell, 1971; Nabeshima, 1971; Heil, 1972). Nelson and co-workers (see also Blinzinger, 1965) observed the active phagocytosis of microorganisms by pial cells. Afterward the pial cells were no longer fixed; these cells detached from the basement membranes when the cytoplasm swelled and the long cytoplasmic processes retracted. As a result, these cells were transformed into motile elements that sometimes exhibited the structural characteristics of macrophages. Due to the phagocytic activity and the tendency toward motility of these pial cover cells, the authors (Nelson et al., 1962c) suggested that at least some of the cover cells must be elements from the reticuloendothelial system. (The question then arises if these cells might be the subpial macrophages mentioned by other authors.) In addition to phagocytes derived from the pia mater, other elements resembling blood monocytes in terms of their ultrastructure were observed during the course of an inflammatory process. These investigations also indicated that phagocytes developed from adventitial cells located on the outer surface of meningeal blood vessels. Only a very small proportion of the cellular elements from the arachnoidea seemed to participate in phagocytic processes and to form infiltrates (Nelson et al., 1962c; Blinzinger, 1965). The Pease and Schultz observations (1958) (see also Matsumoto, 1975), however, did not confirm such an active phagocytic ability on the part of the pial cells.

In addition to the fixed border cells, so-called free cells could be observed within the subarachnoid space, even under normal conditions. In 1875, Key and Retzius had already referred to the unusual "granular" appearance of these cells. On the one hand, these cells can be observed in section preparations with the light microscope (Essick, 1920; Ayer, 1920; Wislocki, 1928; Scharrer, 1936) and with the electron microscope (Pease and Schultz, 1958; Nelson et al., 1962b; Klika, 1967; Frederickson and Haller, 1971; Himango and Low, 1971; Morse and Low, 1972a, b; Fraher and McDougall, 1975). On the other hand, however, the cells can also be observed in the cerebrospinal fluid of living man and living animals following lumbar puncture (Widal et al., 1900; Alzheimer, 1907; Sayk, 1960; for survey of the literature, see Oehmichen, 1976a). Under normal conditions, cerebrospinal fluid cells resemble round cells and macrophage-like elements morphologically. Without anticipating a hematogenesis, almost all authors identified the round cells as "lymphocytes" because of the morphologic similarity to blood lymphocytes (for literature, see Schwarze, 1973). Recently published experiments with immunologic surface markers basically substantiated this assumption (Goasguen and Sabouraud, 1974; Sandberg-Wollheim and Turesson, 1975; Allen et al., 1975, 1976; Levinson et al., 1976; Moser et al., 1976; Naess, 1976; for survey of the literature, see Oehmichen, 1978). Since this cell type exhibits almost no phagocytic activity, it is not dealt with in the following discussion. It cannot be classified as a mononuclear phagocyte.

As mentioned above, mononuclear elements in addition to round cells were observed which resembled macrophages from other regions of the body in terms of light-microscopic (Klima and Beyreder, 1950; Sörnäs, 1971) (cf. Fig. 3C), transmission electron-microscopic (Schmidt and Seifert, 1967; Guseo, 1971), and scanning electron-microscopic criteria (Guseo, 1976). Most authors supported the theory confirmed by Essick (1920) that these "free cells" derived from "fixed" cells by desquamation and proliferative activity (for literature, see Sayk, 1960). Phagocytic activity similar to that of macrophages was demonstrated by in vivo experiments in animals (Kubie and Schultz, 1925) and in vitro experiments in cells from human cerebrospinal fluid (Sörnäs, 1971). A summary of the various terms used for this cell type has been presented by Oehmichen (1976a).

When observed with the light microscope (Fig. 3), the nucleus of free phagocytic cells contains relatively little chromatin. The nucleus itself is often indented, but may also be round to oval. The cytoplasm is usually distended and forms pseudopodialike branches. Vacuoles or microscopic (short-scale contrast) inclusions can frequently be visualized.

When observed with the electron microscope, the nucleus of free cells is usually lobular; clumps of chromatin can be seen in the neighborhood of the nuclear membrane. The cytoplasm contains mitochondria, rough endoplasmatic reticula, and a few lysosomes, as well as vacuoles of varying sizes, shapes, and quantities. Complex inclusions such as phagosomes can be observed in these vacuoles. The plasma membrane is often sharply defined and has longer branches.

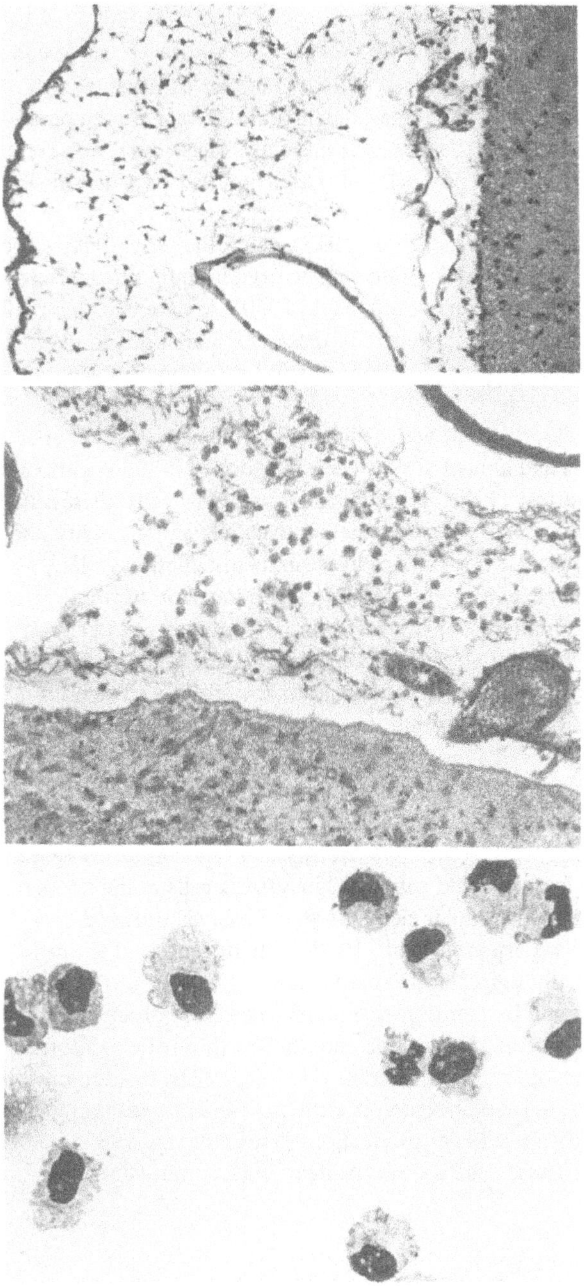

Fig. 3 A–C. Free subarachnoidal cells.
(A) Normal leptomeninx in man with free subarachnoid space.
(B) Increase and activation of free cells inside the subarachnoidal space in man following skull-brain trauma.
(C) Macrophagelike cells in human CSF following ischemic infarct.
[(A and B) HE stain; (C) Pappenheim stain; magnification: (A) x 120; (B) x 200; (C) x 1200]

4. Epiplexus Cells

Kolmer (1921) first investigated the so-called epiplexus cells. He observed macrophagelike cells on the surface epithelium of the choroidal plexus in various kinds of lower vertebrates, particularly amphibians. He referred to this cell as a "wandering cell" and described its motility and phagocytic ability. Later Comini (1929), Vialli (1930), and Scharrer (1936) also demonstrated similar elements in various vertebrates; Schaltenbrand (1955), in various mammals; Chamberlain (1974), in rat fetuses; Merker (1972), in apes; Biondi (1934), in humans.

This cell type was first called the "Kolmer cell." Kappers (1953), however, suggested the term "epiplexus cell" since these cells remained in direct contact with the plexus epithelium for varying periods of time. At the same time, he did not exclude the possibility of their being able to swim freely in the cerebrospinal fluid. He seldom, however, observed the cells on the surface of the ependymal wall. Later other authors described a similar cell on the ependymal wall (Hosoya and Fujita, 1973; Coates, 1972, 1973a, b, 1975; see also Peters, 1974; Allen, 1975; Walsh et al., 1978) which they then referred to as the "supraependymal cell" (Coates, 1973a). Following ventricular punctures, macrophagelike cells were also present in cerebrospinal fluid (Sayk, 1960). Apparently, these cells were one and the same cell type. An increased quantity of these cells was observed in fetal (Chamberlain, 1974) and adult (Schotland et al., 1965) rats following poisoning with the antimetabolite 6-aminonicotinamide.

Kappers (1953), in particular, described the active phagocytic ability of this cell type. He mentioned that epiplexus cells had almost always been overlooked in the traditional microscopic investigations. In contrast to the choroidal and ependymal cells, these cells were first considered to be a separate cell type after their active phagocytic activity had been observed following intraventricular injection of dyes (india ink, methyl violet, trypan blue). Later, cytomorphologic equivalents of this phagocytic activity were found during the course of electron-microscopic investigations (Tennyson and Pappas, 1961, 1964; Carpenter, 1966). Carpenter and co-workers (1967) were able to confirm these observations. With the electron microscope, these authors were able to demonstrate the phagocytosis of intraventricularly administered autologous blood cells by epiplexus cells.

The prevailing opinion for some time was that these cells originated from local connective tissue and then migrated through the choroidal epithelium to reach the ventricle (Vialli, 1930; Biondi, 1934; Kappers, 1953, 1958; Netsky and Shuangshoti, 1970). In 1913, Goldmann had already demonstrated active phagocytizing cells in the stroma of the choroidal plexus. Since, however, similar elements were observed during diapedesis of the choroidal blood vessels (Carpenter et al., 1970), hematogenesis of the cell type, as Kolmer (1921) has originally suggested, was indicated.

Two additional observations should be mentioned: Epiplexus cells are observed primarily on the choroidal plexus of the lateral ventricle and the fourth ventricle, but less frequently on the choroidal plexus of the third ventricle (Merker, 1972). In addition to these macrophagelike cells, isolated lymphocytelike elements were present on the choroidal epithelium, but in significantly lower proportions (Tsusaki et al., 1952; Kappers, 1953; Schwarze, 1975). These cells will not be dealt with in more detail in the context of this study.

Kappers (1953) and Carpenter and co-workers (1970) presented a light-microscopic description of the epiplexus cells (Fig. 4): These cells are relatively polymorphic and

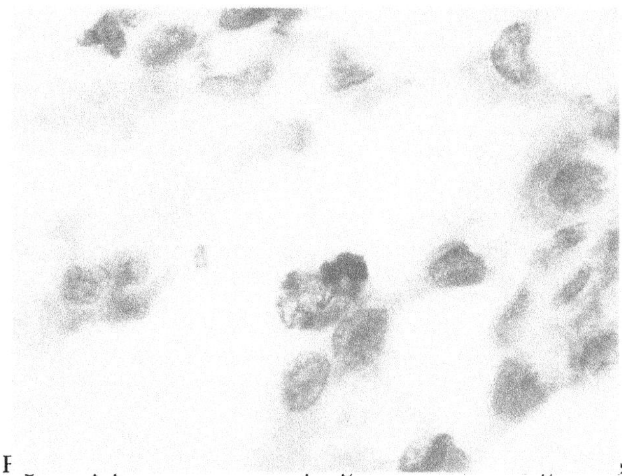

F [illegible] surface of the choroidal plexus in the lateral ventricle of man. (HE stain; magnification: 1200)

possess microvilli as well as pseudopodialike processes. The cytoplasm is slightly basophilic and contains variously sized groups of vacuoles and small granules with differing staining characteristics. The nuclei usually have one or more indentations; some are lobulated. They are frequently located eccentrically. The chromatin is particularly distinct near the nuclear membrane. A nucleolus is seldom present. When observed with the electron microscope (see Santolaya and Echandia, 1968; Carpenter et al., 1970; Merker, 1972; Allen, 1975), the cells are found superimposed on the surface of the plexus cells. Microvilli and cilia from the epithelium infiltrate the cytoplasm, thereby invaginating the epiplexus cells. Mitochondria and endoplasmatic reticula can seldom be demonstrated. Very few free ribosomes, several Golgi apparatuses, microtubules, surface retractions or invaginations, as well as microvesicles and lysosomal dense bodies can be observed. The nucleus is frequently indented.

On the basis of their investigations with the scanning electron microscope, Hosoya and Fujita (1973) distinguished between two cell types [similar observations in regard to "supraependymal cells" have been described by Coates (1975)]: Type I cells contained only fibrous processes originating from a centrally located cell body; Type II cells possessed unusually long, thick pseudopodialike processes. The authors suggested that Type I cells were in a resting phase; Type II cells, in a motile stage. In electron-microscopic investigations of the dog, Allen (1975) also established the polymorphism of this cell type as well as its morphologic similarity to macrophages.

Conclusion

Compared with all cells in the CNS, only four cell types often mentioned in the literature possess an unusual phagocytic ability. The following terms, which we will temporarily refer to as MP (= mononuclear phagocytes) of the CNS, have been applied to these cells based on their differing locations:

1. *Progressive microglia* appear inside the cerebral parenchyma following various types of brain damage. The relationship between progressive microglia and resting microglia is discussed but still unknown.
2. *Perivascular cells* from the intracerebral vessels are characteristically located between the glial and endothelial basement membranes of intracerebral vessels [it is not clear whether this is a separate cell type ("pericyte") or two different cell types].
3. *Free subarachnoidal cells* appear in the subarachnoid space with macrophagelike appearance.
4. *Epiplexus cells* are located primarily on the choroidal epithelium inside the ventricular system.

The question then arises if a similar classification of these four cell types can be found in the literature.

It must be noted that additional cells from other locations with similar function may be present inside the brain. Scharrer (1936) described phagocytes in the paraphysis of amphibians; Goldmann (1913), the so-called pyrrole cells in the connective tissue of the choroidal plexus of rats. There is no need to present a detailed argument at this point since apparently many species-specific differences exist, and in each instance, only groups of local cells of the same type were involved.

III. Considerations on the Origin of Mononuclear Phagocytes in the Central Nervous System

As can be seen from this basically historically oriented survey of the literature, phagocytes in the CNS have been classified in various ways. Even in recent years, totally contradictory and irreconcilable findings and hypotheses have been published, particularly concerning the origin of progressive microglia [see the discussion following the lectures given by Konigsmark and Sidman (1963a) and by Feigin (1969)]. The main reason presented for the divergent findings was the inherent *species-specific differences* (Hain, 1963; Konigsmark, 1969; Terry, 1969; Cammermeyer, 1970b). On the other hand, it was also noted that the various *types of experimental lesions* might well be responsible for the different cell reactions (Stenwig, 1972; Sumner, 1974; Torvik, 1975). In this context, other authors have suggested that the *severity of the experimental lesions* may be an important factor (Kerns and Hinsman, 1973b). The experiments of Ling (1978) tend to indicate age-dependent differences. Finally, similar findings may be *interpreted differently*.

All authors considered those cells designated as MP in the CNS to be highly motile and phagocytically active. On the basis of these criteria, the cells were repeatedly assigned *expressis verbis* to Aschoff's reticuloendothelial system (1924). According to Aschoff, perivascular cells were included in this system (see also Beletzki and Garkawi, 1931; Adams, 1958). Corria (1927) and Asua (1927) were the first to mention the association of microglial cells. This suggestion was later supported by Rio Hortega (1932, 1939), Betletzki and Garkawi (1931), Dunning and Furth (1935), Dougherty (1944), and Horvat and co-workers (1969). Cushing (1925) included free subarachnoidal cells in the reticuloendothelial system; Kappers (1953), epiplexus cells. These suggestions were then, and are now, contradictory. As mentioned above, Aschoff's reticuloendothelial system must be clearly distinguished from the "mononuclear phagocyte system" of Langevoort and co-workers (1970). A survey of these cell types in terms of their cytogenesis and function has not yet been available.

The possibilities for classifying and including MP in the CNS presented in the literature have been summarized here both to illustrate the current problem and to justify the own experiments.

A survey of the literature reveals that the authors can be divided into those who support a homoplastic or heteroplastic genesis or hematogenesis for all or some types of the so-called MP of the CNS. Even though we have referred to the cell types as MP of the CNS, the literature on the origin of resting microglia must be mentioned. A strict differentiation between pericapillarily located pericytes and perivascular cells of intracerebral vessels from other localizations cannot be made since this differentiation is rarely employed in the literature.

1. Homoplastic Genesis

The idea that the same type of local cells proliferated was more easily accepted because the transformation from one cell type to another or the migration through basement membranes (particularly in the presence of an intact blood-brain barrier) was not involved.

a) Resting and Progressive Microglia

With his own staining method, Rio Hortega (1919b) first noted that both "resting" microglia in undamaged animals and "activated" microglia (phagocytes) following stab wound stain selectively. He also observed morphologic transformations from one cell type to another (Rio Hortega and Penfield, 1927; Rio Hortega, 1932). Thereafter, most authors discussed and accepted the possibility of progressive microglial cells originating from resting microglia (see among others Asua, 1927; Russel, 1929; Carmichael, 1929; Kershman, 1939; Glees, 1955; Cammermeyer, 1965c, 1970a, b; Levine et al., 1965, Sjöstrand, 1965; Kreutzberg, 1968b; Feigin, 1969; Brierley, 1972). Those authors considering resting microglia to be ectodermal elements also tended to accept the theory that progressive microglia originated from "resting" prestages (Metz and Spatz, 1924; Vaughn et al., 1970).

The demonstration of cell division was the prerequisite for establishing local proliferation, at least under pathologic conditions (see Penfield, 1925; Metz, 1926; Von Santha, 1932). The mitosis of microglia was observed in retrograde degeneration (Cammermeyer, 1965c, 1967, 1970b; Trumpy, 1971). Under normal conditions (Noetzel and Rox, 1964; Hommes and Leblond, 1967) and following retrograde degeneration (Sjöstrand, 1965b; Kreutzberg, 1968b; Dimova, 1976), local proliferation of microglia could be confirmed by demonstrating the incorporation of the DNS precursor ^{3}H-thymidine in microglial cells. These findings were further substantiated by electron-microscopic investigations (Mori, 1970). Other experiments, in which local irradiation was carried out before inducing the lesion in the CNS (see Hain, 1963; Hopewell and Wright, 1967, 1970a, b) or the peripheral nerves (see Cavanagh, 1968a,b) provided evidence for mitotic division. In these cases the quantity of progressive microglia was significantly lower. It was assumed that the proliferation of local cells was inhibited by irradiation.

Although most authors assumed the mitotic division of microglia, Niessing (1954) suggested the possibility of amitotic division. He had been unable to observe mitoses. Moreover, with the electron microscope, Mori and Leblond (1969) were unable to demonstrate labeled microglial cells in the corpus callosum of undamaged animals following application of ^{3}H-thymidine. One possible explanation for this absence of labeled cells is that too few microglial cells were present to be observed and counted with the electron microscope (cf. p. 112).

Similarly, some authors thought progressive microglia were derived from local microglia and oligodendroglia (Von Santha, 1932; Field, 1957); from resting microglia and perivascular cells (Sasaki, 1955; Brierley, 1972); or from resting microglia, perivascular cells, and oligodendroglia (Bratiano and Llombart, 1929a, b; Davidoff, 1973). Only a few authors rejected the possibility of resting microglia proliferating locally following damage. Instead, they asserted that progressive microglia originated exclusively from perivascular cells (Miyagawa, 1934) or from blood monocytes (Kitamura, 1973; Fujita and Kitamura, 1975, 1976).

b) Perivascular Cells of Intracerebral Vessels

In investigations based on comparative morphology only a few authors have suggested the possibility of the local proliferation of perivascular cells. Majno (1965), for example, stated that no investigations were available on the origin of pericytes and their ability to divide mitotically. Cliff (1963) suggested that pericytes were derived from wandering fibroblastlike cells. As mentioned above, Han and Avery (1963) noted the similarity to fibroblasts. Cervos-Navarro (1963, 1971), however, also described a similarity to endothelial cells which could be observed particularly during the stage of capillary development (Bauer and Vester, 1970).

Cammermeyer (1965a–c, 1970b) was the first to systematically investigate the ability of perivascular cells to divide mitotically. He observed and photographed clear-cut mitoses in PAS-positive and PAS-negative perivascular cells. This finding was then contradicted by the investigations of Kitamura and co-workers (1973, see also Kitamura et al., 1972; Fujita and Kitamura, 1975), in which labeled perivascular cells such as pericytes were not observed following application of ^{3}H-thymidine.

c) Free Subarachnoidal Cells

The theory that phagocytes originate locally in the subarachnoid space is widespread. At first it was only an assumption (Fischer, 1910), but it was later confirmed by Essick's experiments (1920, see also Ayer, 1920; Woollard, 1924). Thereafter the theory of local proliferation of arachnoidal and/or pial elements was generally accepted

(Weigeldt, 1923; Cushing, 1925; Watanabe, 1950; Howarth and Cooper, 1955; Ferner and Kautzky, 1959; Sayk, 1960, 1974; Schönenberg, 1960; Hackenberg, 1967; Wieczorek et al., 1967; Merchant, 1978). The findings were partially confirmed by comparable experiments conducted in conjunction with electron-microscopic investigations (Nelson et al., 1962a, b, c; Blinzinger, 1965; Shabo and Maxwell, 1968a, b; Anderson, 1969; Morse and Low, 1972a, b; Abadia-Fenoll, 1969a). The hypothesis was formulated that cells could detach from the layer lining the cerebrospinal fluid space and then transform into phagocytes. Only a few authors noted that such free cells could also divide mitotically, even though this phenomenon can be observed repeatedly during the cytologic examination of human cerebrospinal fluid (Oehmichen, 1976).

d) Epiplexus Cells

Not one author has demonstrated or even suggested a local proliferation of epiplexus cells on the surface of the choroidal epithelium. It was, however, assumed that these cells originate from the local connective tissue of the tela choroidea; it was suggested that they proliferate locally and migrate into the ventricular cavity (Vialli, 1930; Biondi, 1934). Kappers (1953) thought epiplexus cells were derived from the same connective tissue stroma in which Goldmann (1913) had observed a large number of phagocytizing (pyrrole blue) cells. The migratory ability of these cells could be assumed since they were repeatedly demonstrated between the choroidal epithelia (Tennyson and Pappas, 1964).

2. Local Heteroplastic Genesis

All findings and hypotheses indicating the possibility of a transformation of another (primary, resting) type of local cells into (secondary, activated) phagocytes in the CNS were included in a second group. To some extent, these findings coincide with observations already described concerning "homoplastic genesis" since the authors did not assume a true transformation, e.g., the above-mentioned development and/or migration of epiplexus cells from local connective tissue stroma.

a) Progressive Microglia and Neuroglia

The derivation of progressive microglia (brain phagocytes) from the neuroglia is mentioned again, independent of Rio Hortega's investigations (Spielmeyer, 1922; Metz and Spatz, 1924; Creutzfeld and Metz, 1926; Jakob, 1927; Besta, 1929; Roussy et al., 1930; Rydberg, 1932; Andrew, 1941; Hörstadius, 1950; Robain, 1970). Recently conducted experiments tend to confirm these investigations. These experiments were, however, first intended to demonstrate the origin of resting microglia from the ectoderma and, therefore, the derivation of progressive microglial cells from "multipotential glioblasts" (Vaughn and Peters, 1968; Vaughn, 1969; Peters et al., 1970; Vaughn et al., 1970; Skoff and Vaughn, 1971; Fujita, 1965; see p. 10).

Other authors referred to clear-cut glial types as prestages of progressive microglia. Niessing (1954) thought he observed astroglia transforming into microglia during experimentally induced cerebral edema in mice. On the basis of electron-microscopic investigations, Davidoff (1973) also described the transformation of macroglia into microglia. Several other authors, however, observed continuous transformations of oligodendroglial cells into microglial cells (Pruijs, 1927; Ferraro and Davidoff, 1928; Field, 1957; Takano, 1964; Maxwell and Kruger, 1966; Cook and Wiesniewski, 1973; Davidoff, 1973).

All the investigations cited were basically conducted in regard to comparative morphology and did not agree with the Konigsmark and Sidman findings (1964). Konigsmark and Sidman observed only a few astrocytes that had incorporated ^{3}H-thymidine after a stab wound. The Smith and Walker autoradiographic investigations (1967, see also Murray and Walker, 1973) were also convincing. These authors labeled all neuroglial elements in newborn mice with ^{3}H-thymidine. Two months later the animals were wounded. No labeled blood cells were expected within the peripheral blood vessels. Since no reduction in the number of silver granules per cell was observed, there were no indications for a proliferation of local labeled cells following trauma of the CNS. These authors, therefore, considered a transformation of neuroglial elements into phagocytes of the CNS to be improbable.

b) Microglia and Subependymal Glia

The occurrence of larger quantities of resting microglial cells in the subependymal region (Rio Hortega, 1921 b, c, 1932; Dewulf, 1937; Wislocki and Leduc, 1952, 1954) has been recognized and accepted. Other authors have referred to these cells as "macrophagelike cells" with slender processes between the ependymal cells (Oksche, 1956) or "hypoependymal cells" (Talanti, 1959). Particularly cells phagocytizing protein solution can be found in this region during experimentally induced cerebral edema (Klatzo et al., 1961, 1962). With the silver impregnation technique, Cammermeyer (1965 c; see also Bleier, 1971; Bleier et al., 1975 b) found typical resting microglia in this region of the brain. Other authors reported similar findings from electron-microscopic investigations (Blakemore, 1969; Stensaas and Reichert, 1971; Stensaas and Gilson, 1972; Privat and Leblond, 1972).

Since the subependymal cells were very actively proliferating immature, blastlike cells, Metz and Spatz suggested already in 1924 that microglial cells could originate from the ectodermal matrix cells located in the subependymal region (see also Pruijs, 1927; Jakob, 1927; Schaltenbrand and Bailey, 1928; Rydberg, 1932). Using the hypothesis that microglia originate from matrix cells, Lewis identified multipotential neuroectodermal elements in the subependymal glia which he thought capable of differentiating into microglia as well as neuroglial cells (1968; see also Ling, 1976). The Kerns and Hinsman hypothesis (1973 a) that perineuronal microglia were derived from the ependyma is only slightly different.

Paterson et al. (1973; see also Privat, 1970; Ling et al., 1973) directed their attention exclusively to the type of derivation of microglia. They injected ^{3}H-thymidine intraventricularly and recorded the number of labeled cells contained in semithin sections, in which microglial cells could be identified. No labeled microglial cells were found during the first 2–4 h following the injection. Two days later, however, labeled microglial cells were identified near the subependymal glia and the corpus callosum (see also Lewis, 1968). Most of the labeled microglial cells appeared on the 7th day following the injection; thereafter, the number gradually decreased. Following the intraperitoneal injection of ^{3}H-thymidine, the number of labeled microglial cells, however, was considerably lower at all times; the labeling of all other cell types in brain tissue remained constant (regardless of the method of application). This finding, together with the observations of morphologic transformations in the brain of newborn rats (Ling, 1976), led Paterson and co-workers to suggest that microglia could be derived from subependymal matrix cells.

A series of light-microscopic (Kershman, 1939; Cammermeyer, 1965c) and electron-microscopic (Blakemore, 1969; Stensaas and Reichert, 1971; Stensaas and Gilson, 1972; Blakemore and Jolly, 1972; Matthews, 1974) investigations of comparative morphology yielded contradictory information. These investigations could not provide evidence for the transformation of matrix cells into microglia.

c) Progressive Microglia and Perivascular Cells

The following terms used to describe the perivascular location of microglia reflect the close relationship between progressive microglia and perivascular cells: "vascular satellite" (Rio Hortega, 1920), "perivascular microglia" (Cajal, 1925), "lamellated" microglial element (Rio Hortega, 1932), "juxtavascular cell" (Cammermeyer, 1965a; see below), "pericytial microglia" (Mori and Leblond, 1969a). The derivation of phagocytes from adventitial cells was postulated already in 1902 on the basis of morphologic, functional, and local similarities (Hatai, 1902; see also Alzheimer, 1904; Nissl, 1904; Devaux, 1908; Foot, 1925; Scholz, 1957; Russell, 1962; Vaughn, 1965; Jones, 1970; Baron and Gallego, 1972).

Indications for the similarity were established in a number of different ways. Perivascular cells and microglia could be selectively impregnated by the same method (Mori and Leblond, 1969; see to the contrary, Stensaas, 1975); the phagocytic process in perivascular cells was similar to that in microglial cells (Brichova, 1972; Wagner et al., 1974; see to the contrary Kubie and Schultz, 1925; Cancilla et al., 1972). Biogenetic relationships were found which corresponded closely with the early observation that the occurrence of microglial cells in the embryonic period is dependent on the growth of vessels into the neural tube. In this period, the location of microglial cells was exclusively perivascular; later they migrated into the neuropil (Von Santha, 1932; Juba, 1934a, b; Dunning and Stevenson, 1934; Kershman, 1939; Field, 1955; Baldwin et al., 1969; Jones, 1970; see to the contrary Stensaas, 1975).

For years Cammermeyer's position (1965a, b, 1966, 1970a, b) was relatively independent. Arguing on the basis of light-microscopic investigations of mitotic behavior in CNS cells made during retrograde degeneration, he asserted that microglial cells were derived from elements located on the external surface of the vascular basement membranes of small arteries, capillaries, venules, and small veins. These cells, which he referred to as "juxtavascular," were identical with the perivascular cells of Bennet and co-workers (1959) and Cammermeyer's vascular wall cells (1960), but not with pericytes. The cells underwent mitotic division; a daughter cell could develop into a migrating microglial cell.

The relationship between perivascular cells and progressive microglia was also observed in the most varied experimental and spontaneous lesions in the CNS. The identity of both cell types was mentioned following mechanical brain trauma (Cone, 1928;

Carmichael et al., 1939; Baggenstoss et al., 1943; Dublin, 1945; Silver and Walker, 1947; Kreutzberg and Peters, 1962; Kreutzberg, 1968b; Dimova and Markov, 1974; Boya, 1976), following implantation of foreign bodies (Ischikawa, 1932), following retrograde degeneration (see among others Cammermeyer, 1965c, 1970b; Sjöstrand, 1966b; Wong-Riley, 1972), following chronic lead poisoning (Markov and Dimova, 1974), following high-dosage irradiation (McDonald, 1962; Maxwell and Kruger, 1965; Samorajski et al., 1968), following anoxic-ischemic damage (Hills, 1964), in leukoencephalopathy (Gonatas et al., 1964), in experimental allergic encephalitis and/or neuritis (Lampert, 1969), and following experimental bacterial meningitis (Blinzinger and Hager, 1962, 1964; Blinzinger, 1965; Hager, 1968, 1975). In each case, either a uniform selective reaction was observed on the part of progressive microglia and perivascular cells or the reaction was such that the derivation of reactive microglia from perivascular cells could be assumed.

In the light of findings obtained under pathologic conditions, it was asserted that progressive microglia and perivascular cells were either elements with the same derivation or one cell type was derived from the other. The Mori and Leblond observation (1969a, see also Wendell-Smith et al., 1966b) supported the first assertion. With electron microscopy, they were able to distinguish between two types of microglia cells under normal conditions; so-called pericytial microglia and interstitial microglia. Autoradiographic findings (Kreutzberg, 1966, 1967, 1968b) and light-microscopic observations of the proliferation type were cited especially to support the second assertion (Cammermeyer, 1965a, 1966, 1970b). These authors identified ^{3}H-thymidine-incorporating cells and/or mitotic cells predominantly in elements located in the neuropil in the neighborhood of the vessels. Later, labeled (daughter?) microglialike cells were also observed without any connections to the vessels in the neuropil.

The derivation of progressive microglia from perivascular elements presupposed, at the same time, a diapedesis of the glial basement membrane. Such a process seemed at first inconceivable (Nissl, 1904). Several authors have since been able to observe it with the electron microscope (Maxwell and Kruger, 1965; Bignami and Ralston, 1969; Mori, 1970; Wong-Riley, 1972). As previously mentioned, a few authors asserted that resting microglia originate from the ectoderm. The probability of and possibility for the migration of perivascular cells as well as the ability of perivascular cells to transform into progressive microglia, however, even led some authors to suggest that progressive microglia were derived exclusively from perivascular cells (Schaltenbrand and Bailey, 1928; Miyagawa, 1934; Vaughn, 1965) and not from resting microglia.

Finally one group of authors (see among others Onishi, 1952; Kerns and Hinsman, 1973b, Dodson et al., 1976) rejected the possibility of this kind of related identity or ability for transformation. Cancilla and co-workers (1972; see also Kubie, 1927) were able to observe phagocytic activity in perivascular cells, but not in resting microglia following cerebral edema and intravenous injection of horseradish peroxidase. Kitamura and co-workers (1972, 1973; see also Kitamura, 1973; Fujita and Kitamura, 1975) strictly differentiated between pericytes, microglia, and so-called progressive microglia. They suggested that only migrating monocytes were able to transform into progressive microglia, and depending on the direction of migration, this cell type could also be localized between the basement membranes as are the pericytes.

d) Progressive Microglia and Free Subarachnoidal Cells

The ability for transformation and/or the identity of progressive microglia and free subarachnoidal cells was suggested as early as 1931 for two reasons: During the embryonic period, microglial cells were observed migrating together with ingrowing vessels as well as out of the pial connective tissue (Gozzano, 1931; Beletzky, 1932; Kershman, 1939). Moreover, both cell types exhibited the same degree of phagocytic activity (Blinzinger, 1968a). Cammermeyer (1970b) also noted that, with the same selective staining technique, free subarachnoidal cells were impregnated at the same time as microglial cells.

In addition to the considerations of the related identity of both cell types (see also Takeuchi, 1933), it was also suggested that progressive microglia could be derived from leptomeningeal connective tissue cells (Watanabe, 1950; Bignami and Ralston, 1969). Rydberg (1932), who had suggested an ectodermal origin for progressive microglia, also supported this suggestion. He, however, referred to Harvey and Burr (1926; see above), who asserted that microglia originated from the ectoderm of leptomeningeal tissue (cf. p. 16).

Fujita (1965), in particular, rejected the idea of identity and an ability for transformation on the part of the subarachnoidal cells and microglia during the embryonic period. After injecting ^{3}H-thymidine, he observed that all the pial cells in chick embryos were distinctly labeled after the 3rd–9th embryonic day. Almost no labeling could, however, be demonstrated in the subpial microglial elements. He therefore concluded that these elements must represent a different cell type.

e) Progressive Microglia and Epiplexus Cells

As of the publication of this study, no investigations have been exclusively devoted to the problem of the transformation of progressive microglia into epiplexus cells or vice versa. A few secondary findings and considerations in this direction, however, have been published.

After intracerebral implantation of cryptococcal polysaccharides, Hirano and co-workers (1966) observed subependymally located phagocytes, such as progressive microglia, which seemed to migrate through the ependyma into the ventricular cavity. These cells were apparently "hypoependymal microglia" [see also Cammermeyer's response following the presentation from Hirano and co-workers (1966)]. The above-mentioned finding that branches of subependymally located microglia could be demonstrated between the ependymal cells (Oksche, 1956) tends to provide evidence for the existence of such transformations.

So-called supraependymal cells, which sometimes morphologically resembled epiplexus cells (Coates, 1975), were also observed on the surface of the ependyma (Coates, 1973a, b). Using the Golgi-Cox method, Bleier (1971) observed that supraependymal and subependymal cells stained identically and were similar in structure. The cell types were either microglialike or resembled spider cells. After comparing their own findings with Bleier's photographs, Mestres and Breipohl (1976) suggested that the stained cells were really microglial cells. In 1972, Bleier established that the hypophysiotropic area of the hypothalamus is rich in microglialike cells which invade the overlying ependymal surface. These investigations tended to indicate that intraventricular phagocytes migrated from the neuropil into the ventricular cavity (cf. Hasenjäger and Stroescin, 1939).

It should be noted that Ling (1976) described so-called ameboid microglia not only subependymally, but also in the cavity of the lateral ventricle. He suggested that microglia were derived from subependymal glia, as were cells in the ventricular cavities.

Possible explanations for the above-mentioned (cf. p. 26f.) experimental findings from Paterson and co-workers (1973; see also Watson, 1965) ought to be mentioned at this point. Following intraventricular injection of ^{3}H-thymidine, labeled microglial cells were first observed near the ventricular cavity after a certain waiting period. Among other possibilities, these authors suggested that labeled cerebrospinal fluid cells such as epiplexus cells migrated from the ventricle into the neuropil and there transformed into microglia.

f) Progressive Microglia, Perivascular Cells, and Free Subarachnoidal Cells

Corresponding to Rio Hortega's theory (1932, 1939), mesenchymal cells within the brain were derived from perivascular and pial connective tissue (ameboid cells) during the embryonic period and then invaded the cerebral parenchyma where they appeared as microglia (see also Penfield, 1925, 1928; Kershman, 1939). Other authors, who, like Nissl (1904), assumed a relationship between progressive microglia and adventitial and/or pial cells, based their opinions on the observation of damaged brain tissue. R. D. Adams (1958), therefore, suggested that, in encephalitis, the major portion of so-called microglial cells and/or phagocytes in the brain were derived from adventitial and pial histiocytes. In experimentally induced demyelination, Koenig and co-workers (1962) noted the early appearance of compound granular corpuscles apparently, these corpuscles develop as a result of the proliferation and hypertrophy of adventitial and subarachnoidal cells. Feigin (1969) accepted the theory that these three cell types were related. He stated that the leptomeninges obviously participated in the formation of brain phagocytes in those cases where a destructive process extended to the true cerebral parenchyma. Similarly, cells from tissue associated with intracerebral blood vessels also participated in intracerebral phagocytosis.

These assumptions agreed with the findings obtained from experimentally induced phagocytosis. Using vital stains and implantation of foreign matter, Ishikawa (1932) observed similar behavior on the part of microglial cells as well as of adventitial and free subarachnoidal cells. Blinzinger (1968a, b) also noted that intrathecally applied iron-dextran solution could be demonstrated in free subarachnoidal cells, perivascular cells, progressive microglia, and astrocytes. By comparing the spontaneous fluorescent activity and the PAS reaction, Fleischhauer (1964) observed similarities and differences. He found perivascular cells that should be classified with microglia in terms of nuclear form and structure, but resembled rounded cells found in the leptomenix in terms of cytoplasmic activity.

g) Progressive Microglia, Perivascular Cells, and Epiplexus Cells

After disturbing the blood-brain barrier, Beletzky and Garkawi (1931) injected an iron-dextran solution intravenously. Among other things, they found that iron had been phagocytized by the adventitial cells of the cortical vessels, by the histiocytes of the pia plexus, and by microglial cells. As a result, they suggested that these different cell types should be included in the reticuloendothelial system. They did not, however, mention typical epiplexus cells.

h) Progressive Microglia, Free Subarachnoidal Cells, and Epiplexus Cells

Only a few observations on the possibility of a relationship of these three cell types have been published. On the basis of investigations of human embryos, Kershman (1939) stated that precursor cells of microglial cells are found in the choroidal plexus and in the meninges. He referred to these cells as embryonic wandering cells or histiocytes. After experimentally inducing trauma of adult brain tissue, Macklin and Macklin (1920) observed not only phagocytes (progressive microglia) in the brain, but also similar phagocytes in the leptomeningeal tissue around the trauma site. At the same time, they also found phagocytes from the choroidal plexus which had incorporated increased amounts of hemosiderin after the traumatic event.

i) Perivascular Cells and Free Subarachnoidal Cells

Some authors noted the similarity between perivascular cells and free subarachnoidal cells. These authors distinguished strictly (sometimes *expressis verbis*) between these two cell types and microglia. The possible identity was based on the fact that the subarachnoid space and, therefore, the cells contained in it, continually merged into the perivascular space of the intracerebral vessels. Identical phagocytic activity for both cell types was demonstrated after intrathecal application of dyes (Kubie and Schultz, 1925; Dougherty, 1944; Torack, 1961) and after intravenous application of labeling substances (horseradish peroxidase) following disturbance of the blood-brain barrier (Cancilla et al., 1970, 1972; Baker et al., 1971). The ultrastructural similarity between adventitial cells and cells of the leptomeninges was also demonstrated by studies of comparative morphology (Pease and Schultz, 1958; Hager, 1961). In this case, pericytes occurring between the lamella of the obliterated basement membranes were assumed to be a different cell type (see to the contrary Wagner et al., 1974).

j) Free Subarachnoidal Cells and Epiplexus Cells

Scharrer (1936) considered free cells in the subarachnoid space, epiplexus cells, and phagocytes of local connective tissue (e.g., the choroid tela) to be the same cell type. Kappers (1953) suggested another possible identity. He noted that, biogenetically, the stroma of the choroidal plexus consists of invaginated leptomeningeal connective tissue that had retained its connection with the choroid tela. Given the dynamics of cerebrospinal fluid, Kappers considered a migration of free cells from the subarachnoid space into the ventricular cavity to be highly improbable. He also noted that no open connection existed between the ventricular system and the pericerebral spaces in those amphibians in which an unusually high proportion of epiplexus cells could be demonstrated.

Morse and Low (1972b) noted ultrastructural differences and similarities between the two cell types. According to them, free cells in the subarachnoid space are more polymorphic; their cytoplasm is heavily vacuolated.

k) Epiplexus Cells and Epithelial Cells of the Choroid Plexus

Only one group of authors (Netsky and Shuangshoti, 1970) suggested the possibility that choroidal cells transform into epiplexus cells. These authors observed fat-laden cells within the epithelial layers of the plexus, but were unable to differentiate them from macrophages. It was thought that these cells detached from the stroma and then were transformed into migrating macrophages.

3. Hematogenesis

The possibility of the hematogenesis of cells within brain tissue must be considered a special type of heteroplasia. Since the related literature is so voluminous, this problem will be dealt with separately.

After the phagocytosis experiments of Aschoff and Kiyono (1913), the relation between tissue macrophages and mononuclear blood cells was repeatedly discussed. It is easy to understand why many authors saw a similarity between phagocytically active cells (including those of brain tissue) and these blood cells. The discussion of the problem has intensified since it has been established that macrophages in the body are derived almost exclusively from blood monocytes (see above).

a) Progressive Microglia and Blood Cells

The possible migration and transformation of blood cells into brain phagocytes has been discussed ever since these cells were first demonstrated in brain tissue (Gluge, 1841; Eichenhorst, 1875; Ribbert, 1882; Kolbe, 1889; Stroebe, 1894; Schmaus and Sacki, 1901; Kaufmann, 1904; Schmaus, 1904). Rio Hortega and Asua (1921; see also Asua, 1927; Rio Hortega, 1932) suggested that such a process was only possible under certain conditions. The relationship was obvious after Russell (1929) succeeded in demonstrating the ability of microglia to phagocytize trypan blue and Lebovich (1934) established the presence of bacteria in microglial cells. Other authors (Costero, 1930, 1931; Wells and Carmichael, 1930; von Mihalik, 1935) demonstrated the phagocytic ability of microglial cells in brain-cell cultures. On the other hand, tissue macrophages from other organs were also stained with Hortega's method for the selective demonstration of microglia (Asua, 1927; Visintini, 1931; Dunning and Stevenson, 1934; Dunning and Furth, 1935; see to the contrary, Miyagawa, 1934). The von Santha and Juba (1933) and Juba (1934b) investigations of embryos provided similar indications. Since the microglia are located in the neighborhood of the vessels during the embryonic period, these authors suggested that blood cells migrated out of the vessels via diapedesis. Dunning and Furth (1935) summarized the then available findings in order to establish the related identity of blood monocytes, histiocytes (tissue macrophages), and microglia. Since then electron-microscopic investigations of the comparative morphology have tended to confirm the similarity between progressive microglia and blood monocytes (Schultz and Pease, 1959; Gonatas et al., 1964; Lampert and Carpenter, 1965; Blakemore, 1972, 1975; Anker, 1975; Das, 1976a, b; Persson, 1976).

The kinetic method of autoradiography developed in the 1950s made important new insights possible. The method of "cumulative labeling" (cf. p. 41 f) has proved to be particularly valuable for cytogenetic problems. Using this particular method, Konigsmark and Sidman (1963a, b) found indications for a hematogenesis of progressive microglia. Intending to investigate similar problems, Roessmann and Friede (1968) injected in vivo and in vitro labeled bone marrow cells. They interpreted the occurrence of isolated labeled cells in the neuropil of normal and traumatized receiver animals to be indicative of their hematogenesis.

Some of the authors cited here also established the proliferation of local cells via ^{3}H-thymidine autoradiography ("pulse labeling," see below). It was suggested that the majority of the invaded mononuclear blood cells also proliferate locally (Konigsmark and Sidman, 1963a, b; Adrian and Smothermon, 1970; Smith and Adrian, 1972; Kitamura et al., 1972, 1973; Fujita and Kitamura, 1975; see also Watson, 1965; Hopewell and Wright, 1970a). The possibilities of simultaneous transformation of migrating blood cells and local division were discussed prior to the development of autoradiographic techniques (Achucarro, 1904; Forster, 1908; Marchand, 1909; Merzbacher, 1910). With electron-microscopic observations, it was established that progressive microglia originated in these two ways (Gonatas et al., 1964; Herndon, 1968).

b) Progressive Microglia, Perivascular Cells, and Blood Cells

As mentioned above, the embryologic investigations conducted in the 1930s indicated that perivascular cells accompanying ingrowing vessels were blood monocytes that may be transformed into microglial cells. Cammermeyer (1970b), among others, considered the possibilities of perivascular cells transforming into progressive microglia and blood cells invading the damaged adult brain under certain pathologic conditions. On the basis of investigations with electron-microscopic autoradiographic methods, Kitamura and co-workers (1972, 1973; Kitamura, 1973, 1975; Fujita and Kitamura, 1975) considered the migration of blood monocytes to be possible under *all* those pathologic conditions that lead to an increase in progressive microglia. These authors assumed that progressive microglia were derived exclusively from blood monocytes that had invaded the brain tissue. It is possible that the blood monocytes arbitrarily lie inside the basement membrane sheaths during their migration; they could not be distinguished from local pericytes with the light microscope. As a result, these authors suggested that progressive microglia were not true pericytes and that true pericytes were not derived from blood monocytes.

c) Progressive Microglia, Perivascular Cells, Free Subarachnoidal Cells, and Blood Cells

Rio Hortega (1932, 1939) as well as Schaltenbrand and Bailey (1928) suggested that progressive microglia might be composed of various types of cells, such as activated resting microglia, perivascular cells, free subarachnoidal cells, and blood monocytes. Privat (1975) questioned if the typical microglia found in Wallarian degeneration originated from the mesenchyma of the nerve tissue, i.e., from meningeal and perivascular cells. In a study published together with Paterson (1973), Privat cited an observation from Herndon and Johnson (1970) to establish the hematogenesis of free subarachnoidal cells.

Subsequently Matthews (1974) referred to the possible identity of these four cell types. He summarized that, according to Morse and Low (1972a, b), elements originating in the blood and adventitial tissue were distributed in the subarachnoid space. Many of these mesenchymal elements on the brain surface as well as long the vessels inside the brain were capable of a reactive transformation that included the enrichment of fat vacuoles and an increase in the number of dense bodies (Morse and Low, 1972b). During their transition from a relatively quiete to a reactive phase, these cells are extremely similar to microglial cells in morphology and in the mode of transformation. The arbitrary movement of microglia from the edges of the vessels or leptomeninges into the neuropil and their possible reactive transformation could also explain their functional morphology. Herrlinger and co-workers (1977) in their electron-microscopic studies of the brains of mice with experimentally induced yellow fever encephalitis supported an identity of these cell types (cf. p. 92f.). The observed peroidase-positive cells (derived from monocytes) juxtavascularly located in the neuropil (sometimes in "satellite" formation) and inside the subarachnoid space. They could not find peroxidase-positive resting microglia. They did note, however, that peroidase-positive granules rapidly disappear after monocytes have left the blood stream.

d) Free Subarachnoidal Cells and Blood Cells

The cytomorphologic similarity between free cells of the subarachnoid space and blood monocytes was noted early since both cell types (free subarachnoidal cells such as cerebrospinal fluid cells following lumbar puncture) could be demonstrated in easily comparable smears and stains. These cells were cytomorphologically similar (Nissl, 1904; Merzbacher, 1904; Andernach, 1910; Klima and Beyreder, 1950; Sörnäs, 1971). Kubie and Schultz (1925; in contrast to Essick, 1920, and others; see p. 17) had observed the phagocytic ability of free cells, but not of the border cells, in in vivo experiments with vital stains. They thought that the free cells were invaded blood monocytes. Using comparative electron-microscopic investigations, other authors were able to establish the similarity between blood monocytes (and/or macrophages in other regions of the body) and cerebrospinal fluid cells (Schmidt and Seifert, 1967; Wender and Sniatala, 1969; Herndon, 1969; Herndon and Johnson, 1970; Guseo, 1971; 1976) and/or free cells in situ within the subarachnoid space (Frederickson and Haller, 1971; Himango and Low, 1971; Morse and Low, 1972a, b; Cloyd and Low, 1974; Allen and Didio, 1977; Merchant and Low, 1977a, b).

Several other authors found indication for an invasion of blood monocytes into the subarachnoid space as well as for a desquamation of local cells; the cells reacted like macrophages (Rehm, 1910, 1931; Szecsi, 1911; Rotstadt, 1916; Wislocki, 1928; Weed, 1932, Bannwarth, 1933, 1944a, b; Huebschmann, 1956; Schmidt, 1968; Morgan et al., 1974). Electron-microscopic investigations conducted by Nelson and co-workers (1960c) and Blinzinger (1965) confirmed this assumption. These authors observed active phagocytosis of microorganisms and motile elements by pial cells. The ultrastructure of these motile elements resembled that of hematogenic monocytes.

e) Free Subarachnoidal Cells, Epiplexus Cells, and Blood Cells

Malloy and Low (1976) used transmission and scanning electron microscopy to examine the spinal cord and choroid plexus in dogs; special emphasis was placed on the study of free cells. Investigations of the comparative morphology confirmed that the free cells in both cavities were identical. The internal morphology of these cells corresponded to that of macrophages from other regions of the body. This assumption was further confirmed by demonstrating the ability of these cells to phagocytize horseradish peroxidase or red blood cells.

f) Epiplexus Cells and Blood Cells

Kolmer (1921) indicated that epiplexus cells were actually invaded blood cells that might react to a stimulus from endogenous particles in the ventricular fluid. Even though almost all the other authors investigating this cell type repeatedly described macrophages in the choroidal stroma and sometimes between the epithelia (Vialli, 1930; Biondi, 1934; Tennyson and Pappas, 1964), they still considered migration to be highly improbable. Using the electron microscope, Carpenter and co-workers (1970) and Merker (1972) as well as Allen (1975) observed and described a similarity between this cell type and macrophages from other organs. They suggested that blood monocytes reached the ventricle by migrating through the choroidal vessels and epithelium of the choroidal plexus. During the last few years, a similarity with macrophages from other organs and/or blood monocytes was established with the scanning electron microscope (Chamberlain, 1974) and enzyme-histochemical studies (Schwarze, 1975). With the use of the scanning electron microscope, supraependymal cells were also described (Bleier, 1975; Bleier et al., 1975; Coates, 1975) as being macrophagelike (i.e., monocyte derived).

Conclusion

This survey of the literature on the origin, identity, and classification of all those mononuclear phagocytes in the CNS considered to be important (progressive microglia, perivascular cells of intracerebral vessels, free subarachnoidal cells, and epiplexus cells) revealed that almost every conceivable, or at least hypothetical, classification has already been proposed. Most authors considered these four cell types to be mesenchymal cells. More recent investigations have tended to indicate that these cells may be derived from blood monocytes. The absence of definitive results motivated the author to investigate the problem further.

B. Author's Investigation

The author's investigations were conducted with the following question in mind: Under normal or pathologic conditions, are cells actually present in the nervous system which can, on the basis of identical criteria, be compared with the so-called mononuclear phagocytes described by hematologists, immunologists, and pathologists? For this reason, the investigations were concentrated particularly on the origin and functional potential of the four cell types which, according to the literature, are most probably MP of the CNS, namely, progressive microglia, perivascular cells of intracerebral vessels, free subarachnoidal cells, and epiplexus cells. The experimental procedure is determined partially by the kinetic methods and partially by comparable functional methods. The possibility of radioactively labeled mononuclear phagocytes from the peripheral blood *invading* the nervous system, the *transformability* of the cells inside the nervous system, as well as their *possible fate* were investigated in detail. Various modes of *function* were compared. The results, of course, can be evaluated only in terms of the limitations of each respective method.

The number of figures was intentionally kept to a minimum since the photographs are intended only to help visually clarify the formulation of the problem in terms of comparative (light-microscopic)morphology (Figs. 1-4). A reproduction of the morphologic equivalents of the results described by the author (Figs. 7-36) also aid the understanding of these and other methods applied.

Since the author's results are based primarily on *qualitative* cytologic investigations, it was possible to record findings after a particular method had been applied about which no quantitative statements could be made regarding its frequency. The figures, therefore, are intended to substantiate the results described, without, of course, verifying them.

Materials and Methods Consistently Used

Since this investigation was conducted over a period of several years, there is some variation in the experimental models and methods for each experimental procedure, although they may seem to be quite similar. The similar materials and methods used to approach the problem are presented here. The description of these experiments provides the experimental procedure as well as the detailed methodological data valid for each experiment.

The following *cytokinetic techniques* were used: pulse labeling; parabiosis; and transfusion experiments with in vivo labeled blood cells using ^{3}H-thymidine (^{3}H-TdR), with in vitro labeled blood cells and/or peritoneal macrophages using ^{3}H-diisopropyl fluorophosphate (^{3}H-DFP), with in vitro labeled lymphocytes using ^{3}H-cytidine and erythrocytes using ^{51}chromium (^{51}Cr). The radioactive substances were acquired from Amersham Buchler Co. (Braunschweig/FRG). Specific activity for the labeling substances was: ^{3}H-TdR=5.0 Ci/mmol; ^{3}H-DFP=10 Ci/mmol; ^{3}H-cytidine=2.5 Ci/mmol; ^{51}Cr ($Na_2{}^{51}CrO_4$)=100-420 μCi/μg. Each respective dose was different and is, therefore, always given separately.

A number of *experimental disorders* were induced to generate an increase of MP in the nervous system. They included stab wounds, glass implantation, herpesvirus meningoencephalitis, experimental storage of golactocerebroside, retrograde nerve cell degeneration in the facial nucleus, and Wallerian (orthograde) degeneration in the sciatic nerve.

The disorders will be described in detail below. All surgical procedures were carried out under ether anesthesia.

Rabbits (German giant breed) of both sexes and female rats [breed: A S-2 Max (Max Planck Institute for Immunobiology, Freiburg/FRG)] were used as *experimental animals.* Most of the rabbits were 5–10 months old and weighed 1500–3500 g. The rats were 1–2 months old and weighed 100–200 g. All animals were fed with Altromin (Altromin GmbH, 4937 Lage/FRG) and were given water ad libitum.

In several of the experiments, it was necessary to stimulate proliferation and isolate the *peritoneal macrophages.* The methodological procedure used here was very similar to that published by Gesner and Howard (1967). Each rabbit was injected with 50 ml sterile paraffin oil intraperitoneally. After 5 days, the peritoneal cavity was washed with 200 ml warm Hank's balanced salt solution containing 20 U.S.P. heparin/ml. Due to the relatively high-fat content of the suspension, it was seldom necessary to filter the cells through a gauze net. In rabbits the cell yield was $\sim 2 \times 10^6 - 1 \times 10^7$ cells. About 90% of the cells obtained could definitely be identified on the basis of their morphologic criteria as cells from the monocyte-macrophage series. The viability of the cells in the suspension was tested with 0.5% trypan blue solution.

Different solutions [Hank's balanced salt solution and Medium Tc 199 (Fa. Serva Feinbiochemica, Heidelberg/FRG)] had to be used for the cell washing and for a number of other experiments. Two types of buffers were also used: phosphate buffered saline (PBS: 0.15 mol, pH 7.4) and veronal buffered saline (VBS: 0.15 mol, pH 7.4).

The *immunologic labeling method* was used only in the last test series; it will be thoroughly described in this context.

The *histologic treatment* was carried out as follows: Under ether anesthesia, the animals were perfused through the descending aorta or the heart with ~200 ml warm 4% formalin. After removing the tissue, it was fixed for several days and then routinely embedded in paraffin. Sections of 5-μ thickness were prepared and stained with hematoxylin-eosin (H&E). If necessary, they were also stained with Giemsa solution, cresyl violet, or via the Klüver-Barrera technique. When additional special stains were used, they are mentioned in the text.

Certain *enzymes* were repeatedly demonstrated in one series of experiments via histochemical techniques. For these experiments, the tissue was frozen in liquid nitrogen or in dry ice immediately after it was removed and was then sectioned on a standard cryostat (SLEE Co., Mainz/FRG). For the most part, the enzymes demonstrated were acid phosphatase (Löffler and Berghoff, 1962), α-naphthyl acetate esterase (Nachlas and Seligman, 1949), naphthol AS acetate esterase (Löffler, 1961), and naphthol AS-D chloroacetate esterase (Leder, 1964). Each respective enzyme was then also demonstrated in the cytologic smear specimen.

Autoradiographic treatment was carried out via the dipping method (Kopriwa and Leblond, 1962), either in Kodak NTB3 emulsion or in Ilford K2 emulsion. The Ilford K2 emulsion was diluted 1:2 with distilled water. The coated specimens were exposed in darkness using silicate gel at 4° C for varying time periods. They were developed with a Kodak D19 developer at 18° C for 6 min. The sections were then routinely stained with H&E.

Each cell type was classified according to the following criteria:

1. Considered so-called resting or progressive *microglia* were those cells that could be selectively stained in frozen sections fixed in formalin according to the techniques of Rio Hortega (1919), Tsusiyama (1963), or Weil and Davenport (1933) and stained in paraffin sections according to the technique of Naoumenko and Feigin (1963).
   The author modified the Weil and Davenport method (1933) and occasionally employed this modification. The brain tissue was stored in formalin for 24 h and then cut in 0.5-cm frontal sections. These sections were stored in a solution of 6% dextran [mol.wt. 20000 (100 ml)], 40% formalin (4 ml), and potassium chloride (2 g) for 48 h at 4° C. They were then stained according to the methods described by Weil and Davenport (1933).
   The identification of autoradiographically labeled cells on the section subjected to a silver impregnation technique (see Hommes and Leblond, 1967; Mori and Leblond, 1969) could not be used for quantitative investigations (see also Kreutzberg, 1968a). For the most part, H&E-stained sections were then used for the identification. On the H&E-stained sections, those cells were considered to be microglia which, because of their localization, could not possibly be vascular wall cells or nerve cells. Microglial cells were, therefore, either sought in the white matter or were identified, on the basis of their localization, as satellite cells (perineuronal microglial cells) in the gray matter. In contrast to the astrocytes and oligodendrocytes (both classified as neuroglia), microglia cells were identified on the basis of the darkly staining and sometimes spindle-shaped and/or indented nucleus. In the neuropil, those cells were considered progressive microglial cells which, because of their macrophagelike appearance, could not be neuroglial cells and which possessed a nuclear structure identical with that of resting microglia. Errors in the quantitative evaluation were, therefore, unavoidable.
   Another problem was the differentiation of resting microglial cells from progressive microglial cells. Differentiation was often impossible because the H&E solution provided only morphologic criteria. Microglial cells in damaged brain tissue were considered to be progressive microglial cells; microglial cells in undamaged brain tissue, resting microglial cells. Sometimes both cell types had to be considered undiffentiable (as in the literature) and were classified only as "microglial cells."
2. All those cells were considered to be *perivascular cells* which were in direct contact with intracerebral vessels. Important here was that the cells were not vascular wall cells (endothelial cells, smooth muscle cells) or cells from the neuropil. A perivascular concentration in the Virchow-Robin space was often seen, particularly around the somewhat larger vessels. In the smaller vessels, definite identification was sometimes complicated because the basement membrane could not always be demonstrated. Differentiation of pericytes (mesenchymal cells between the two sheaths of the basement membrane surrounding the capillaries) from perivascular cells of other types was, therefore, not carried out.
3. Those cells were identified as *free subarachnoidal cells* which were located within the trabecular network of the subarachnoid space. Using purely histomorphological criteria it was possible to differentiate adventitical cells, pial cells, and arachnoid cover cells from free subarachnoidal cells because of their localization.

4. All those macrophagelike cells within the ventricular system which were in direct contact with the choroidal cells or were located in the neighborhood of the choroidal cells were classified as *epiplexus cells.*

In most cases, differentiating these four cell types was relatively simple in the undamaged animal. After damage had been inflicted and the cells activated, the cells could no longer be differentiated cytomorphologically. In addition, the boundaries of the brain compartments (subarachnoid space, perivascular space, ventricle, neuropil) were frequently obliterated in the formation of a continuous transition from the leptomeningeal tissue to the damaged neuropil and then to the ventricular system following, for example, a stab wound. Under these conditions, the only valid criterion was to assume that the structure present under normal conditions was also present under pathologic conditions. It should be noted that, under pathologic conditions, all cell types mentioned could often no longer be definitely distinguished from activated macrophages in other body regions, not even cytomorphologically. The cells usually have an indented, round to oval or kidney-shaped nucleus with a looser chromatin structure. Nucleoli can seldom be demonstrated with routine staining. Sometimes two or more nuclei are present. The cytoplasm is usually extended; the nucleus, often marginal. The cytoplasm frequently contains vacuoles or substances such as fat and siderin that can be demonstrated only via special histochemical methods (cf. Figs. 1C, 2D, 3C, 4C).

I. Origin of Mononuclear Phagocytes of the Nervous System

The development of autoradiographic methods made it possible to investigate cytokinetics and, therefore, also the origin of cells. The use of ^{3}H-TdR as tracer has proved to be particularly effective (Hughes et al., 1958; Cronkite et al., 1959; Gall and Johnson, 1960) in the following ways:

a) Since ^{3}H-TdR is almost exclusively incorporated in desoxyribonucleic acid (DNA), it can then be incorporated by cells synthesizing DNA, i.e., cells in the process of mitosis.
b) Since there is only a short period in which thymidine is available [40–60 min (Hughes et al., 1958; Koburg and Maurer, 1962)], the moment of DNA synthesis can be determined fairly accurately.
c) Radioactive labeling is maintained throughout the life of the cell; half the amount is then found in daughter cells each time cell division occurs.

Three different experimental models were frequently applied, particularly to investigate the origin of cells. These methods are pulse labeling, cumulative labeling, and the transfusion method. For *pulse labeling,* one dose of ^{3}H-TdR is administered intravenously or intraperitoneally. The animal is then killed 40, 60, or 120 min later. The labeling index can be determined with this method. This index indicates the amount of cells present at this time in the DNA synthesis phase (S-phase). *Cumulative labeling* has proved successful as a second method (see Bintliff and Walker, 1960). The ^{3}H-TdR dosage is applied either in one dose, repeatedly at intervals of 4, 6, or 8 h, or via a continuous infusion. The animal is killed after 24, 48, (etc.) h after the first injection. In this way, a high proportion of rapidly proliferating cell systems (e.g., blood cells) in particular is labeled. After a lesion has been induced in slowly proliferating tissue (e.g., muscle tissue or brain tissue), the appearance of a great number of labeled cells can provide evidence for the migration of blood cells into the lesion area. Finally, the *transfusion method* and/or its variants (e.g., parabiotic technique) have proved valuable. In vitro or in vivo labeled blood cells are applied to receiver animals and the fate of these cells is observed.

Various authors have determined the origin and the kinetics of the peritoneal macrophages with these labeling methods. Using pulse labeling, it could be established that the labeling index for peritoneal macrophages in in vivo experiments was low (Van Furth and Cohn, 1968). The proliferative activity of local resting alveolar macrophages and Kupffer's cells in the liver (Van Furth, 1970b) is similar. Following nonspecific stimuli (e.g., through the intraperitoneal injection of fetal calf serum or glycogen), the number of peritoneal macrophages marcedly increases, but not the labeling index (Volkman, 1966; Van Furth and Cohn, 1968). With cumulative labeling, a pronounced increase in the amount of labeled cells in the peritoneal cavity was established. This was then interpreted as evidence for the migration of cells from the blood. The parabiotic experiments of Volkman and Gowans (1965a, b), as variants of the transfusion of labeled cells, were also convincing. Only one parabiont was repeatedly injected with ^{3}H-TdR so that all rapidly proliferating cells were labeled with ^{3}H-TdR. These cells were, for the most part, blood cells. Labeled blood cells could invade the other parabiont by vascular anastomosis. The appearance of labeled macrophages after nonspecific stimulation of peritoneal macrophages in the receiver animals served as evidence for the migration of blood cells.

Similar methods were also used by neuropathologists to investigate the origin of microglia (see pp. 112ff.). The author's investigations with a modified experimental model were carried out because the findings obtained tended, at least in part, to show contradictory results. In addition, no experiments had been carried out with rabbits. Since most of the experiments have been limited to progressive or resting microglia, comparable investigations of other cell types (here designated MP of the CNS) are not available.

The following questions, however, remained unanswered and deserve further discussion:

a) The evidence presented in the literature for hematogenesis of MP of the CNS was acquired by cumulative labeling (see in particular, Konigsmark and Sidman, 1963) or by injecting labeled bone marrow cells (Roessmann and Friede, 1968) using ^{3}H-TdR as a tracer. The validity of these results can be called into question since, in each case, a considerable amount of ^{3}H-TdR was freed during the course of the experiment, which then could be reutilized by local proliferating cells (see Feinendegen, 1967; Stöcker and Pfeifer, 1967; Rafferty and Gfeller, 1969; Sidman, 1970; Helpap et al., 1971; Myers and Feinendegen, 1975; Gerecke and Gross, 1976). A high degree of reutilization is found particularly during the course of the enucleation of labeled erythroblasts.

b) At present, clear-cut investigations providing evidence of the type of hematogenic precursor cells are not available. The migration of blood lymphocytes (Kosunen et al., 1963; Waksman, 1965) or blood monocytes (Roessmann and Friede, 1968) thought to transform into phagocytes is a possibility that should be discussed.

The cytokinetic experiments are presented in the following section. The intention, special modification of the method, as well as the material and/or experimental model are given for each experiment. The results are recorded under a separate rubric and followed by a conclusion.

1. Local Proliferation

The proliferative capacity of local cells can be determined via pulse labeling with ^{3}H-TdR, since few labeled blood cells appear in the peripheral blood during a 1- or 2-h period; any appreciable migration of these cells into the tissue is highly improbable. If the MP of the NS are not migrated blood cells, but rather locally proliferating cells, labeled cells in particular should be found that, under normal circumstances or after induction of a nonspecific stimulus, morphologically resemble MP. Reutilization of ^{3}H-TdR is impossible in the short survival time following the injection.

The results obtained in the peripheral nerves with the methods described are presented in the following text. It should be noted that, in addition to isolated fibroblasts and perivascular cells, only Schwann cells are present in normal peripheral nerves without lesions. These Schwann cells can be explained as possibly local phagocytes after a lesion. In the literature, Schwann cells, in particular, have been considered extremely active phagocytically (Guth, 1956; Wechsler and Hager, 1962; Holtzman and Nivikoff, 1965; O'Daly and Imaeda, 1967; Cravioto, 1969; Williams and Hall, 1971; Morris et al., 1972). On the other hand, a hematogenous origin of phagocytes in damaged peripheral nerves (Olsson and Sjöstrand, 1969; Bradley and Asbury, 1970) has been postulated (Stenwig, 1972; Berner et al., 1973; Torvik, 1975). It, therefore, seems justified to report our observations.

Material and Methods

Animals: Three undamaged rabbits and four rabbits with intracerebral stab wounds were examined. In four additional rabbits, the left sciatic nerve was ligated, thereby producing Wallerian degeneration. The right (undamaged) sciatic nerve served as a control in these four animals.

Stab wound: After the calotte was exposed, a hole ~0.1 cm in diameter was bored with a dental drill about 0.3 cm from the sagittal suture and behind the lambdoid suture; the inner osseous lamellae were preserved. The lamellae were then pierced with a sterile No. 2 needle. The needle was then introduced perpendicularly into the brain tissue until opposition was encountered with the basal bones of the brain. This ensured that the lateral ventricles were also pierced. Finally, the galea aponeurotica was sutured under sterile conditions.

Ligation of the nerve: The sciatic nerve was sought under the gluteus maximus muscle and exposed. It was ligated with surgical silk in the middle between the ramification of the common peroneal nerve and the sural nerve as well as at its exit from the lesser pelvis, thereby producing paralysis of the hind leg.

Experimental procedure: After the stab wound, the four animals were allowed to survive for 24 h. Following ligation of the nerve, the animals were allowed to survive for 5 days. Each animal received ^{3}H-TdR (2.0 μCi/g body wt.) intravenously 1 h before it was killed. Except for one animal with a stab wound, all animals were killed with the above-mentioned fixation method; the tissue was routinely treated and then stained. One animal was exsanguinated, and the brain was removed immediately. Approximately 0.5-cm-thick slices were frozen in liquid nitrogen and sectioned on the cryostat. Before the sections were autoradiographically prepared by coating them with Kodak NTB3 emulsion, the activity of nonspecific esterases (α-naphthyl acetate esterase and naphthol AS acetate esterase) and of naphthol AS-D chloroacetate esterase were demonstrated on the sections (Oehmichen and Saebisch, 1971). All sections taken from the undamaged animals and from animals with stab wounds were exposed for 14 days. The sections of the damaged and undamaged sciatic nerves were exposed for 28 days.

Evaluation: The quantitative evaluation of the labelling index was conducted exclusively with material embedded in paraffin. One thousand each of microglialike cellular elements of the cortex, perivascular cells, and free subarachnoidal cells as well as 100 epiplexus cells were identified in the brain sections. One hundred spindle cells (probably Schwann cells) were located in undamaged nerves. One hundred spindle cells as well as 100 round cells with abundant cytoplasm (phagocytes) were counted in the damaged nerve in the area of the orthograde degeneration (at the distal nerve stump). In all cases those cells were considered labeled which demonstrated five or more reduced silver granules per nucleus. Due to the short exposure time, background correction was not necessary.

Results

The labeling indexes for the various intracerebral cell types before and after the stab wound are presented in Table 1. Table 2 lists the percentage of labeled cells in undamaged sciatic nerves as well as in the peripheral stump of ligated sciatic nerves. On the basis of these results, it can be concluded that the rate of DNA-synthesizing, nonactivated cells in the central and peripheral NS is extremely low.

The proliferation of cell types from identical locations, however, obviously can be stimulated by nonspecific mechanical irritation. After stimulation the percentage of labeled cells is increased for all cells counted. The significant increase of cells in the respective lesion areas cannot, however, be explained satisfactorily by the proliferation of local cells. After autoradiographic preparation of sections pretreated with enzyme-histochemical methods, a portion of the labeled cells in the stab wound showed clear-cut nonspecific esterase activity (Fig. 16A), an enzyme used to identify monocytes. The increased number of DNA-synthesizing spindle cells (Schwann cells) in the area of the peripheral nerves subsequent to stimulation is conspicuous. Cells such as the so-called round cells appear for which there are no true precursor cells in the undamaged nerves, if the possibility of the transformation of Schwann cells into phagocytes is excluded (see Palmer et al., 1961; Spencer and Thomas, 1974).

2. Hematogenesis

Since virtually only mature labeled blood cells [and in very slight amounts also precursor cells (see Seno et al., 1976)] reach the receiver animals, parabiotic experiments were

Table 1. Labeling index of MP of the CNS in three undamaged rabbits and in three rabbits 24 h after stab wound[a]

	Undamaged animals				24 h after stab wound			
Cell type	LI	M	SD	VC	LI	M	SD	VC
Resting and/or progressive Microglia (1000 cells counted)	0.1 0.3 0.2	0.2	±0.1	±50.0%	0.6 2.3 3.4	2.1	±1.4	± 67.1%
Perivascular cells (1000 cells counted)	0.4 0.3 0.2	0.3	±0.1	±33.3%	1.2 0.8 1.9	1.3	±0.5	± 42.3%
Free subarachnoidal cells (1000 cells counted)	0.1 0.2 0.4	0.2	±0.1	±60.8%	1.2 1.8 2.4	1.8	±0.6	± 33.3%
Epiplexus cells (100 cells counted)	0.0 0.0 0.0	0.0	–	–	1.0 0.0 2.0	1.0	±1.0	±100.0%

[a] LI: Labeling index; M: Mean; SD: Standard deviation; VC: Variability coefficient.

Table 2. Labeling index of cells in the left sciatic nerve (undamaged) and in the right sciatic nerve (ligated 5 days previously–Wallerian degeneration) of four rabbits[a]

	Undamaged (left) nerve		Nerve (right) ligated 5 days previously (Wallerian degeneration)			
Cell types	LI	M	LI	M	SD	VC
Spindel cells–probably Schwann cells (100 cells counted)	0 0 0 0	0	4 2 3 0	2.2	±1.7	±75.5%
Round cells–probably mononuclear phagocytes (100 cells counted)	0 0 0 0	0	5 2 3 1	2.7	±1.7	±61.8%

[a] LI: Labeling index; M: Mean; SD: Standard deviation; VC: Variability coefficient.

conducted to establish the hematogenesis of MP of the NS. The possibility of a reutilization of DNA following the degeneration of cells in the area of the lesion cannot be definitely excluded with this experimental model, even though reutilization here is significantly lower than after the injection of bone marrow cells (cf. Roessmann and Friede, 1968).

Materials and Methods

Animals: There were 18 rats included in the parabiotic experiments. In each case one parabiont (receiver animal) was damaged by inflicting a cerebral lesion; the other parabiont (donor animal) remained undamaged. Intracerebral stab wounds were inflicted in six receiver animals (series 1), meningoencephalitis was induced in six animals (series 2), and cerebral storage of galactocerebroside was induced in the remaining six animals (series 3).

Stab wounds: See above.

Meningoencephalitis: This disease was induced by intracerebral injection of a virus suspension (herpesvirus simplex hominis I: strain Thea; titer: $\sim 6 \times 10^6/0.25$ infectious units). The virus was cultured in a mouse brain. After centrifugation, a 2% suspension of the supernatant was diluted with physiologic saline solution (1:10). The dose per animal was 0.05 ml suspension (virus suspension provided by Prof. H.-J. Gerth, Hygiene Institute, University of Tübingen, Tübingen/FRG).

Experimental storage of galactocerebroside: This procedure was carried out according to data cited by Austin and Lehfeld (1965) and Anzil et al. (1972). A suspension of 15 mg purified crystalline galactocerebroside (bovine galactocerebroside: Applied Sciences Lab. Inc., State College, Pa/USA) dissolved in physiologic saline was applied to induce globoid cell production.

Parabiotic suturing and treatment (cf. Figs. 5 and 6): According to data published by the author elsewhere (Grüninger and Oehmichen, 1972), the skins of two rats were laterally incised and then sutured together. To prevent the sutures from tearing, the animals were kept in a special cage constructed for this purpose. Ten days after the operation, one of the animals was irradiated to destroy the blood-forming bone marrow (see also Tyler and Everett, 1966, 1972). Only the two hind legs were exposed to x-irradiation. X-irradiation was carried out with a Siemens apparatus (Type: Stabilipan SRW x-ray apparatus, 200 kV and 16 mA; dosage: 800 R. The beam was directed from a distance of 60 cm for 11.2 min with the aperture wide open). The rest of the animal's body as well as the body of the parabiotic neighbor animal was covered with a 10-cm-thick lead block. The irradiated animal was designated as the "receiver" animal because its blood supply had to be partially taken over by the nonirradiated parabiont animal (i.e., "donor" animal). (Irradiation of the animals was made possible by Prof. G. Breitling, Institute for Medical Radiology, University of Tübingen, Tübingen/FRG.)

Thymidine application: In the first two experimental series (stab wound and meningoencephalitis), ^{3}H-TdR was administered to the donor animals intraperitoneally for a period of 96 h (0.5 μCi/g body wt./8 h). In the third experimental series (experimentally induced storage of galactocerebroside), ^{3}H-TdR (1 μCi/g body wt.) was given two times in 24 h for a period of 11 days.

The thymidine itself was applied according to the plan presented in Fig. 5. The parabiotic suture was clamped with an intestinal clamp; 5-mg nonlabeled ("cold") thymi-

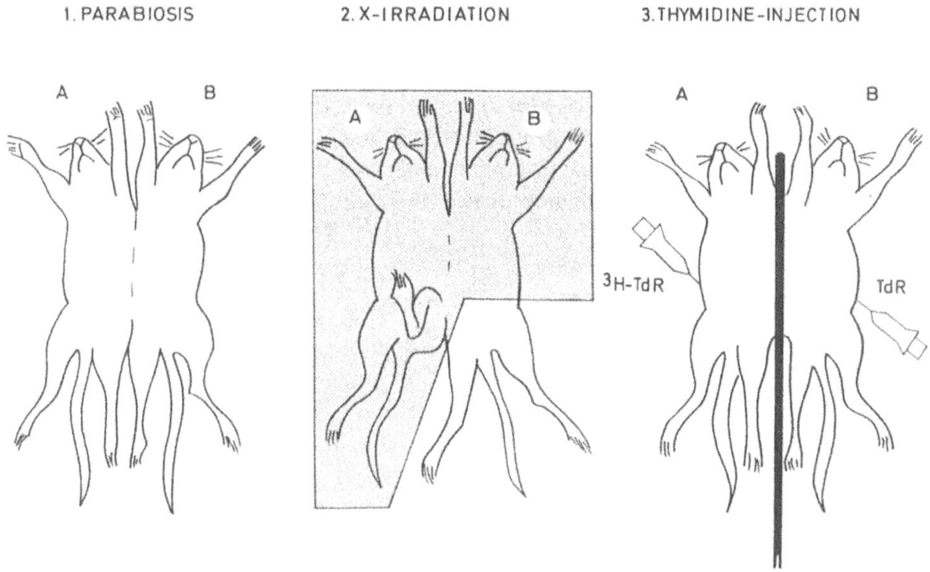

Fig. 5. Parabiotic experiments: Schematic representation of the experimental procedure modified according to Tyler and Everett (1966). It applies for all parabiotic experiments described. *1.* Parabiosis: Suture; *2.* X-irradiation: Lead shield for body regions which are not to be irradiated; *3.* Thymidine injection: Injection procedure for labeled and non-labeled thymidine (for details, see text)

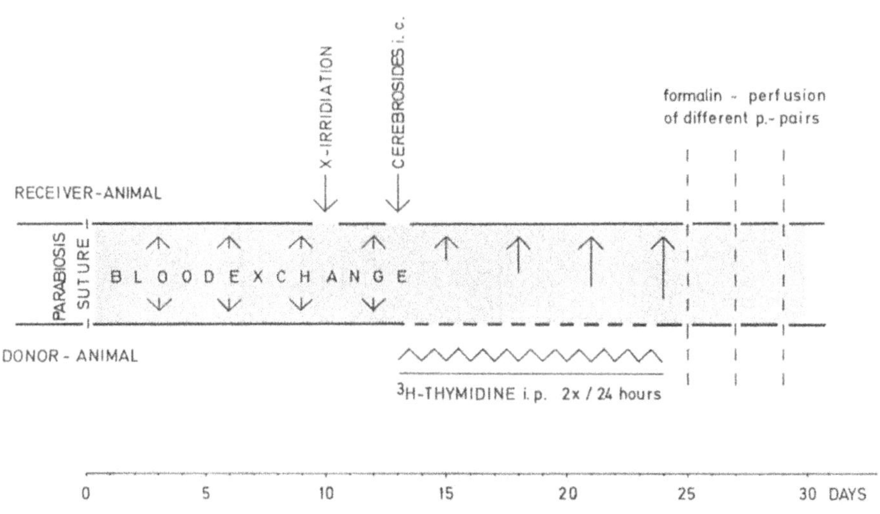

Fig. 6. Sequence of experimental procedure for parabiotic experiments, demonstrated in the experiments with galactocerebroside storage

dine (Serva Feinbiochemica, Heidelberg/FRG) dissolved in physiologic saline solution was administered intraperitoneally to the receiver animal to cover its thymidine requirements. The donor animal then received an injection of radioactively labeled thymidine. The clamp was left in place for 20 min in order to adjust for the time that dissolved, incorporated ^{3}H-TdR was still present in the peripheral blood. Before loosening the clamp, the receiver animal received enough cold thymidine to fill up its thymidine pool. The clamp was then removed. The labeling type of the intestine is used as a control (cf. Figs. 7 A and B).

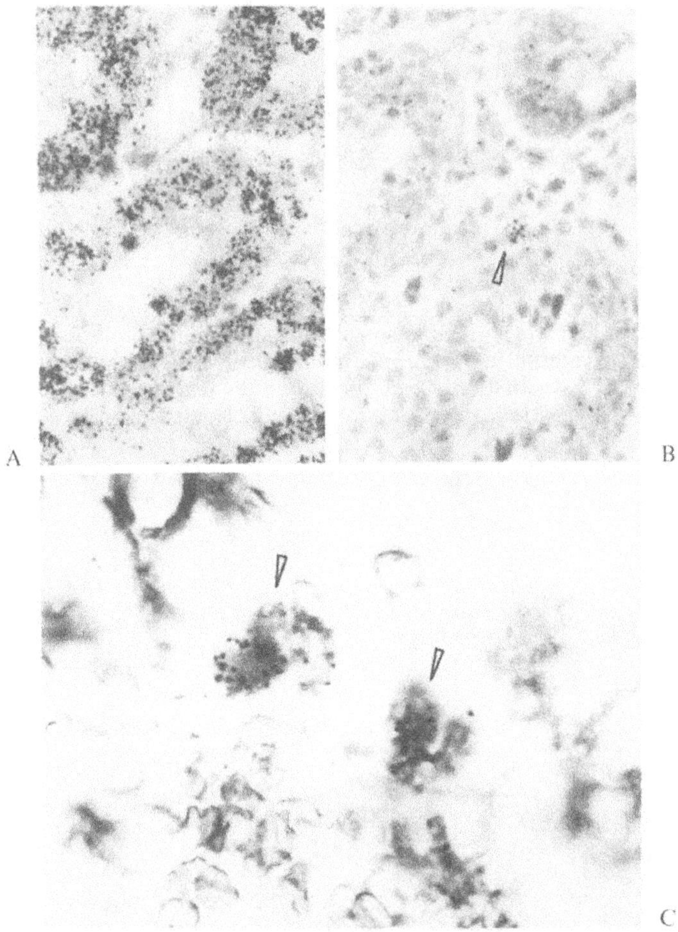

Fig. 7 A–C. Parabiotic experiments to demonstrate the migration of mononuclear blood cells in damaged brain tissue of rat. Intestinal tissue was examined as a control: (A) The nucleus of almost every cell in the intestinal epithelia is loaded with labeled thymidine in the so-called donor parabiont. (B) single labeled cells can be observed in the stroma (intravascular mononuclear cells of the donor animals) of the receptor parabiont. (C) The fact that macrophagelike cells could always be observed in the receptor parabiont following intracerebral stab wounds indicated that mononuclear blood cells of the donor animal migrated into the damaged neuropil of the receptor animal. [(A–C) hemalum stain; magnification: (A and B)x 500, (C)x 1200] (Fig. 7 A and B after Oehmichen, 1973)

Experimental procedure (cf. Fig. 6): Ten days after parabiotic suturing, the receiver animal was x-irradiated. The experimental procedure varied according to the experimental series.

The animals in the series with stab wound and meningoencephalitis received the first thymidine injection 3 days after irradiation; 24 h later, a brain lesion was inflicted in the receiver animal. Thymidine was applied for 2 additional days, and the animals were killed 36 h after the final application.

The animals with experimental storage of galactocerebroside (cf. Fig. 6) also received their first injection of thymidine 3 days after irradiation. Here the lesion was applied on the same day because cerebroside-storing globoid cells have a relatively long formation period. Thymidine injections, therefore, were extended over 11 days. Two parabiotic pairs were killed at intervals of 1, 3, and 5 days after the final thymidine injection.

Autoradiographic treatment: The organs as well as some of the prepared blood smears from series 1 and 2 were coated with Kodak NTB3 and exposed for 14 days. The organ sections from series-3 animals were coated with Ilford K2 emulsion and exposed for 28 days.

Results

Blood smears from receiver and donor animals were prepared at various times during the experiments with stab wounds and meningoencephalitis. After the blood smears were fixed with methanol, they were treated autoradiographically. The results presented in Table 3 show that blood cells do actually migrate from one animal to the other.

Table 3. Median percentage of labeled mononuclear blood cells in 12 parabiotic rats after 100 cells of each cell type were counted in blood smears of so-called donor and receiver animals (in parabiotic experiments)

Time (in days) after the first injection of ^{3}H-TdR	Donor animals		Receiver animals	
	Lymphocytes	Monocytes	Lymphocytes	Monocytes
1	0	17	0	1
2	16	53	2	4
3	31	83	5	19
4	52	100	10	22

Following the stab wound, individual labeled mononuclear cells were found in the brain tissue, neuropil, and subarachnoid space of the receiver animals. The quantity was usually low: approximately two labeled cells per section. Cells were seldom found perivascularly. Labeled cells containing isolated erythrocytes and vacuoles (indicating dissolved fat) were repeatedly found. In the meningoencephalitis experiments, many labeled cells were found distributed diffusely in the neuropil. Most of the labeled cells were migrated monocytes (Figs. 7C, 8A, 16B, C). In addition, a dense mixed cell population consisting of lymphocytes and monocytes was found in the leptomeningeal, ventricular, and vascular spaces. Some of these cells were labeled.

In the globoid cell experiments, a large number of mononucleated and polynucated cells containing PAS-positive material was found in the area of the cerebroside injection. Cytomorphologically, these cells could be classified as globoid cells (see Figs. 8, 16B, C). Labeled cells were repeatedly found here (approximately two–eight per section). Binucleated and polynucleated cells were found with only one labeled nucleus (Figs. 8B, C, D). After the complete autoradiographic treatment, H&E-staining, and photographing, the labeled cells were tested for the PAS reaction. As a result of the PAS-reaction test, the number of reduced silver granules was decreased. With the demonstrable content of PAS-positive substances at this time, the cells could, however, definitely be classified as experimentally induced globoid cells. Although isolated labeled cells were found in the leptomeninges and perivascularly in these experiments, they were not found in the vicinity of the plexus because the ventricle had not been directly damaged by the injection.

It can, therefore, be concluded that in the presence of cerebral damage blood cells can migrate into the brain. At the same time it was established that migrated blood cells are capable of forming polynuclear giant cells through apposition (fusion?).

In select experiments, the animals were decapitated and cerebroside was injected. The brain tissue from some of the animals was immediately frozen for 10 and/or 30 days and then sliced on the cryostat. In this way, the enzyme activity of acidic phosphatase, α-naphthyl acetate esterase, naphthol AS acetate esterase, naphthol AS-D chloroacetate esterase was observed. A comparable activity of these enzymes in mononuclear blood cells can be demonstrated only in monocytes.

3. Monocytic Origin

The aim of the transfusion experiments was the same as that of the parabiotic experiments were to provide the same evidence (i.e., that blood cells can migrate into the nervous system), but in another species. The experiments were also conducted to obtain additional information regarding the types of hematogenic precursor cells for MP. Construction of an experimental model that would eliminate the reutilization of labeled tracers under every circumstance presented a problem in itself.

Three experiments were then carried out, each geared to a different formulation of the problem.

a) Investigations of the Hematogenesis of Mononuclear Phagocytes in the Central Nervous System of Rabbits

Monocytosis was induced in the peripheral blood of each of the three so-called donor animals (cf. the experimental procedure shown in Fig. 9) by repeated intraperitoneal injection of carmine (4x/3 days; individual dosage: 2.5 ml/kg body weight of saturated sterile solution (see also Komiya et al., 1961; Oehmichen et al., 1972). The percentage of monocytes was, therefore, increased from 3–4 relative percent up to 10–20 relative percent in each animal.

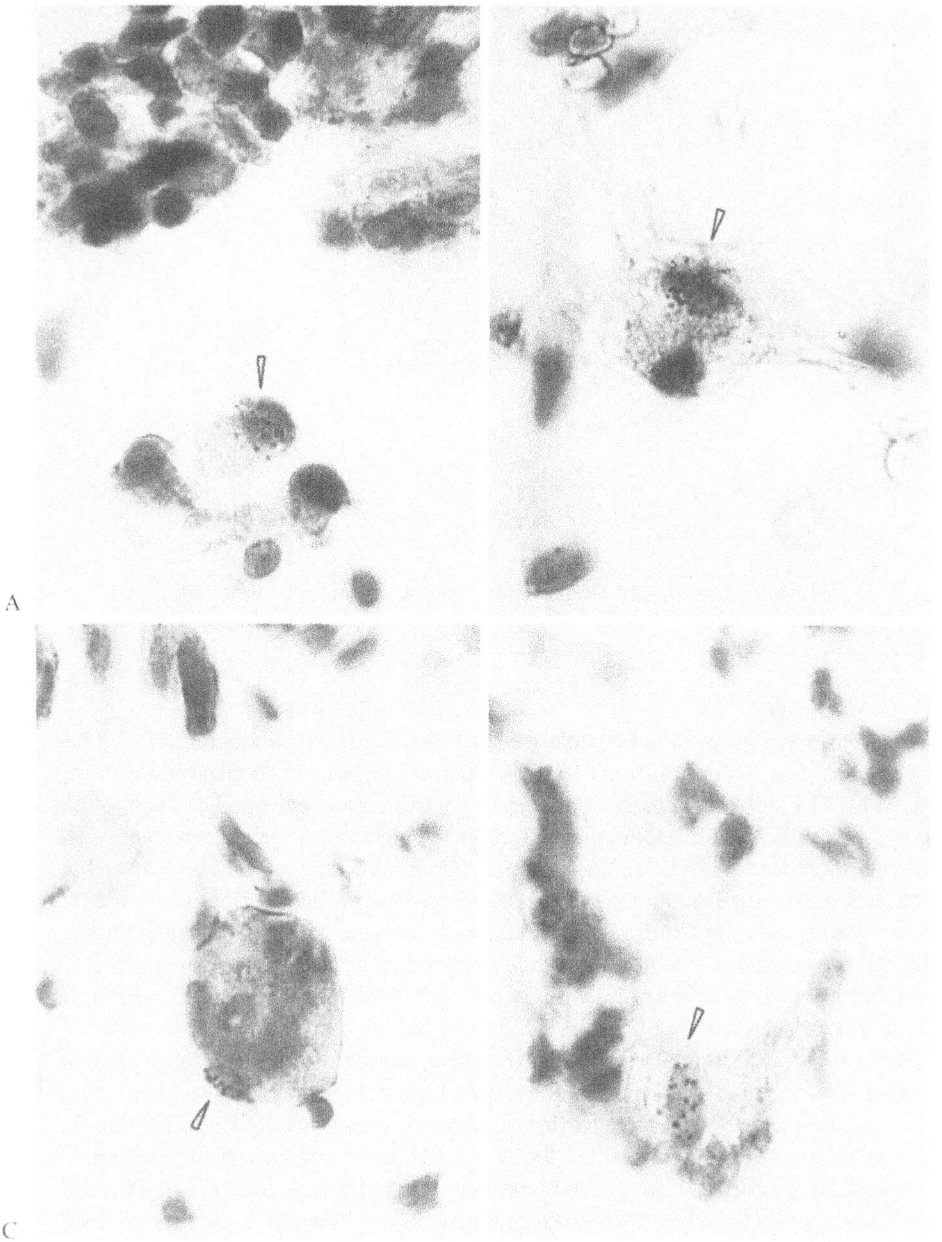

Fig. 8 A–D. Parabiotic experiments with storage of galactocerebroside to establish the origin of PAS-positive, macrophagelike elements and/or mononuclear and polynuclear globoidlike elements from mononuclear blood cells (cf. also Fig. 15 B and C). Labeled (i.e., migrated via the blood stream) isolated cell nuclei are found in the mononuclear (A), binuclear (B), and polynuclear (C and D) PAS-positive cells in the brain tissue of so-called receptor parabionts. This indicates the development of polynuclear cells by superimposition (fusion?) of mononuclear blood cells. [(A–D) H&E stain; magnification: (A–D) x 1200] (Fig. 8 A, C, and D after Oehmichen, 1974)

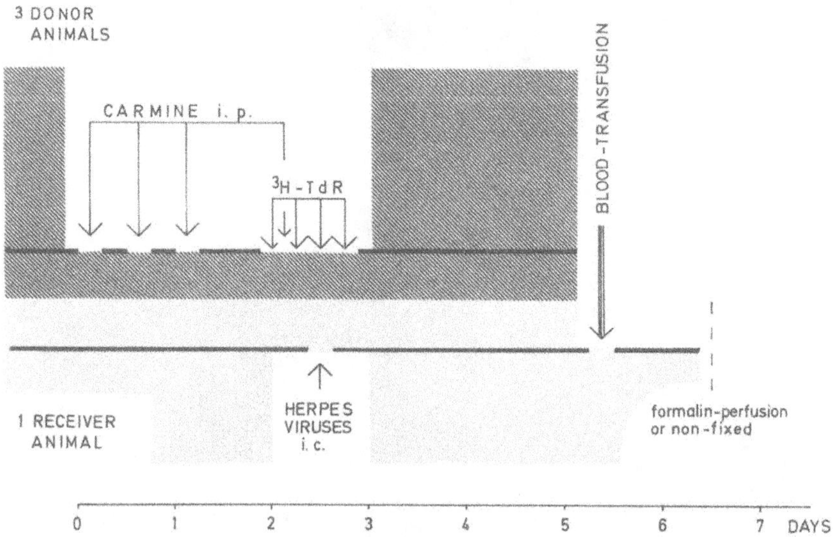

Fig. 9. Transfusion experiments. Course of an experimental series in which monocytosis was induced by injecting carmine into the donor animals while meningoencephalitis was induced in the receiver animals

An attempt was made to use cumulative labeling to label all monocytes. At 18 h before the final injection of carmine, ^{3}H-TdR was repeatedly injected intravenously (4x/24 h). The individual dosage consisted of 1.0 μCi/g body weight. The upper limits for the relative percent of monocytes as well as the peak for the relative percent of labeled cells was reached 3 days later, almost 100%. At this time, blood was removed from each of the three animals via cardial puncture under ether anesthesia and artificial ventilation. After the thoracic cavity had been opened, 2500 U.S.P. heparin was injected intracardially. The blood was then removed under negative pressure of the heart and stored in 120 ml bottles with 24 ml ACD Biostabilizer (Biotest Serum Institute, Frankfurt/Main, ACD-Stabilizer U.S.P. XVII B).

The total blood volume (average: 80–100 ml) from each of the three donor animals was immediately transfused over a 6–8 h period into the so-called receiver animals via the ear vein. Tolerance tests were carried out prior to each transfusion. Each animal was injected with a total of $1 \times 10^6 - 1.5 \times 10^7$ labeled blood monocytes. At the same time, granulocytes (100% labeled) and lymphocytes (~20% labeled) were also transfused. The animals were killed via aortal perfusion of 4% formalin, 24 h after the transfusion had started. The receiver animal either remained undamaged (four animals) or received an intracerebral stab wound 3 days prior to the transfusion (four animals), or an experimentally induced meningoencephalitis (herpesvirus suspension IC; individual dosage: 0.2 ml/animal; four animals). The autoradiograms were coated with Kodak NTB emulsion and exposed for 14 and/or 28 days.

Results

In two undamaged animals, isolated labeled cells were found inside the neuropil. A definite localization in relation to the vessels was not observed (Fig. 10) and no labeled

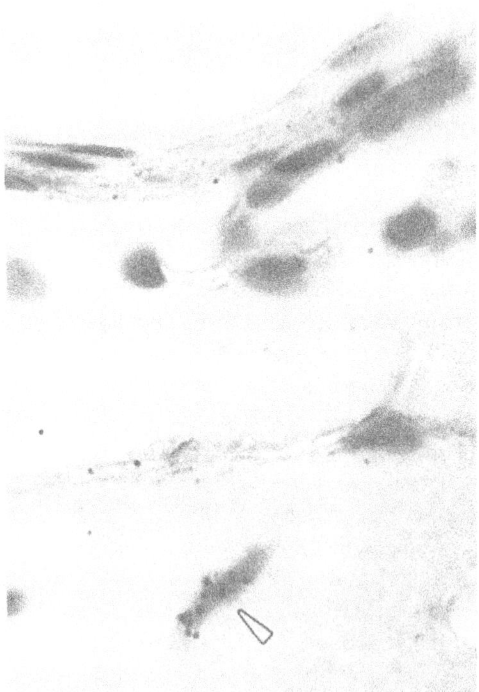

Fig. 10. Transfusion experiments to establish hematogenesis of mononuclear cells in undamaged neuropil. One labeled cell can be seen subpially (questionable resting microglia). (H&E stain; magnification: x 1200)

cells could be definitely identified in the other two undamaged animals. The varying findings could not be attributed to the experimental procedure. No labeled cells were found in the leptomeninges, in the ventricle, or localized perivascularly in the undamaged animals.

After the stab wounds, isolated labeled mononuclear cells (i.e., phagocytes) were found adjacent to the puncture channel in the leptomeninges, neuropil, and ventricle. In the ventricle, some adhered to the surface of the ependyma and choroidal plexus. Some of the cells contained erythrocytes or nuclear debris. The presence of vacuoles in the cytoplasm was interpreted as an indication of dissolved droplets of fat *(Fettkörnchenzellen).*

The most pronounced alterations occurred in the series with experimental herpesvirus meningoencephalitis. A relatively dense cellular infiltrate was found, particularly in the leptomeninges, which extended into the most superficial cortical segments and as far as the perivascular spaces. Fewer labeled lymphocytes were also found among the labeled cells here, sometimes in a proportion of 1 : 1000. Frequently, macrophage-like cells could be recognized by virtue of their nuclear structure and light, distended body of cytoplasm. Thus, a labeled cell with a relatively loosely structured nucleus was observed migrating through a vascular wall into the leptomeninges (Fig. 11 A). Increased quantities of labeled cells were found deposited near the outer wall of small leptomeningeal vessels. Sometimes labeled cells were also concentrated at the level of the pial cells (Fig. 12); here they assumed the shape of spindle cells. Sometimes, however, the cells could not be distinguished from local pial cells. Since they were seldom also found at the level of the inner layer of the arachnoidal cover cells, the cells seemed to be identical to these cover cells. The cells were also drawn into the trabecular network in those areas containing only loose cell infiltrates. They were located on the collagenous fibers of the trabecular network and could not be distinguished from the trabecular cells normally found here (Figs. 11 B and C).

Limited clumps of microglia were observed subpially in the neuropil at the outermost cortical layers. The direction of the cells tended to indicate that the increased amount of cellular elements found here had migrated from the pia (Figs. 12 and 13). Each respective serial section was treated autoradiographically (Fig. 13 C), on the parallel section, the microglia were selectively impregnated with silver (Fig. 13 A). Increased quantities of labeled cells were found in those areas where a clear-cut increase in progressive microglia was observed (Fig. 13 B). The labeled cells were identified morphologically as progressive microglia.

No cellular infiltrate was recognized in the more deeply lying cortical sections. Labeled cells were repeatedly found attached externally to individual vessels the size of capillaries, arterioles, and/or venules as well as arteries and/or veins (Fig. 14). Some of these cells possessed a spindle-shaped nucleus and, therefore, closely resembled pericytes (cf. Figs. 14 A, B, and 16 F, G, H). The nucleus was more indented in some of the cells and, therefore, the cells bore a closer resemblance to monocytes. Just as frequently labeled cells in the medullary layer were also often found located in the neighborhood of the vessels, even though they no longer had any direct contact to a particular vessel (Figs. 12 and 14 c). Here, a migration was sometimes apparent. Only isolated labeled cells were observed in the ventricle itself, and then in those animals in which the herpesvirus had been deeply injected intracerebrally into the medullary layer. The labeled cells identified here were almost exclusively macrophagelike cells (Fig. 15).

b) Investigations of the Monocytic Origin of Mononuclear Phagocytes in the Central Nervous System

Basically, the transfusion experiments for this particular approach to the problem correspond methodologically to the experiments described above. For the new formulation of the problem three receiver animals were examined which had received an experimentally induced meningoencephalitis prior to the transfusion. The only difference between this experiment and the previous experiments was the method of fixing the brain tissue. Instead of using formalin, the animals were perfused via the aorta with 200 ml

Fig. 11 A–C. Transfusion experiment to establish hematogenesis of cells of the subarachnoid space in experimentally induced meningeoencephalitis. (A) One labeled mononuclear cells can be seen migrating through vascular wall *(arrow)*. (B and C) Labeled cells inside trabecular network *(arrow)*, and [(A–C) H&E stain; magnification: (A)x750; (B and C)x1500]

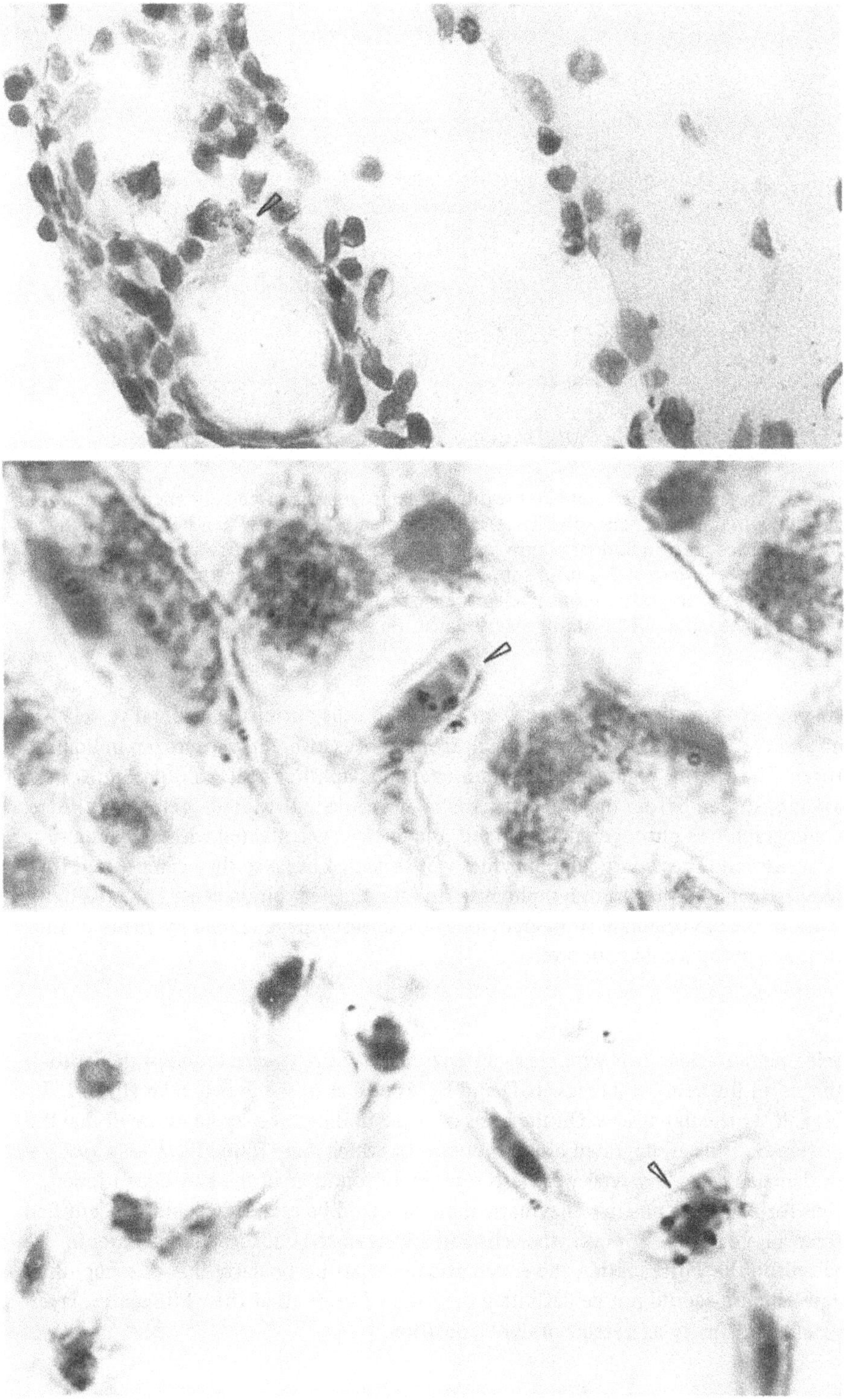

A

B

C

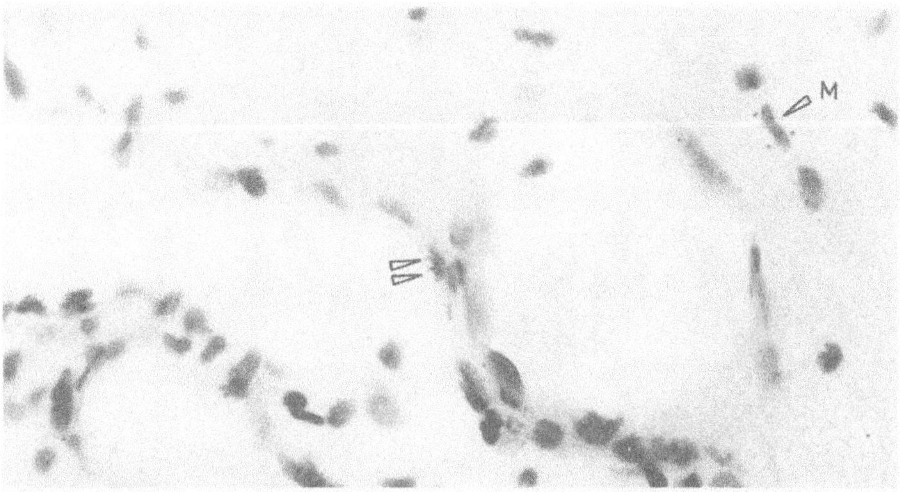

Fig. 12. Transfusion experiment to establish hematogenesis of cells of the subarachnoid space following meningoencephalitis. One labeled cell *(2 arrows)* can be seen which, because of its localization and structure, cannot be distinguished from a pial cell. One other labeled cell *(arrow)* is found subpially inside the neuropil, in the vicinity of the vein. This cell is a migrated mononuclear cell which has assumed the characteristics of progressive microglia. (H&E stain; magnification: x 1000)

warm physiologic saline solution to wash the blood cells out of the cerebral vessels. The brain was then exposed, and 0.5-cm-thick frontal slices of brain were frozen in liquid nitrogen. The activity of nonspecific esterases and of naphthol AS-D chloroacetate esterase was demonstrated before the cryostat sections were treated autoradiographically. After the radiograph was photographically fixed, the nucleus was stained with hemalum or nuclear fast red. These particular enzymes were selected because they can be used to differentiate monocytes from lymphocytes in mononuclear blood cells. The possibility that MP of the NS originate from granulocytes can easily be excluded by virtue of the nuclear and cytoplasmic structure.

Results

Labeled mononuclear cells with clear-cut enzymatic activity were found in the leptomeninges, in the neurophil (Figs. 16D and E), as well as in the perivascular (Figs. 16F, G, H) and ventricular spaces. On the basis of these findings, it may be assumed that the cells were transfused, migrated blood monocytes, which were found in various localizations. Labaled cells, however, were also repeatedly found in all the above-mentioned regions for which no positive enzymatic material could be established and/or identified. Cytomorphologically, however, the cells still appeared to be macrophages. Later in isolated cells in the white matter, the enzymatic material–particularly that of α-naphthyl acetate esterase–could not be definitely determined since all of the white matter layer was stained diffusely as a result of dye deposition.

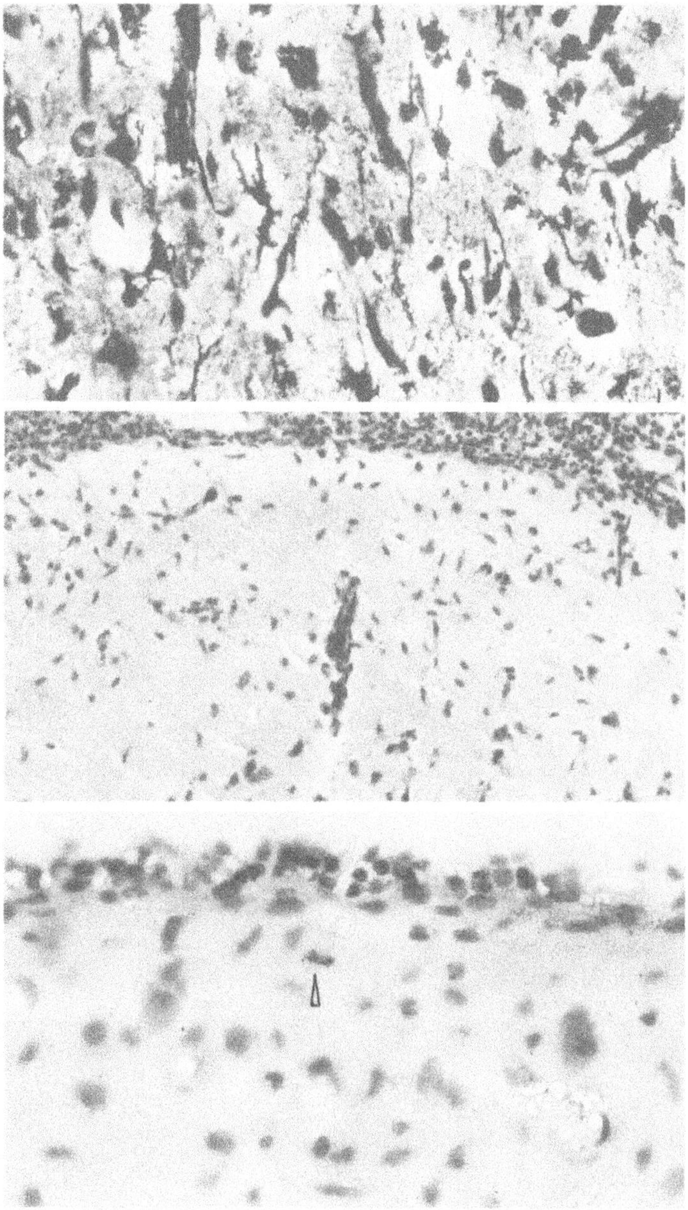

Fig. 13A–C. Transfusion experiment to establish hematogenesis of progressive microglia in experimentally induced meningoencephalitis. (A) Silver impregnation to demonstrate progressive microglia. (B) H&E stain. (C) Autoradiograph to establish labeled cells undertaken in serial sections. A distinctly increased number of progressive microglia is seen in the region near the pia mater. Isolated migrated blood cells *(arrow)*, (C) are seen. [(A) silver impregnation according to Tsusijama (1962); (B and C) H&E stain; magnification: (A)x300, (B)x200, (C)x500] (Fig. 13C after Oehmichen, 1975)

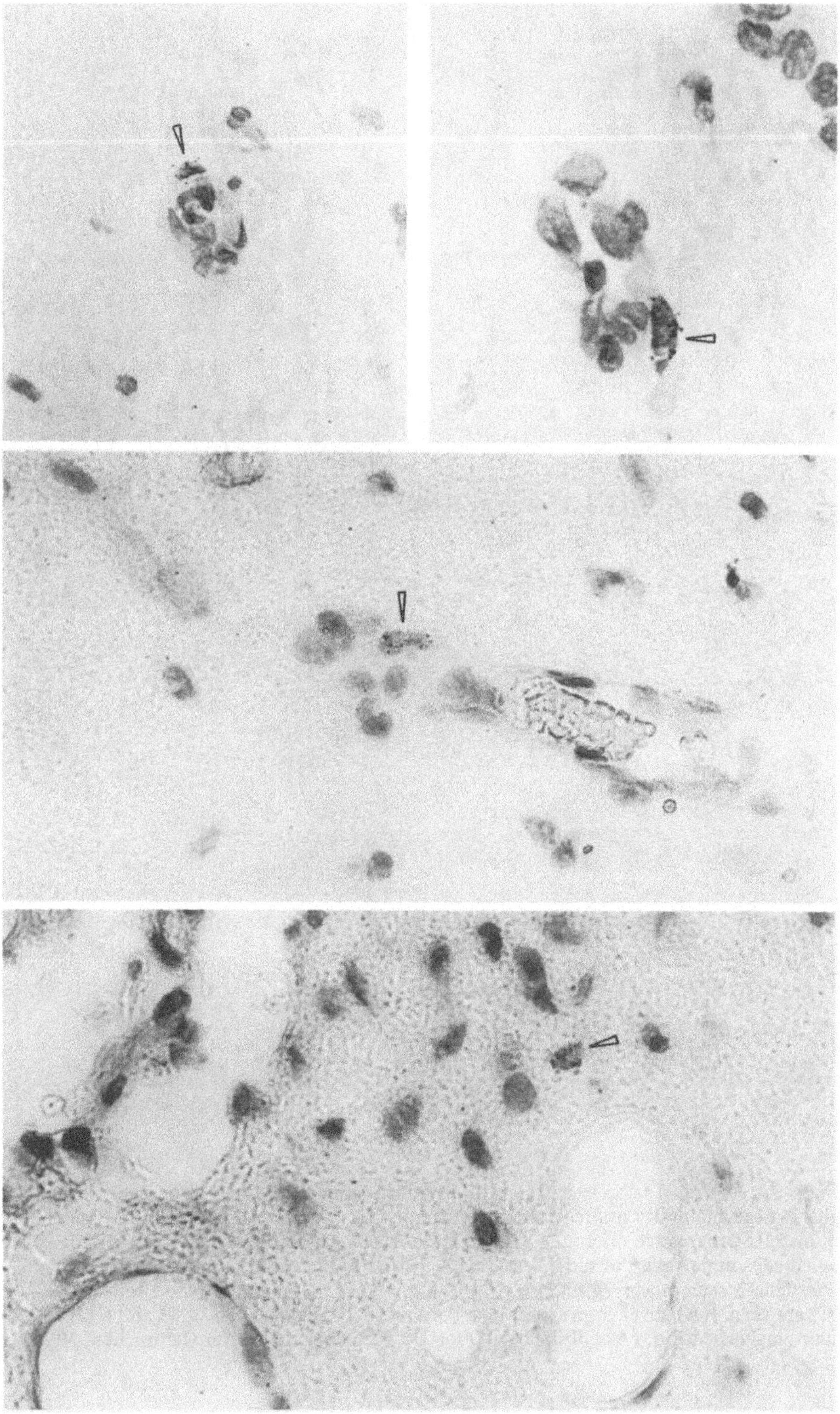

A

B

C

D

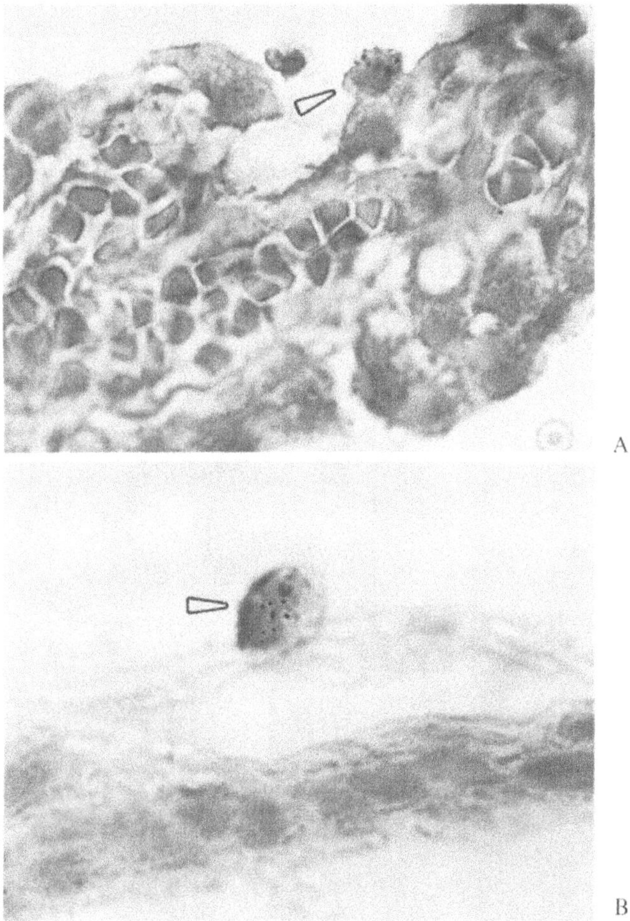

Fig. 15 A and B. Transfusion experiment to establish hematogenesis of epiplexus cells following meningoencephalitis. Labeled mononuclear blood cells *(arrows)* adherent to the surface of the choroidal plexus resembling epiplexus cells. [(A and B) H&E stain; magnification: x 1200]

c) Investigations of the Monocytic Origin of Mononuclear Phagocytes in the Nervous System which Avoid Tracer Reutilization

This investigation required application of a radioactive substance that was not utilized in cellular metabolism during cell degeneration. Tritium-labeled diisopropyl fluorophos-

---

Fig. 14 A–D. Transfusion experiments to establish hematogenesis of perivascular cells from intracerebral vessels following meningoencephalitis. (A–C) Labeled cells in perivascular connective tissue of small arteries. (D) Labeled cells in the vicinity of a vein of the subpial neuropil. (A and B) naphthol AS-D chloroacetateesterase/hemalum stain; C and D: H&E stain; magnification: [(A) x 500, (B–D x 1200] (Fig. 14 A and B after Oehmichen, 1973; Fig. 14 D after Oehmichen, 1975)

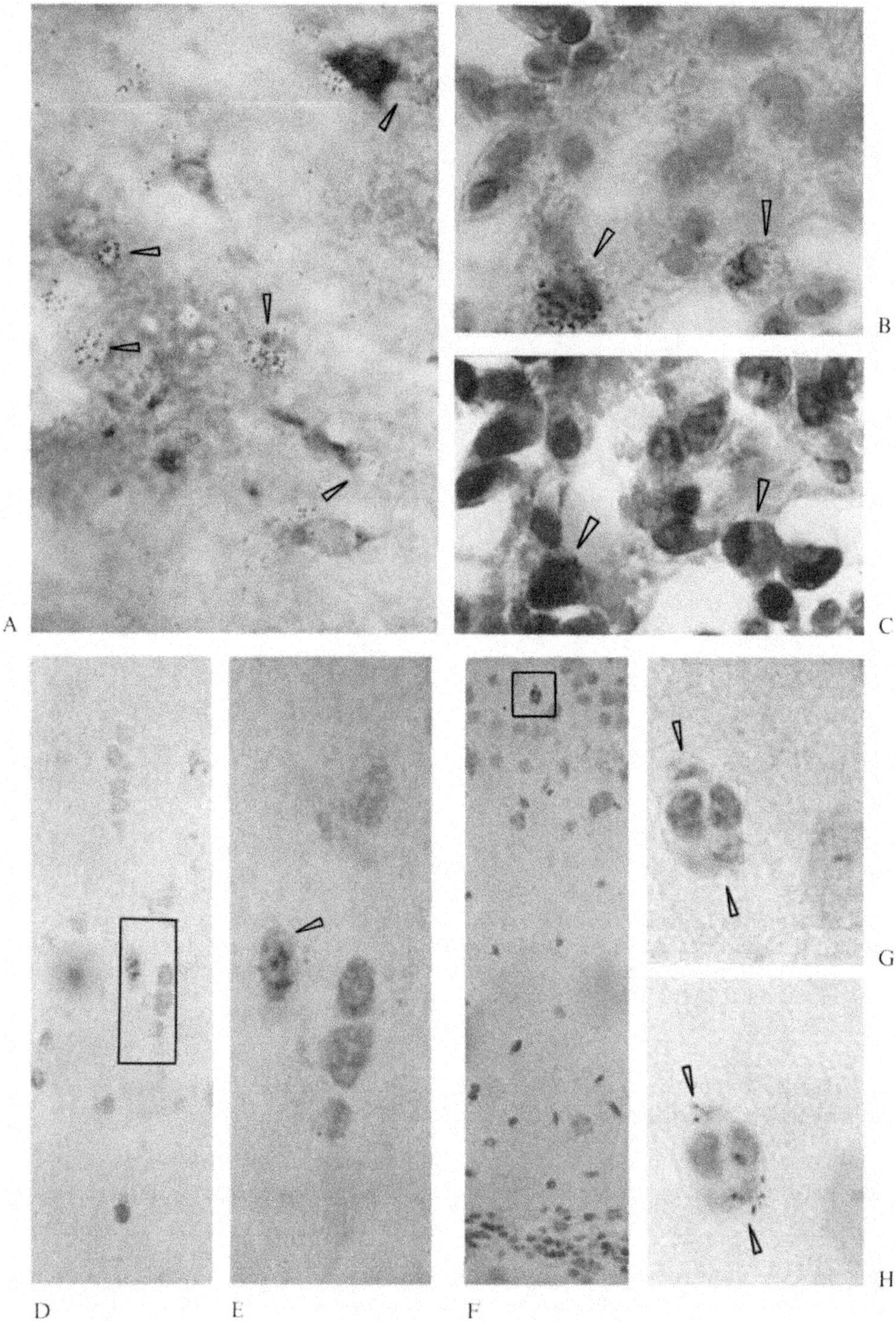
A
B
C
D
E
F
G
H

phate (^{3}H-DFP) is particularly well suited for experiments with blood monocytes (see also Van Hasselt, 1970; Meuret and Hoffmann, 1973) because it is irreversibly bound to esterases. Athens and co-workers (1959) were successful in obtaining a bond with leukocytes but not with lymphocytes. We used the following two experimental procedures:

1. Blood was collected via cardiac puncture from two and/or three untreated rabbits. To this blood was added 2 μCi/ml ^{3}H-DFP dissolved in propylene glycol. The blood was then mixed periodically, incubated at room temperature for 1 h, and then transfused into a receiver animal. Herpesvirus had been applied intracerebrally to these receiver animals (total: three rabbits) 4 days prior to the transfusion. The receiver animals were killed 24 h later. The brain tissue was embedded in paraffin; the slices were then coated with Ilford K2 emulsion and exposed for 28 days.
2. Peritoneal macrophages were labeled instead of blood cells. The collection of these cells from the abdominal cavity has already been described (see p. 39). The washed cells were labeled in vitro with ^{3}H-DFP in the same way as the blood cells had been labeled. The cells were washed one more time in Hank's balanced salt solution and then intravenously applied in the form of a 10 ml cell suspension (total: 2×10^6 bis 1×10^7 cells).
   Two different types of injuries had been inflicted in each of the receiver animals (total: four rabbits) 4 days prior to the application: The right sciatic nerve had been ligated (see above) and the left facial nerve had been removed. In the latter procedure, a small incision was made under the ear of the rabbit to expose the nerve. The nerve was then resected and the proximal segment removed from the stylomastoid foramen. The purpose of this procedure was to increase the quantity of perineuronal microglial cells via the subsequent retrograde degeneration of nerve cells in the area of the facial nerve nucleus.

Results

After transfusion of blood labeled with ^{3}H-DFP, labeled mononuclear cells were found inside the neuropil, in the leptomeninges, and around the individual vessels in those receiver animals with meningoencephalitis (Fig. 17). These cells should only have been migrated, extravascular, labeled blood monocytes since the lymphocytes possessed no identifiable labeling either here or in the blood smears examined. Monocytes in the

◁

Fig. 16A–H. Hematogenesis or monocytic origin of cells in the central nervous system. (A) Three days following intracerebral stab wound and 1 h after intravenous injection of ^{3}H-thymidine, labeled, α-naphthyl-acetateesterase-positive cells are seen [indication of a local proliferation of monocytic cells. (B) Following intracerebral injection of galactocerebroside, macrophagelike, labeled cells with clear-cut positive PAS reaction (C); compare (B and C) identical cells from the same section after different treatment] are found in the so-called receptor parabiont (indication of hematogenesis of cerebroside-storing cells). (D–H) Labeled naphthol-AS-D-chloroacetateesterase-positive cells in the neurophil (D and E) same cells in different magnification and perivascularly around a capillary. (F–H) Same cells with different magnification and fucosing; indication of monocytic origin in experimentally induced meningoencephalitis following transfusion of labeled blood monocytes. [(A) α-naphthyl acetateesterase; (B and C) hemalum stain; (C) PAS reaction; (D–H) naphthol AS-D chloroacetateesterase/hemalum; magnification: (A) x620; (B and C) x1200; (D) x500; (F) x200; (E, G, H) x1200]

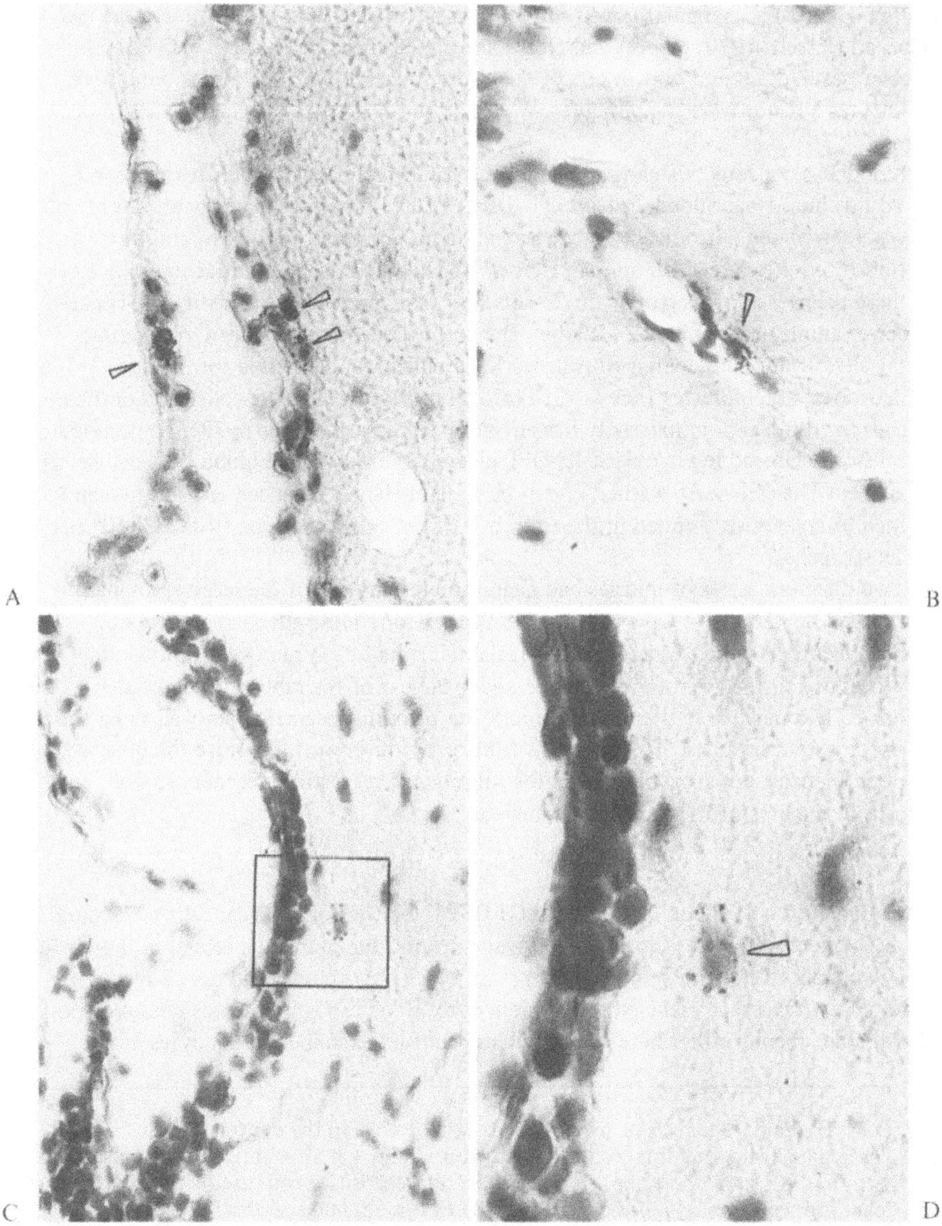

Fig. 17A–D. Transfusion experiment avoiding reutilization by intravenous injection of blood monocytes labeled with ^{3}H-DFP in receptor animals with experimentally induced meningoencephalitis. Labeled mononuclear cells are seen in the subarachnoid space (A), in the perivascular space of an intracerebral vessel (B), and/or in the neuropil (C and D), same cell in different magnifications, subependymal. [(A–D) H&E stain; magnification: (A–C) x500, (D) x1200]

blood smears from the transfused blood were 100% labeled. Although we looked carefully for labeled cells, we were unable to observe any in the ventricular system. This finding was not too surprising since, in each case, the inflammatory reaction was localized superficially and remained limited to the leptomeninges of the hemispheres and the superficial cortical sections. Compared with the transfusion experiments utilizing ^{3}H-TdR as a tracer and in vivo labeling, the number of labeled cells was, on the whole, lower in those experiments with ^{3}H-DFP. Since only monocytes and granulocytes (but not lymphocytes) are labeled with ^{3}H-DFP, an increased number of monocytes in the donor animals was avoided in the transfusion experiments. For this reason, the total amount of injected labeled monocytes was distinctly lowered (reduced to 50% or 20%). A valid methodological comparison, particularly in regard to the frequency of reutilization with ^{3}H-TdR labeling, was, therefore, impossible.

In the second experimental series (injection of labeled peritoneal macrophages), the total number of injected labeled cells was as high as in the experiments described above. The cells, however, were not infused over a period of several hours, but rather injected within a few seconds. The type of lesions in the receiver animals differed somewhat from those in the similar transfusion experiments described above.

Labeled cells were found particularly in the periportal fields of the liver (after counting 1000 Kupffer cells: 0.3%) and isolated in the spleen in the receiver animals. The cells were also repeatedly observed in the area of the traumatically damaged segments of the sciatic nerve (ligature region: ~0.1%). No labeled cells were found, however, in the area of Wallerian degeneration at the distal nerve stump or in the area of retrograde degeneration at the facial nerve nucleus. On serial sections, a slight increase in cells was observed in both regions. These cells were primarily phagocytes and/or also microglialike elements. The question remains whether the increase in cells was too low to stimulate especially the injected labeled cells to leave the vascular system in the area of the lesion investigated or the cells in this kind of lesion react only by local proliferation and not by extravasation.

4. Lymphocytic Origin

Even though some of the experiments described above have provided indications both for the possibility of a migration of monocytes out of the blood vessels and for the ability of these cells to transform into mononuclear phagocytes of different localizations in the central and peripheral nervous systems (at least under pathologic conditions), *negative evidence* has been absent up to now. Establishing such negative evidence seems appropriate since further clarification is, in any case, needed as to whether or not lymphocytes (e.g., in resting microglia) could transform in the normal, undamaged central nervous system. On the other hand, however, it should be established if lymphocytes could also migrate into the CNS, at least under pathologic conditions.

Material and Methods

Transfusion experiments were carried out with in vitro labeled cells. The blood for these experiments was collected from untreated donor rabbits via cardial puncture.

After tolerance tests were carried out, ^{3}H-cytidine (dosage: 1 μCi/ml) was added to the blood (for methods see Bremer and Fliedner, 1971). After incubation at room temperature for more than 3 h, 1000 times the amount of nonlabeled (cold) cytidine was added in order to hold the incorporation of labeled cytidine per cell to a minimum after the injection into a receiver animal. Molecules of ^{3}H-cytidine are incorporated in the RNA and, therefore, also in the lymphocytes. Almost all normal lymphocytes and monocytes were labeled after 3 h in vitro incubation. Since the average differential blood count for the rabbit contains 3%–4% monocytes and 40–60% granulocytes, labeled lymphocytes were primarily transfused (2×10^{7}-3×10^{7} for each receiver animal). The number of transfused monocytes labeled at the same time could, therefore, be disregarded in each case.

Blood from each of two donor animals was transfused into two undamaged receiver animals and two animals with meningoencephalitis induced 4 days prior to the transfusion. Each of the brains was fixed with formalin in the usual way and embedded in paraffin. The sections were coated with Kodak NTB emulsion and exposed for 14 and/or 28 days.

Results

No labeled cells were found in the undamaged receiver animals. After experimental meningoencephalitis, however, typical labeled lymphocytes, each with a rounded nucleus and narrow, distended body of cytoplasm, were observed in the leptomeninges and also perivascularly, close to the surface of the cortical vessels. Under the specified experimental conditions, no labeled cells were observed in the neuropil or inside the ventricular system.

Conclusion

The cytokinetic investigations provided the following information:

1. Local MP inside undamaged CNS and peripheral nervous system exhibit their own proliferative ability, even if only a very slight one. Under pathologic conditions, this proliferative ability can be increased three–fivefold. Those cells proliferating under pathologic conditions are, in part, esterase positive. On the basis of this enzymatic activity, they can, therefore, be compared with monocytes from the peripheral blood.
2. Under pathologic conditions, hematogenic-monocytic cells can migrate into the brain tissue where they are found with the appearance and localization of progressive microglia, perivascular cells, free subarachnoidal cells, and epiplexus cells.
3. Under pathologic conditions, lymphocytes can also migrate into the CNS. They do not, however, assume the form of macrophages and certainly not the form of microglial cells, either at this time or under normal conditions. They, therefore, are not to be considered hematogenic precursor cells.
4. Migrated blood cells, erythrophages, fatty granule cells *(Fettkörnchenzellen)*, and also polynucleated giant cells can be found in the CNS. Apparently, polynucleated giant cells did not develop from modified, atypical divisions, but rather from the fusion of migrated blood cells that were originally mononuclear cells.

5. Isolated migrated (hematogenic) cells also found in the neuropil of undamaged animals should possibly be interpreted as resting microglia. The findings, however, are not relevant since only two labeled cells were observed within the neuropil of two animals.
6. By excluding the possibility of the reutilization of radioactive markers, it was established that a portion of the MP found extravascularly inside the CNS was composed of hematogenic-monocytic elements.
7. Negative findings were observed only under two pathologic conditions: Wallerian (anterograde) degeneration in the sciatic nerve and retrograde degeneration in the nucleus of the facial nerve. Since the increase in reactive cells was relatively low in both conditions, it could not be definitely established if this negative finding was related to the method or if this type of lesion possibly stimulated a proliferation [but not a migration (!)] of local cells.

II. Mode of Distribution and Possible Lymphatic Efflux of Intracerebrally Injected Corpuscular Particles and Cellular Elements

Only a few studies are available at present on the fate of macrophages in the body. With the use of radioactive gold, a survival time of at least 2 months was established for macrophages in the liver and spleen (Roser, 1970a, b). Since alveolar macrophages are located on the boundaries of the body, it was logical to assume that this was the normal way in which macrophages were removed from the body (Eliot, 1926; Nicol and Bilbey, 1958; Spritzer et al., 1968). Conclusive studies dealing with this question are not yet available.

A few statements can, however, be made in regard to whether or not tissue macrophages are able to recirculate, i.e., whether or not they are transported from the tissue via the circulatory or lymphatic systems into other areas of the body. After intraperitoneal injection of labeled peritoneal macrophages, these cells were observed migrating to distant lymph nodes, the spleen, the liver, and into the subcutaneous fatty tissue (Vernon-Roberts, 1969a, b; Roser, 1968, 1970a, b; Gilette and Lance, 1971; Langhammer et al., 1973). Individual studies are available in which macrophages were observed inside the lymphatic and/or the circulatory system (Benested et al., 1971).

Only hypotheses on the fate of intracerebral mononuclear phagocytes have been presented. The observation of only one macrophage in the lumen of an intracerebral vessel was presented by different investigators as an indication of hematogenic removal (Tani and Evans, 1965; Luse, 1968). Luse considers this hypothesis questionable.

A number of earlier investigations indicated the possible existence of connecting passages between the subarachnoid space and the cervical lymph nodes (Schwalbe, 1869; Key and Retzius, 1875; for surveys see Scheid, 1941; Bowsher, 1957; Millen and Woollam, 1962; Földi, 1972; Kozma et al., 1972). The morphology of the assumed anatomic connecting passages and/or spaces between the subarachnoid space and the extracerebral tissue are described with the aid electron-microscopic techniques. Openings have been observed in the pial cell layer which lead from the subarachnoid space to the subpial space. This space merges into the open-ended perineurial space, which runs along the nerve fiber exiting from the CNS, and facilitates the transition to extracerebral tissue (see p. 16).

The author's experiments described below were carried out to investigate intracerebral distribution and morphology as well as to provide information regarding the lymphogenic efflux of intracerebrally injected macrophages. The dye experiments described below should be understood as preliminary experiments. They were carried out to reconfirm the possibility of an anatomic and/or functional *connection between the cerebrum and the cervical lymph nodes* in the rabbit, but they will also provide supporting evidence for the *phagocytic ability* of certain types of cells inside the CNS. Finally, the *time interval* required for dye removal, the point in time when the dyes can be found in the lymph nodes, and the lymph nodes involved will be established. Almost no information on this matter has been available. Information on the time aspect was important because it could then be used to set up the more elaborate experiments for investigating the location of the cells.

Cellular elements were injected in a second series of experiments. These cellular elements were labeled erythrocytes, labeled lymphocytes, and labeled peritoneal macrophages. The *intracerebral distribution* and the *location of these cells in the lymph nodes* was to be investigated. Another question involved the *morphologic structures* that *macrophages* are able to assume when they appear *inside brain tissue.*

The following procedure was used for all experiments. The corpuscular or cellular remnants were injected intracerebrally (in the region also selected for the stab wounds). Since an accompanying destruction of nerve tissue was always present, dyes as well as cells were also located intraventricularly, subarachnoidally, and inside the brain tissue itself. The same amount of the substance and/or the same cell suspension was also administered intravenously to control animals in order either to exclude the possibility of or to observe distribution via the blood stream. All experiments were carried out with rabbits.

1. Corpuscular Particles

The questions considered here are: How and where are the intracerebrally injected corpuscular particles of various sizes and types to be found inside the brain? At what point can they first be recognized in the cervical lymph nodes? In which cervical lymph nodes are they distributed? And do the methods applied here provide any indications for a perineurial drainage of the tracer?

Material and Methods

Two different types of corpuscular particles were injected intracerebrally:

a) *Ferritin* (crystalized twice, 10% sterile aqueous solution, cadmium-free, equine spleen [Serva Feinbiochemica Heidelberg/FRG]) is a protein (apoferritin) with a molecular weight of 445 000 and a diameter of 120 Å bound to the average 250 Fe molecules (Wetz and Crichton, 1973). Ferritin was confirmed with the prussian blue reaction and nuclear staining with nuclear fast red.

b) *Colloidal carbon* (Günther Wagner, Pelikan Werke, Hannover, FRG, Suspension No. C 11/1431 a) solution was diluted with watered gelatin according to Biozzi and co-workers (1953). The final suspension contained 16 mg carbon and 1% gelatin. The size of the colloidal carbon particles in solution pretreated in this way is 250–500 Å (Biozzi et al., 1953). The sections were then stained with nuclear fast red.

Ferritin was selected because it is more easily demonstrated and is well tolerated by the animals. In addition, it is an aqueous solution of a protein with average molecular weight and average diameter. Colloidal carbon was also used for control since phagocytosis of colloidal particles is considered to be specific for cells in the reticuloendothelial system (Biozzi et al., 1953), particularly the macrophages (Gosselin, 1956; Roser, 1965; Luk and Simon, 1974). Moreover, the particles have a diameter more than twice that of ferritin.

After injection of the 0.1 ml dose, the skull was closed with sealing wax to prevent an outflow of tracer. The intracerebral injection of ferritin was well tolerated by all animals. Following intracerebral injection of carbon, a few of the animals died; the exact cause of death could not be determined.

The animals were killed at various time intervals following the injection via cardial perfusion of formalin. Different specimens were investigated: frontal sections of the brain, longitudinal sections through the optic nerve with sections of the orbis, regional cervical lymph nodes, isolated inguinal lymph nodes, spleen, and liver.

A bilateral preparation was made of three easily located lymph nodes (LN) in the cervical region (cf. Fig. 18). These lymph nodes were numbered consecutively for the purpose of simplification.

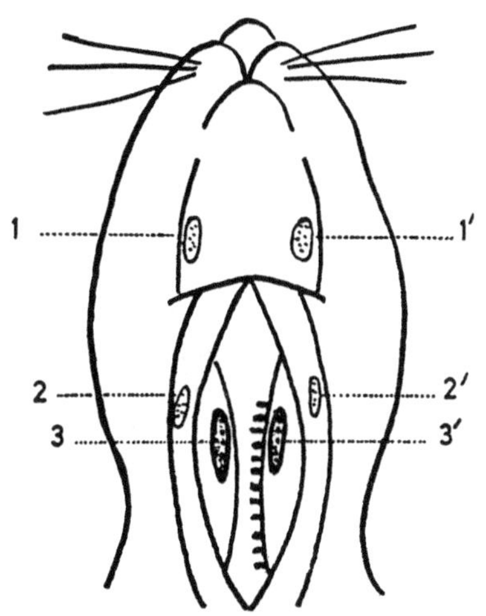

Fig. 18. Localization of those lymph nodes in the neck of rabbit which were investigated during the course of intracerebral injection of corpuscular particles and cellular elements: 1 and *1′*=submandibular lymph nodes; 2 and 2′= superficial cervical lymph nodes; 3 and *3′*=deep peritracheal lymph nodes

The cranial portion of the LN was marked with a silk thread. The tissue specimens were cut into only 5-μ-thick slices on the cryostat. For control, the same amount of labeling material was administered intravenously via the ear vein in one animal that was allowed to survive for the same period of time. The quantity of labeling substances after staining (color intensity) in the LN was assessed semiquantitatively via compartive microscopy (see also Fig. 21).

Following injection of the two tracers, the animals were killed at intervals of 10 and 30 min, 1, 3, and 8 h; 1, 2, 3, and 4 days; 1 and 2 months. Two animals were used to study the distribution of intracerebrally injected ferritin for each interval. One animal was used to study the distribution of intracerebrally injected carbon for each interval.

Results

Up to 3 h after *intracerebral injection* of ferritin, the tracer was still found filling the preformed CSF spaces (Fig. 19A). Moreover, diffusely homogeneous and granular ferritin was demonstrated intracellularly. The labeling material was diffusely homogeneous and was observed exclusively in cells in the region of the damaged neuropil. Here the cells could definitely be identified as astrocytes, sometimes on the basis of the processes containing ferritin (Fig. 20A). Some of these cell projections led to clumps of deposited tracer, from which the diffuse staining seemed to radiate; other processes led to vessels. It was, therefore, possible to suggest a transport mechanism. Diffuse deposits of ferritin were also found in isolated perivascular cells, isolated nerve cells, and in the perikaryon of cells that could not be definitely identified on the basis of their processes or their localization. A homogeneously stained space was found around the optic nerve (perineurial space) and around individual vessels inside the nerve itself.

Ferritin particles in all areas described were also found deposited intracellularly in granular form (Figs. 19B, C, and 20C, D). The fine granules were located almost exclusively in the subarachnoidal (trabecularly located) cells, in perivascularly located cells of the neuropil, and in epiplexus cells. Reaction products were sometimes found between the ependymal cells, particularly in the area of the third ventricle. Here the tracer apparently passed through the intercellular spaces and into the neuropil. These tracer paths appeared to extend toward subependymally located cells. Inside the neuropil, astrocytelike cells containing granular deposits of ferritin were not found on any sections. Finally, intracellular deposits of granular ferritin were also found in isolated cells of the perineurium of the optic nerve.

These findings were demonstrated within the first 3 h at all times selected for study; a few quantitative differences were evident. The quantity of cells with granular labeling material was directly related to the length of time between injection and examination. The tracer was increasingly pronounced at the base of the brain–in the subarachnoid space as well as in the perivascular spaces of basal intracerebral vessels. First a diffuse, space-filling deposit was identified. It was later also found in granular form within different cell types in direct relationship to the length of time between injection and examination.

Comparable differences in cellular deposits were not found, however, after intracerebral application of carbon. The carbon was always identified in granular form. It was never found in astrocytelike cells or between ependymal cells. For the most part, the behavior of carbon was similar to that of ferritin. This observation is particularly valid for the longest time span between injection and examination.

The type of intracerebral distribution of labeling material 8–96 h after injection was similar for all animals. Only a few quantitative differences were observed. Both tracers were found only in granular form and intracellularly localized. The free subarachnoidal cells (Fig. 19B), perivascularly located cells (Fig. 19C), and epiplexus cells were all

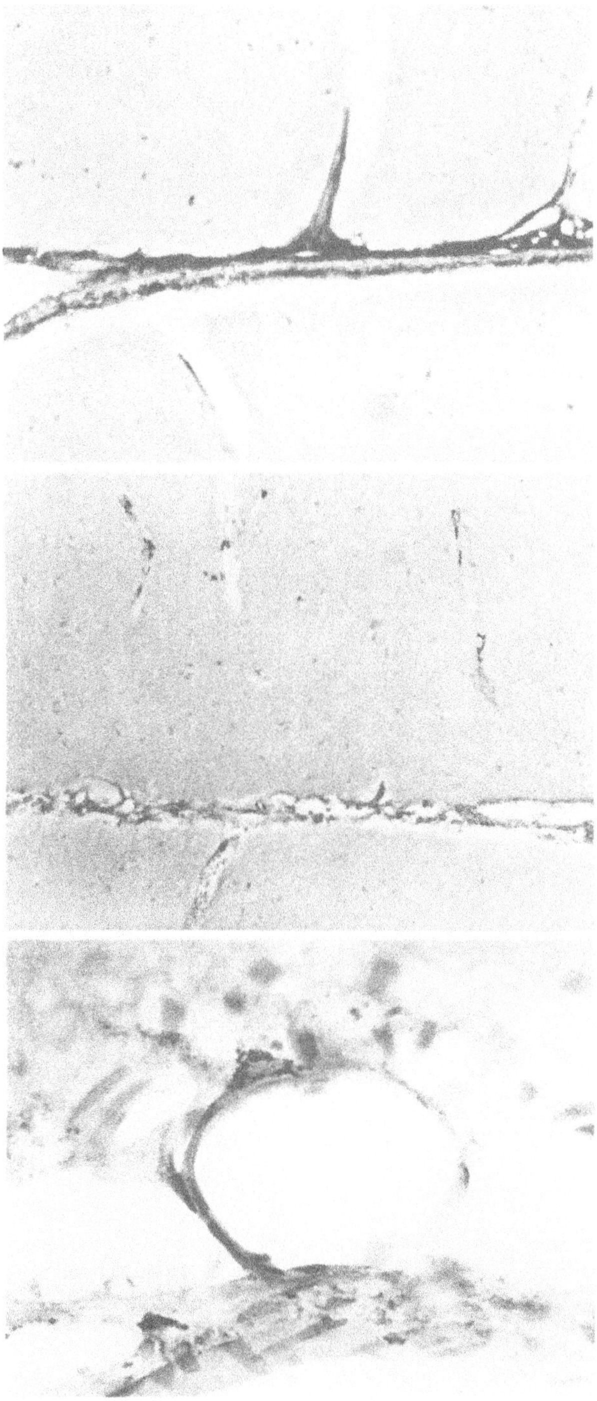

A

B

C

Fig. 19 A–C. Distribution of intracerebrally applied ferritin in the subarachnoid space. Within the first few hours [(A) 3 h], the subarachnoid space as well as the perivascular spaces may still be filled with homogeneous staining reaction products. Later [(B) 8 h], ferritin is only found intracellularly in the cells of the subarachnoid space and of the perivascular space. Fine granular tracer is found loosely distributed in almost all cells bordering the CSF spaces (C). A distinct increase is observed only in macrophage-like cells that are distributed both perivascularly and independent of the vessels (i.e., free subarachnoid cells) in the subarachnoid space. [(A–C) nuclear red stain, prussian blue reaction; magnification: (A and B) x 120; (C) x 500]

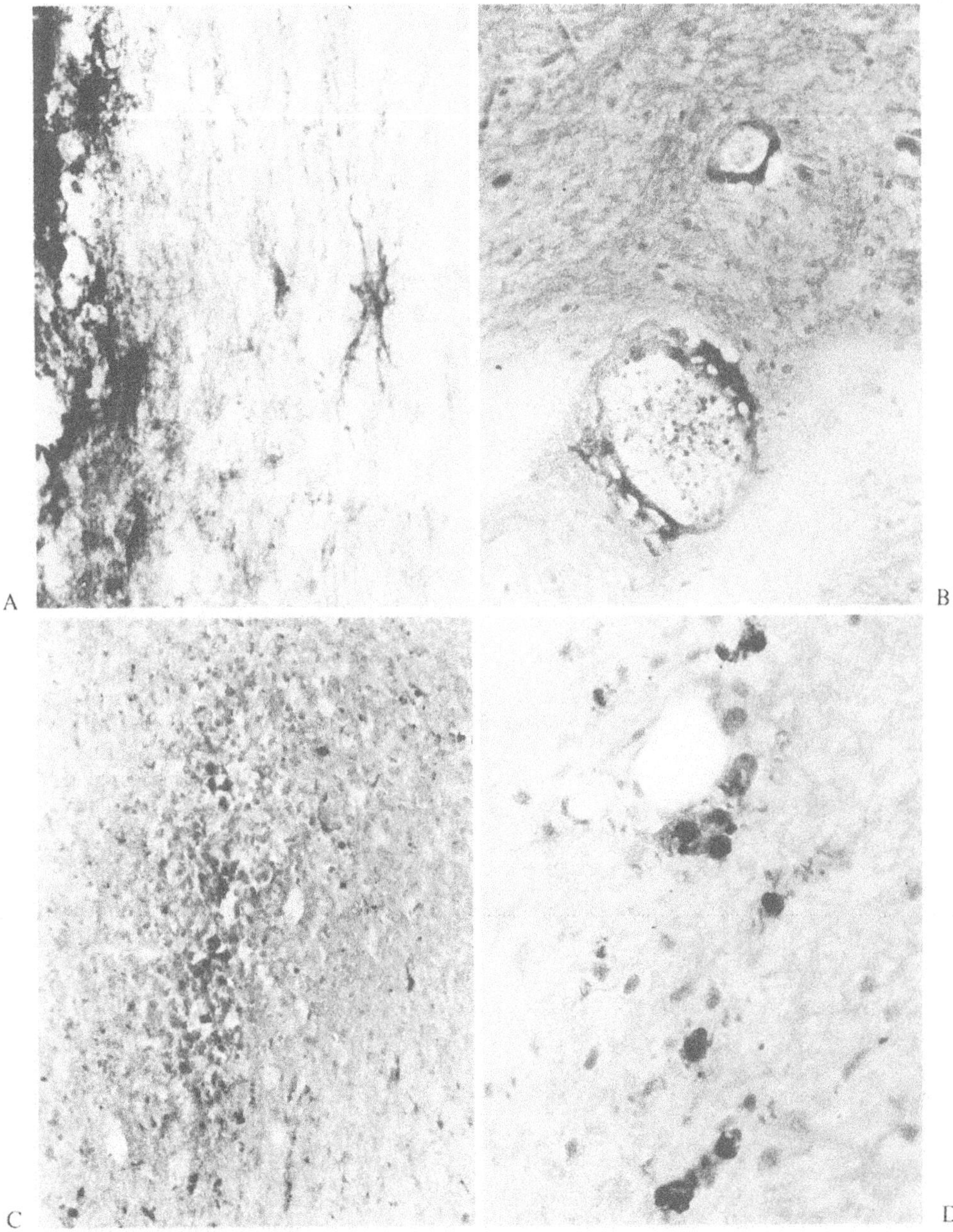

Fig. 20 A–D. Distribution of intracerebrally applied ferritin in the neuropil of the injection site as well as in the perivascular spaces of intracerebral vessels. Ferritin is seen staining diffusely in a matter of minutes or hours [(A) 10 min] in the area of the injection site. It is finally seen just as diffusely in the adjacent astrocytes. In the same period [(B) 60 min], the tracer is demonstrated in the perivascular spaces of adjacent cerebral vessels. Ferritin is also demonstrated intracellularly in the area of the injection site, 24 h at the latest after injection [(C) 4 days]. Progressive microglia as well as perivascular cells of adjacent vessels are predominantly (and most clearly) loaded. [(A–D) nuclear red stain, prussian blue reaction; magnification: (A and D) x 500; (B) x 300; (C) x 200]

heavily laden with tracer particles. A large number of macrophagelike cells, some with pseudopodialike processes such as those found with progressive microglia (Fig. 20B and C), were also found in the area of the intracerebral puncture site (puncture channel). All these cells contained the same amount of tracer particles. Isolated cells with dense granular deposits of ferritin (not carbon) were, however, found at considerable distance from the puncture site in the subependymal zone.

The diffuse staining of isolated astrocytes containing ferritin, which was observed within the first 3 h, could rarely be demonstrated later. In all of the animals, most of the basal intracerebral vessels in the right hemisphere (side of intracerebral injection) at this point possessed unusually large quantities of perivascularly located cells with dense deposits of tracer. More tracer-positive cells inside the loose connective tissue were present on both sides around the eyeball at this particular time than had been observed during the short intervals of time at the beginning. Deposits of tracer in the cells of endoneurial connective tissue were now demonstrable only in granular form. Even if clear-cut criteria for assessing the quantitative differences for tracer-containing cells in the optic nerve were not given, the nerve ipsilateral to the hemisphere injected appeared, nevertheless, to be more involved than the contralateral nerve.

In addition to these different deposits (some of which were even demonstrable with a magnifying glass), all other cells bordering the cerebrospinal fluid space (e.g., pial, arachnoidal, ependymal, and plexus cells) also contained tracer granules that appeared to be loosely structured and finely distributed in the cytoplasm. Labeling material was also found deposited in isolated cells in the neuropil. These cells were found in the neighborhood of the puncture channel (edematous zone?) and within the subependymal zone. The type of cells, however, could not always be definitely identified.

After a survival period of 4–8 weeks, intracellular particles of tracer were still identifiable. Now, however, they were deposited predominantly in the form of coarse clumps (Fig. 20D). As a whole, the number of tracer-containing cells was distinctly reduced; cells with intracellularly located tracer were no longer found close to each other. At this time, isolated, loosely distributed tracer particles were still found in cells bordering the cerebrospinal fluid space.

Astrocytes diffusely stained with prussian blue were also found in one animal that had been allowed to survive for 8 weeks after intracerebral injection of ferritin. Some of these astrocytes were located subpially; some, around the vessels in the neighborhood of the cortex. They were demonstrated over the same hemisphere only in the vicinity of the puncture channel. These cells gave the typical picture of a so-called border zone siderosis *(Randzonensiderose)*.

Following *intravenous administration* of an equal amount of ferritin and/or colloidal carbon, no tracer was found in the above-mentioned brain tissue cells. Only isolated endothelials from intracerebral vessels contained tracer granules. These granules were seldom definitely differentiable from artifacts. Tracer deposits were, however, definitely found in the Kupffer cells of the liver, isolated cells of the spleen (carbon), and also on rare occasions in isolated cells from the cervical lymph nodes. Some of the particle-containing cells were elements that were definitely identifiable as endothelials or, occasionally, as macrophages (e.g., in the liver). Even if a clear-cut quantitative difference related to the injection time can be established, the cell type containing tracer is still the same. After the intravenous application of tracer, the tracer was found intracellularly within 10 min in all cell types described. The quantity of tracer-containing cells increased after an 1-h survival period; the same amount was demonstrated in each of the animals allowed to survive for up to 96 h. On the whole, the quantity of tracer-containing cells seemed to decrease quantitatively in those animals allowed to survive 4 and/or 8 weeks.

No tracer was found in the inguinal *lymph nodes* of the control animals after intracerebral injection of tracer. The distribution of both tracers in the cervical lymph nodes (here considered as regional) was identical for both labeling materials (Fig. 21). The semiquantitative results for ferritin are presented in Fig. 22. These findings can be summarized as follows: Light-microscopy could not demonstrate the tracer in the cervical lymph nodes 10 and/or 30 min after the intracerebral injection. In each case, tracer was also observed after 1 h at the earliest in the cervical lymph nodes and predominantly (as well as most pronouncedly) in the homolateral deep (peritracheal) lymph nodes. Compared with the other lymph nodes, these nodes were also the most heavily laden with labeling materials at all other investigated times. The amount of tracer after 1 h, however, was slight. The sinusoids were partially filled with homogeneous staining material exhibiting a slight iron-positive reaction. Some of the bordering sinusal cells contained iron-positive granules of about the same size. Here, as well as in other lymph node regions, isolated, tracer-containing cells were found to resemble macrophages.

At all of the following time periods examined, tracer was demonstrated in the cells bordering the sinus as well as in the macrophages of the lymph node. The ipsilateral lymph nodes contained considerably larger quantities of tracer particles than the contralateral lymph nodes (each from the same location). The deep cervical lymph nodes were the first of the lymph nodes on each side to be laden with tracer; they were also the most intensively laden. The least amount of labeling material was found relatively late in the submandibular cervical lymph nodes.

After an 8-h survival period, the tracer distribution in the lymph nodes remained relatively constant for the next few days. After 4–8 weeks, a noticeable reduction in tracer was first observed in the lymph nodes. This reduction affected all lymph nodes equally.

One unanswered question was if, in each case, the cranial portions of the lymph nodes were laden first and most intensively with labeling material. This hypothesis was substantiated by examining the deep cervical lymph nodes from animals allowed to survive for only brief periods of time (1 and/or 3 h). The same amount of tracer deposition was found in the basal and cranial portions of the lymph nodes for all other cervical lymph nodes and all other time intervals. Sometimes a regionally localized deposition was also found at this particular time. The system of distribution could not, however, be established.

Another complex of questions was if labeling materials appeared in the spleen, and if so, when could they be found. Since normally the spleen contains a large quantity of iron-positive cells, ferritin was not suitable as a tracer. Colloidal carbon was observed in the spleen in only 3 of 11 animals following intracerebral injection of separate cell-bound granules. These animals survived 96 h and/or 4–8 weeks.

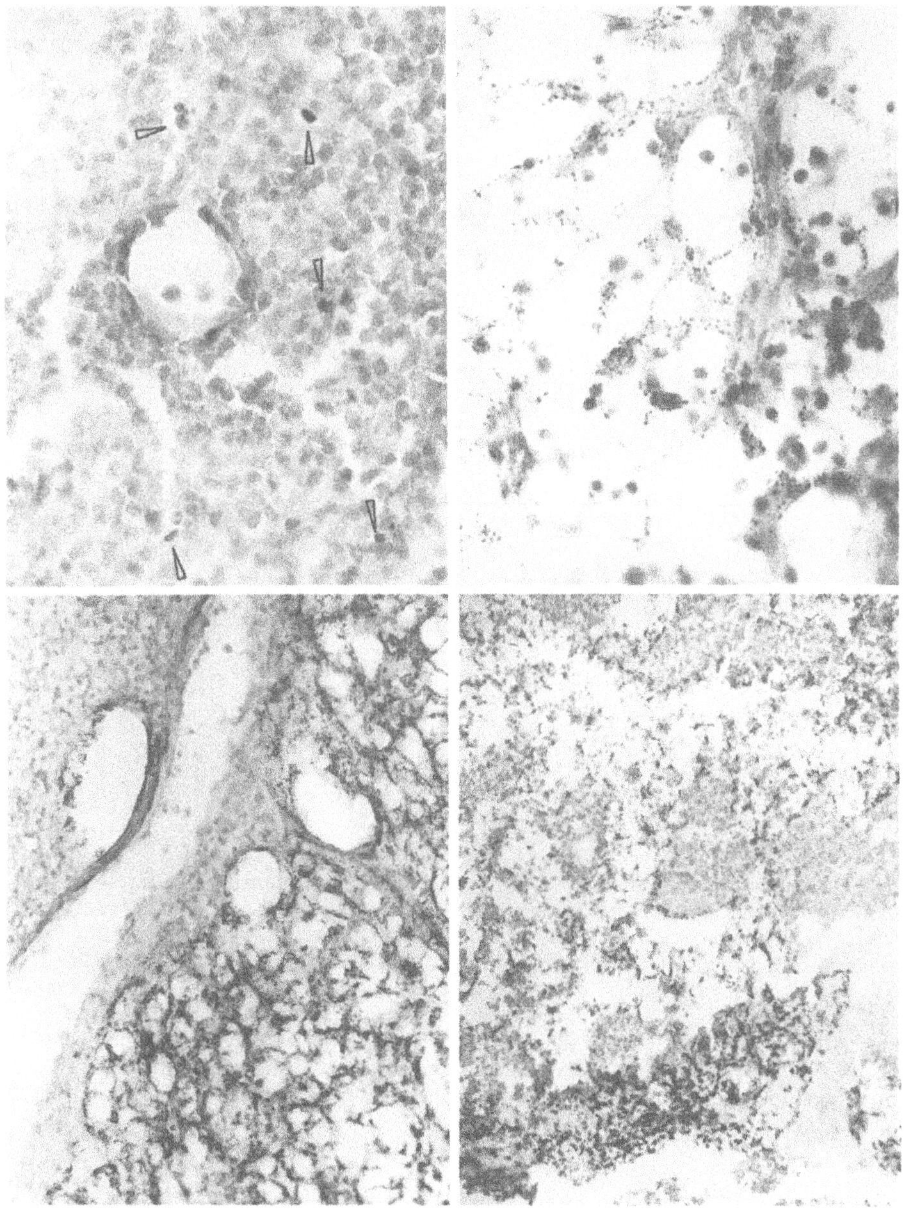

A B C D

Fig. 21 A–D. Lymph drainage of intracerebrally applied ferritin. Depending on the time, the tracer is found in various quantities in the deep (peritracheal) ipsilateral cervical lymph nodes. (A) Individual, intracellularly located ferritin particles, after 60 min *(arrow)*; (B) Locally limited, slight ferritin concentration after 2 h; (C) Locally limited, distinct concentrations of ferritin after 3 h; (D) Distinct concentration of ferritin in all lymph node regions after 24 h. [(A–D) nuclear red stain, prussian blue reaction; magnification: (A and B) x500; (C) x300; (D) x200]

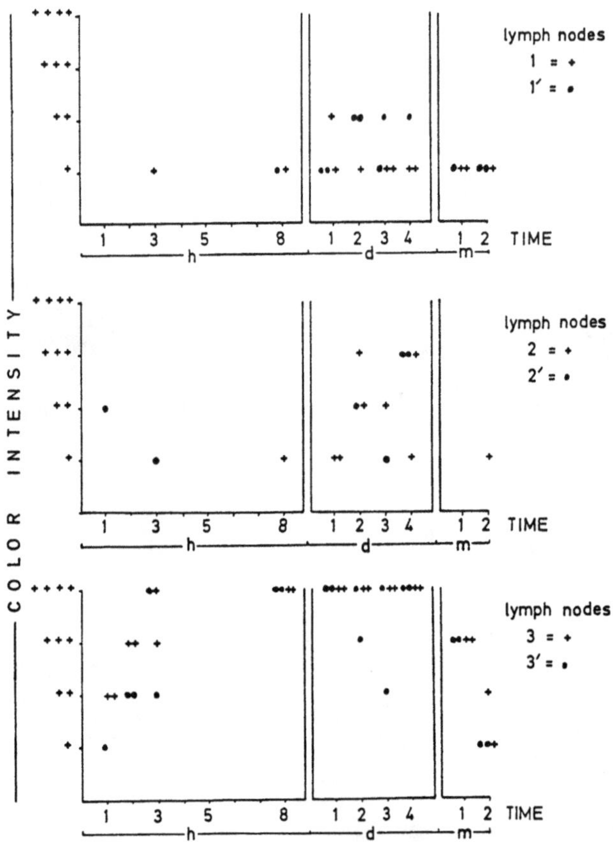

Fig. 22. Semiquantitative analysis of time-dependent color intensity in various cervical lymph nodes after intracerebral injection of ferritin (right hemisphere) using prussian blue reaction. Time dependency was an indication of the relative amount of drained tracer particles/time unit. Compare the color intensity in *right (1, 2, 3)* and *left (1', 2', 3')* lymph nodes from various locations (*1* and *1'*: Submandibular LN; *2* and *2'*: Superficial peritracheal LN; *3* and *3'*: Deep peritracheal LN). ϕ = Tracer particles not demonstrated; + = Isolated cells present containing tracer; ++ = Many tracer-laden cells in focal location; +++ = Locally limited tracer-positive cells; quantity of tracer slight; ++++ = As in +++, quantity of tracer pronounced; compare Fig. 21

2. Cellular Elements

To demonstrate a connecting passage for cells between the subarachnoid space and the cervical lymph nodes, labeled erythrocytes and lymphocytes were first applied intracerebrally. Only at the end of this experiment were labeled peritoneal macrophages also injected intracerebrally to investigate the intracerebral distribution and morphologic transformation of macrophages following intracerebral injection and the possible efflux of these cells into the cervical lymph nodes. One animal was used as a control for each to survive for the same period of time following intravenous injection of labeled cells with the same cell suspension.

Material and Methods

1. *Injection of erythrocytes:* 5 ml blood was removed from the ear vein of each laboratory animal (rabbit). The blood was washed three times in PBS and then centrifuged at 450 *g* for 15 min; a 5% erythrocyte suspension was derived (1 ml). The erythrocytes were incubated with ^{51}Cr (470 μCi) at room temperature for 45 min. This tracer has proved suitable for labeling erythrocytes (Ebauch et al., 1953; Lilien et al., 1970; Eyre et al., 1970). The erythrocytes were then washed four times, and a suspension of erythrocytes (final concentration: 5%) was obtained. Intracerebral application of 0.1 ml suspension followed; one animal received an intravenous injection of autologous erythrocytes. For technical reasons, the animals were allowed to survive for only 3 h; they were killed via aortal formalin perfusion. The possibility of and the technique for autoradiographic demonstration of ^{51}Cr has already been described (Ronai, 1968; see also Forberg et al., 1964). The material (brain tissue, optic nerve, liver, spleen, inguinal lymph nodes, cervical lymph nodes) was embedded in paraffin. The specimens were then sliced, coated with Ilford K2 emulsion, and exposed for 28 days.
2. *Injection of lymphocytes:* After heparinization, 30–50 ml blood was removed via cardial puncture from one rabbit in each series. Lymphocytes were isolated from the blood by the method described by C. Huber and co-workers (1974). Since rabbit blood has an extremely low sedimentation rate, the blood was run through a column of nylon batting. The erythrocytes were then destroyed by adding sterile distilled water. This suspension then contained ~90% lymphocytes. Lymphocyte viability exceeded 95%. The suspension was washed three times in Tc 199 culture medium centrifuged at 450 *g* for 10 min. It was then adjusted to 2×10^7 cells/ml and incubated together with ^3H-cytidine (1 μCi/ml) at room temperature for 3 h. The cell suspension was then washed three times with PBS and adjusted to 2×10^7 cells/ml. The suspension (0.1 ml) was administered intracerebrally to two rabbits and intravenously to one rabbit. Each animal was allowed to survive for 24 h and then killed via formalin perfusion. Specimens from the brain, optic nerve, inguinal lymph nodes, cervical lymph nodes, liver, and spleen were embedded in paraffin. The specimens were treated autoradiographically in the manner described in the preceding experiment.
3. *Injection of macrophages:* Peritoneal macrophages were collected via the previously described methods and labeled in vitro with ^3H-DFP (p. 61). A 0.1 ml suspension adjusted to 2×10^7 cells/ml was then injected intracerebrally. The survival periods varied; 2, 24, and 48 h; 6 and 60 days. Following intracerebral injection, two animals in each series were allowed to survive for each respective time period. The same amount of labeled macrophages was administered intravenously to five animals. Specimens from the brain, optic nerve, liver, spleen, inguinal lymph nodes, and cervical lymph nodes were embedded in paraffin. The specimens were treated autoradiographically in the manner described above.

Results

Each *red blood cell* was labeled on the smear specimens of the in vitro labeled erythrocytes; the smears were prepared prior to the injection of erythrocytes into the animal. Isolated labeled erythrocytes were found in the spleen after the intravenous injection, but not in the liver or cervical lymph nodes. A labeled erythrocyte was seldom found (~1 : 8000) on smear specimens of peripheral blood made before the host animals were killed.

Following intracerebral injection, large numbers of labeled erythrocytes were identified in the subarachnoid space. Here they were clearly distinguishable from the nonlabeled erythrocytes that had apparently been effluxed into the subarachnoid space as a result of the traumatic injury and/or are localized within the vessels (Fig. 23 A). Labeled erythrocytes were also observed in the perivascular spaces of basal vessels (particularly around the veins) as well as in the ventricle in the injection area. One isolated

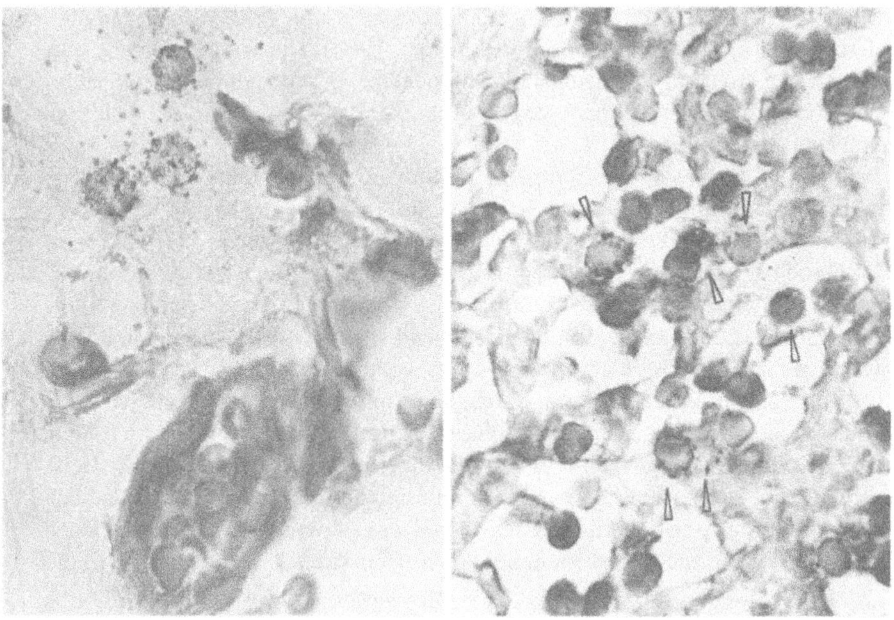

A B

Fig. 23 A and B. Migration of intracerebrally injected ^{51}Cr labeled autologous erythrocytes in the lymph note. (A) Labeled erythrocytes next to nonlabeled, autologous intravascular erythrocytes in the leptomeningeal network, 3 h following intracerebral injection. (B) Labeled erythrocytes in ipsilateral cervical lymph nodes, 3 h following intracerebral injection [(A and B) H&E stain; magnification: (A and B) x 1200]

labeled erythrocyte was also found in the perineurial space of the optic nerve. A careful study of the 3-h period revealed no phagocytized erythrocytes, neither labeled nor unlabeled.

Isolated groups of clearly labeled, but unphagocytized erythrocytes were found in the cervical lymph node sinusoids (Fig. 23 B). The erythrocytes were demonstrable only in the deep cervical lymph nodes on the ipsilateral side of the injected hemisphere. No labeled cells were found in the spleen, liver, and/or in blood smears taken from these two animals.

The smear specimens after in vitro labeling of *lymphocytes* contained only labeled lymphocytes. At 24 h after the intravenous injection, only slightly labeled cells were observed in the splenic tissue. A localization preference could not be established. No labeled cells were identified in the blood smear, the cervical lymph nodes, or liver of these animals.

Following intracerebral injection, labeled cells were found inside the CNS in the same localization as those found following the injection of erythrocytes. All cell nuclei retained their distinctly rounded shape. Lymphocytes were definitely identified in the H&E-stained specimen as clearly defined cells. Only isolated lymphocytes were identified in the ipsilateral deep cervical lymph nodes. Here it was also impossible to determine the localization preference. No labeled cells were observed in the spleen, in the liver, or on blood smears.

The autoradiographically treated smear specimens of *macrophages* made prior to the injection of macrophages were 100% labeled (Fig. 24A). At all time intervals investigated, isolated labeled elements were found after intravenous injection of the suspension, particularly in the liver but also occasionally in the spleen. One labeled cell was observed in a cervical lymph node 24-h after the injection in only one animal that had received the macrophages intravenously. The possibility of an intravascular localization could not definitely be excluded here. No labeled cells were found in blood smears from host animals.

After intracerebral injection of macrophages, clearly labeled cells were found in the preformed spaces of the leptomenix (Fig. 24B), in the ventricular cavity (Fig. 24C), as well as around the vessels (Fig. 25B). Since the labeled cells inside the ventricles tended to attach to the choroidal epithelium, they resembled epiplexus cells. During the first 6 days, the number of labeled cells was high. After 60 days, however, only isolated labeled cells were found in the CNS, and they were demonstrated exclusively in the subarachnoid space and the ventricles.

The distribution pattern and the changing morphology of the macrophages inside the neuropil were conspicuous (Fig. 25). Isolated labeled cells were identified perivascularly around vessels the size of venules and arterioles. Some of the cells were located longitudinally on the surface of the vessels. Labeled cells were found diffusely scattered in the area of the injection site as well as in the surrounding edematous region of the neuropil.

Two methods were used to identify the type of labeled cells more exactly:

1. Serial sections were prepared: One section was coated with film; the other underwent microglial staining (Naoumenko and Feigin, 1963).
2. The section was first stained (microglia) and then coated with film.

In the first series, an increased quantity of labeled cells as well as progressive microglia (Figs. 25A and 26) was found in the same region. It was not possible to identify positively the isolated labeled cells on the one section. Labeled microglialike cells were found in the sections treated according to the second method (Fig. 25C). In addition to microglia, a large number of perivascular cells as well as subarachnoidal cells and cells in the ventricular system all proved to be argentophilic.

Labeled macrophages were recognized bilaterally in the deep peritracheal cervical lymph nodes (ipsilateral more frequently than contralateral) (Fig. 27). These cells appeared at all investigated time periods following intracerebral injection; significant

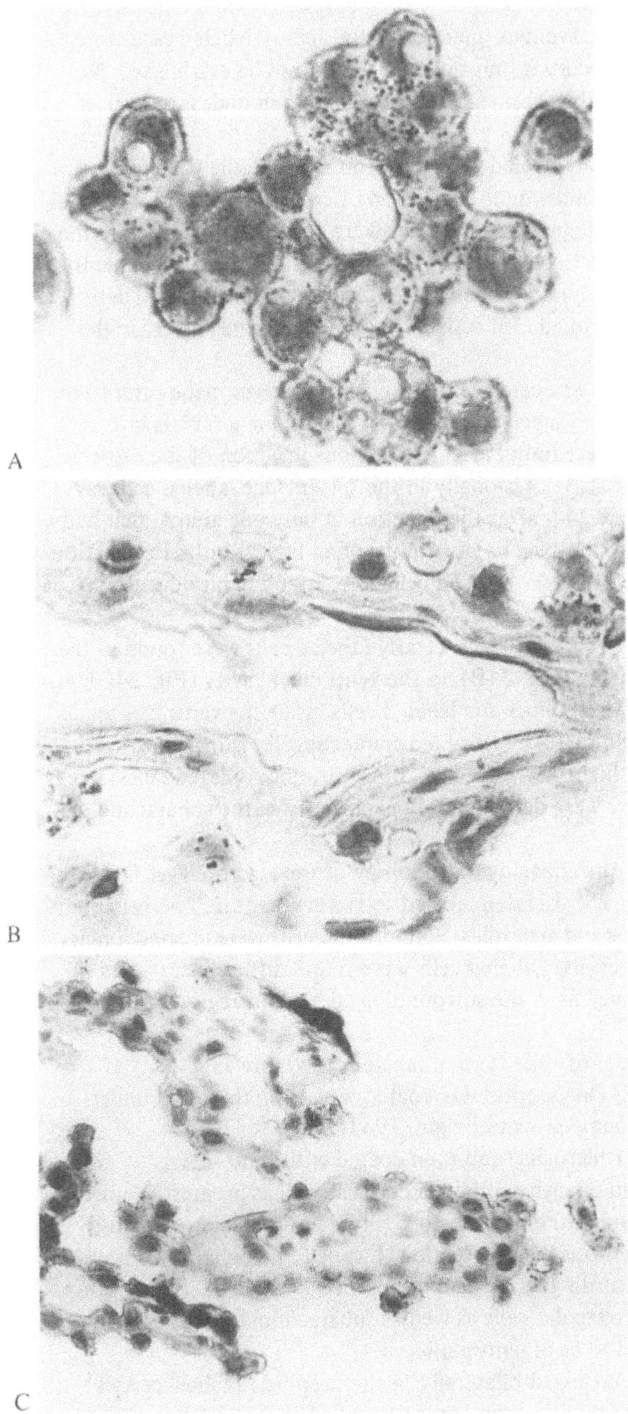

Fig. 24A–C. Intracerebral distribution of intracerebrally injected ^{3}H-DFP labeled peritoneal macrophages.
(A) Smear of labeled cells prior to injection.
(B) Labeled cells in subarachnoid space; (C) Labeled cells in the vicinity of the choroidal plexus, partially adhering to choroidal epithelium.
[(A–C) H&E stain; magnification: (A and B) x 1200; (C) x 500]

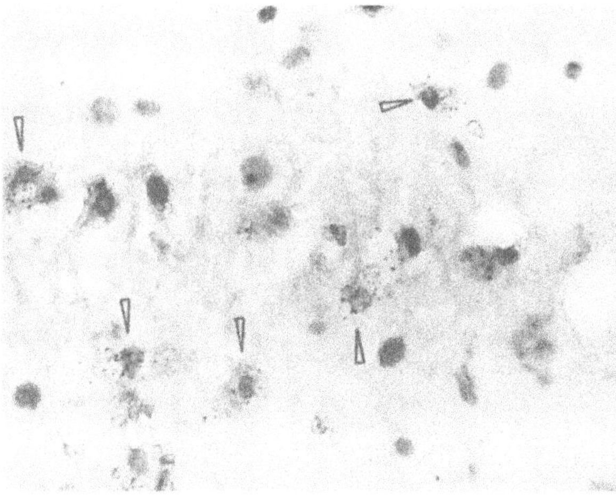
A

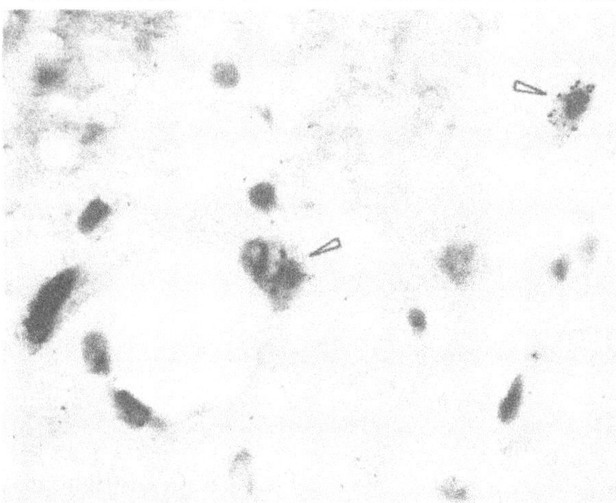
B

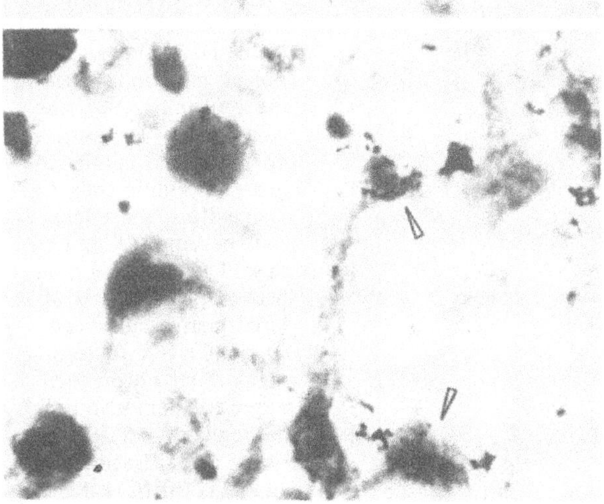
C

Fig. 25 A–C. Distribution of intracerebrally injected ^{3}H-DFP labeled peritoneal macrophages in the neuropil.
(A and B) Arrows point to labeled cells which are seen within the neuropil and/or perivascularly.
(C) Isolated argentophilic cells with reduced silver granules in the overlying layer of film *(arrows)* on the sections treated consecutively with the Naoumenko and Feigin technique for demonstrating microglia and then autoradiographically.
[(A and B) H&E stain; C: demonstration of microglia according to Naumenco and Feigin, additionally treated autoradiographically; magnification: (A) x 500; (B and C) x 1200]

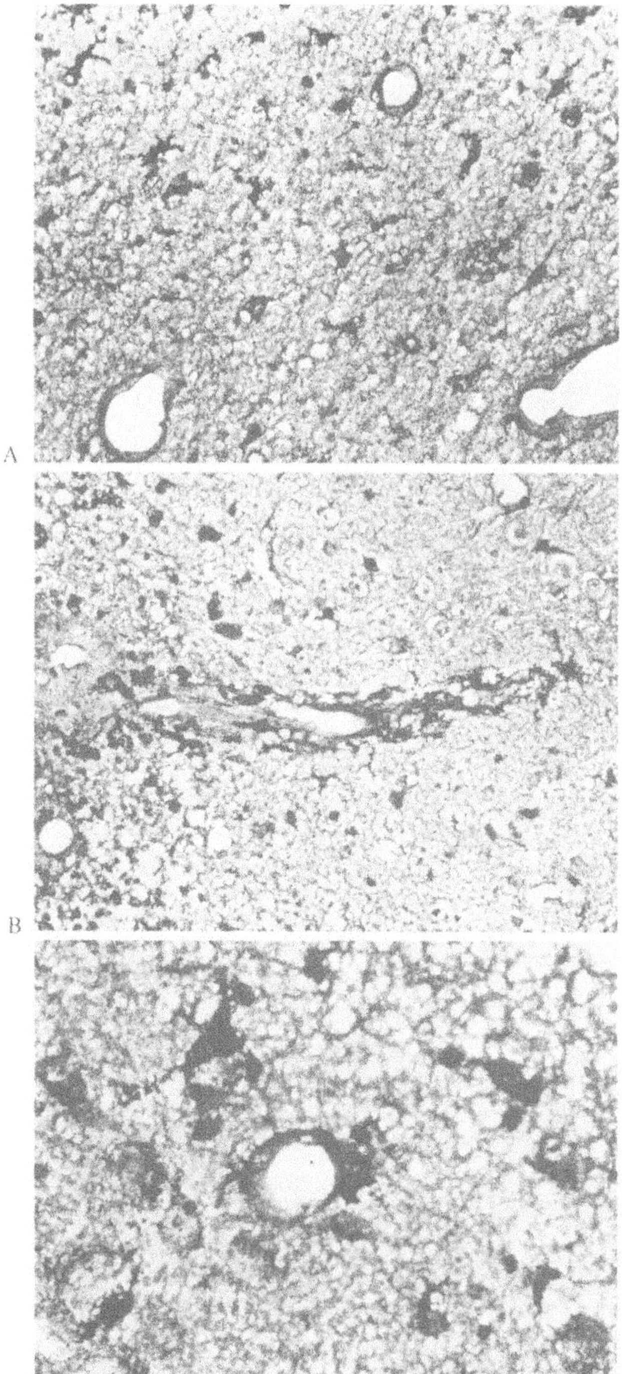

Fig. 26 A–C. Distribution of intracerebrally injected ^{3}H-DFP labeled peritoneal macrophages in the neuropil and perivascular spaces. Progressive microglia and comparable argentophilic cells are seen within the edematous neuropil (A and C) as well as increased numbers of progressively altered perivascular cells (B and C). [(A–C) Naoumenko and Feigin technique for demonstrating microglia on paraffin sections; magnification: (A and B) x 500; (C) x 1200]

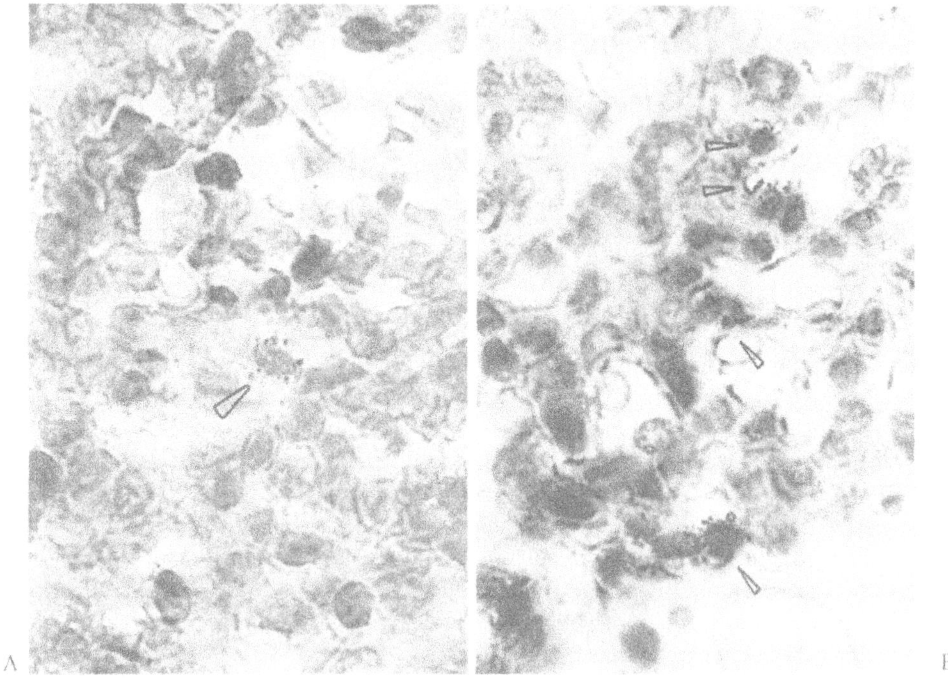

Fig. 27 A and B. Appearance of labeled mononuclear cells *(arrows)* in the cervical lymph nodes following intracerebral injection of ^{3}H-DFP labeled peritoneal macrophages (H&E stain; magnification: x 1200)

quantitative differences were confirmed, i.e., the quantity of cells was distinctly reduced 60 days later. Most of the cells were located on the border between the sinus and the follicles. A preferred cranial and/or caudal localization was not observed. On the average, two labeled macrophages were found in the ipsilateral lymph nodes for each longitudinal section. Isolated labeled cells were found in the spleen of these animals, but never in the liver.

Conclusion

The methods described above provided the following information:

1. Intracerebrally injected corpuscular material and cellular elements are distributed similarly inside the CNS. They are primarily found in the preformed spaces of the leptomeninx, in the ventricular cavities, and in the perivascular spaces.
2. Some of the corpuscular particles were found intracellularly within 10 min; at this time (and particularly later), certain cell types are more heavily laden with labeling material than are the other elements. These cell types are free elements inside the subarachnoid space, epiplexus cells in the ventricular cavity, and perivascular cells in the neuropil. Several hours after the injection, progressive microglia can be found

in the area of the puncture site. During the first 3 h following intracerebral injection of ferritin, considerably less labeling material could be found in the other cells bordering the cerebrospinal fluid space and in astrocytes around the puncture site. Eight weeks after the intracerebral injection, the labeling material was demonstrated in a few cells in the form of clumps.

3. The labeled peritoneal macrophages that were intracerebrally injected were distributed around the puncture site in the edematous, spongy neuropil. Here, they were localized, structured, and stained like progressive microglia and perivascular cells of intracerebral vessels as well as epiplexus cells.
4. Following intracerebral injection, particles of staining material were found in the perineurial space of the optic nerve. After 10 min, they can be identified in the connective tissue around the eyeball.
5. Following intracerebral injection of corpuscular elements in one hemisphere, the tracer reached the homolateral, deep (peritracheal) cervical lymph nodes first (and most distinctly for all investigated time periods). Somewhat less tracer was found in the contralateral deep cervical lymph nodes. In descending order, tracer was then found in homolateral superficial cervical lymph nodes, contralateral superficial cervical lymph nodes, and finally homolateral and contralateral submandibular lymph nodes. The same quantity of intravenously injected labeling material was identified at all time periods in all cervical lymph nodes examined. The amount of labeling substance found here at all time periods was always less than that following intracerebral injection. Finally, the intravenously applied tracer is also found in other organs (e.g., spleen and liver). Only very small quantities can be demonstrated in the spleen (bound to individual cells) after intracerebral injection.
6. After intravenous injection of labeled cells, only a few erythrocytes, lymphocytes, and peritoneal macrophages could be demonstrated in the spleen. The frequency of peritoneal macrophages in the periportal fields of the liver is higher in these experiments. Following intracerebral injection of cells, the above-mentioned cell types can also be found occasionally in clusters, but more frequently singly in the cervical lymph nodes. Cells and corpuscular particles were particularly observed in the ipsilateral deep cervical lymph nodes. Labeled macrophages were still found inside the CNS and in the cervical lymph nodes after an 8-week survival period.

III. Functional Activity of Mononuclear Phagocytes of the Central Nervous System

The common criterium for all cells belonging to the mononuclear phagocyte system (see above) is the *high degree of phagocytic activity* for these cells. Already for Aschoff (1924, see also Kiyono, 1914), the determining factor for classifying cells in the reticuloendothelial system was the capacity for assimilating vital stains. This phagocytic activity is also a common characteristic of the four cell types described here. In the literature, almost author questions this phagocytic activity.

To a certain extent, the *enzymatic activity* of mononuclear phagocytes should also be understood in relationship to phagocytosis. When acid phosphatase is used as marker enzyme for lysosome, its activity increases in the presence of phagocytic processes (Cohn, 1970). Numerous investigations have been conducted on the enzymatic activity of cells in the monocyte-macrophage series (for survey, see Leder, 1967; Braunsteiner and Schmalzl, 1970; Roos, 1970). The function of each individual enzyme can vary considerably; this variation is apparently due to different functional conditions (Oehmichen, 1973b; Kaplow, 1975; Walker, 1976). On the other hand, a few scattered studies have been published about the activity of these similar enzymes on mesenchymal cells of the CNS. A similar enzyme pattern for cells from the monocyte-macrophage series and some mesenchymal cells of the CNS would tend to indicate that the cells have an identical function.

Characteristic of the cells of the monocyte-macrophage series are the *surface receptors* for IgG (Lobuglio et al., 1967; Huber and Fudenberg, 1968; Huber et al., 1971), the third component of the complement (Huber et al., 1968) and anti monocyte sera (Greaves et al., 1975). These receptors can partly be demonstrated with sheep erythrocyte antibody complexes. With this method, demonstration of the receptors is specific for the cells of the monocyte-macrophage series (LoBuglio et al., 1967; Shevach et al., 1973). The suggestion has been made (see Mantovani et al., 1972; Huber and Holm, 1975) that, in the course of the immune response, complement receptors force immune complexes to remain in such a position on the cell membrane that the complexes stimulate immune competent cells. During the course of the secondary immune response, the IgG receptor is thought to mediate rapid intracellular assimilation, and as a result, the immune complex is destroyed. In addition to nonspecific phagocytosis (scavenger type), the surface receptors also permit a specific immunologic phagocytosis (Mariano et al., 1976; Kaplan, 1977).

The identical receptors demonstrated on the surface of CNS cells were attributed to the fact that the cells function similarly in immunologic processes, which might possibly provide additional evidence for the interrelationship of the cells. Experiments demonstrating the phagocytic behavior as well as enzymatic and receptor activity of NS cells from laboratory animals and also of human cerebrospinal fluid cells are described below.

1. Phagocytosis Experiments

The following experimental series were carried out to show a possible phagocytic activity of CNS cells:

a) Animal experiments (rabbit) were conducted in which tracers such as ferritin and colloidal carbon were injected.
b) Animal experiments (rats) were conducted in which cerebroside was injected.
c) In vitro experiments with human spinal fluid cells were carried out using latex (polystyrene) particles.

Since the first two experimental series have already been described in another context (see pages 66–74), only the simultaneously observed phenomenon of phagocytosis will be discussed here. At this point, a detailed report should be presented of the third experimental series, "Phagocytic Reaction of Human Cerebrospinal Fluid Cells" (see below).

a) Phagocytic Reaction of Local Cells Following Intracerebral Application of Labeling Material

After intracerebral application of ferritin (cf. text pp. 68–72), two different conditions were observed regarding the assimilation of tracer by the cells: a diffuse homogeneous distribution throughout the whole cell body and a granular deposit.

The homogeneous distribution was usually found within the first few hours after the injection. It was present only in those cells in the area of the puncture channel, i.e., astrocytes, isolated nerve cells, and perivascular cells. Usually this type of distribution could no longer be demonstrated after 1–2 days. In three animals, however, a diffuse distribution was found in subpial astrocytes 2 months later.

A granular deposit of tracer was found in single cells already 10 min after the application. The frequency and the amount of the deposit was directly related to the time interval between injection and examination. Several hours after the injection, labeling material in coarse-grained, form was demonstrated almost exclusively in subarachnoidal phagocytes, perivascular cells, and epiplexus cells. Isolated cells with coarse tracer granules were also found in the subependymal layer. Isolated, fine tracer granules were observed in pial and arachnoidal cells as well as in choroidal and ependymal cells after 8 h; later the amount increased. On the 3rd–4th day after the injection, increased amounts of macrophagelike progressive microglial cells containing granular ferritin were found in the area of the puncture channel.

The colloidal carbon experiments showed only a granular deposit, which sometimes was so heavy that the whole body of cytoplasm was filled with carbon. The astrocytelike cells never contained carbon. Isolated carbon granules were found in single endothelial cells and fibroblastlike cells. For the most part, inclusions were found only in the leptomeningeal macrophages, perivascular cells, epiplexus cells, and several days later, in progressive microglia. The time period required for this incorporation was roughly the same as that for ferritin deposition.

The homogeneous ferritin deposits during the first few hours following the injection are probably the result of passive diffusion due to damage to the cell and/or cell membrane. The possibility of a pinocytotic process cannot be excluded with light microscopy. Diffuse deposits appearing later may be the result of intracellular transport activity. The transport activity may result from the fact that the tracer, which has apparently already been incorporated once by other cells, had a different state of solvency. Another type of intracerebral deposit may, therefore, have been produced.

b) Giant Cell Formation

Polynucleated PAS-positive giant cells appear in rats and in rabbit brains after intracerebral injection of galactocerebroside (cf. pp. 49–50). These cells resemble the so-called globoid cells in Krabbe's disease and/or foreign body giant cells and were always found in the area of the injection. A few isolated mononuclear and binuclear PAS-positive cells were still found in more distant regions, particularly in the subarachnoid and perivascular spaces.

The stimulation of giant cell formation depends on the size of the particle that the phagocyte acknowledges as foreign and, therefore, as something to be phagocytized (among others, see Nelson, 1969; Roos, 1970). Since one phagocyte alone cannot assimilate these large particles, many cells assemble around the particle. During the course of phagocytosis, the cells fuse and a polynuclear giant cell is formed. Other factors probably also play a role here since giant cells are also formed during the phagocytosis of small particles. Phagocytic activity, however, is always a prerequisite for polynuclear giant cell formation.

The parabiotic experiments indicated that experimentally induced giant cells in brain tissue were produced basically by an assembling (fusion?) of migrated mononuclear blood cells. At this particular time, DNA synthesis can be demonstrated in only a relatively few local cells with pulse labeling method.

Globoid cells and/or foreign body giant cells each form their own respective cell type. In the literature dealing with Krabbe's disease, they have, for example, been classified as a variety of intracerebral cell types [microglial cells, perivascular cells, astrocytes, etc. (for survey, see Oehmichen and Grüninger, 1974)]. Since a definite classification cannot be made on the basis of the morphology of spontaneous or experimentally induced diseases, we carried out our own investigation.

In this experimental series, polynuclear cells were formed by migrated blood cells which, on the basis of their enzyme activity (α-naphthyl acetate esterase, naphthol AS acetate esterase, naphthol AS-D chloroacetate esterase and acid phosphatase) were most likely derived from monocytes. If the hypothesis is correct that subarachnoidal phagocytes, perivascular cells, epiplexus cells, and progressive microglia are derived from blood monocytes, this giant cell formation can be easily included in the system of MP of the CNS. It is, however, not clear if the mechanism for the development of giant cells after injection of cerebroside can be compared with the mechanism for the development of foreign body giant cells. It is highly probable that other factors play a role here. The results from the demonstration of receptors described below tend to support this suggestion (see pp. 102-107). Glass splinters were implanted intracerebrally. After the splinters were removed, polynuclear giant cells were found adhering to them. Receptors for IgG and for the complement could be demonstrated on the surface of these cells. With the technique used here, these receptors can be demonstrated only in cells of the monocyte-macrophage series. After the cells were incubated in vitro with colloidal carbon, the giant cells exhibited distinct phagocytic activity.

c) *Phagocytic Reaction of Human Cerebrospinal Fluid Cells*

Since all the cell types described, which were considered to be MP of the CNS, are localized only in spaces where CSF is present, it should be possible to obtain the same cells via a cerebrospinal fluid (CSF) puncture in living humans. Approximately 4000 cells/ml are found in CSF. One-half of these cells are similar to lymphocytes; the other half bear considerable resemblance to monocytes and macrophages. It must be assumed that, in terms of the macrophages, these elements are similar to those found inside the subarachnoid space in the animal experiments.

The following experimental investigators were carried out because of the differing findings on phagocytic behavior of monocytelike and macrophagelike cells of cerebrospinal fluid (see Schönenberg, 1952; Sörnäs, 1971). The second aspect was whether or not the cells were still capable of phagocytosis after they had been removed via lumbar puncture.

Material and Methods

One drop/ml of a 0.02% mixture of polystyrene particles (Difco-Latex: ϕ 0.79 μ, dialyzed 71 h at 4° C against distilled water; Dow Chemical Co., Midland/Michigan, USA) and physiologic saline solution was added (see also Joos et al., 1969) to at least 2 ml fresh CSF acquired via lumbar puncture and incubated on a vibrator for 30 min at room temperature. The CSF was then allowed to settle for 30 min/ml at 4° C in a Sayk chamber, and the material was stained according to Pappenheim.

Those mononuclear cells containing at least five latex particles in the cytoplasm were considered phagocytic positive. After counting at least 100 monocytelike and/or macrophagelike cells per specimen, the percentage was determined.

The CSF specimens were obtained from 200 patients suffering from a variety of diseases. No significant alterations in the CNS region and/or the dura or pia mater could be found in 50 patients. No qualitative or quantitative pathologic findings were evident in the biochemical, serologic, and cytologic composition of the CSF. This group was considered the "normal population" or "control group." The remainder of the patients suffered from diseases with inflammatory or reactive alterations in the region of the leptomeninges.

Results

Latex particles were observed as uniform light vacuoles in the gray-blue stained cytoplasm of monocytelike and macrophagelike cells (Fig. 28). These vacuoles could be distinguished from vacuoles of other origins because of their uniformity. Phagocytes containing latex particles were observed in 29.5% (= M; SD = ±1.2%) of the mononuclear phagocytes found in the CSF of the control group. The number of phagocytically active elements from this cell type as significantly decreased in inflammatory alterations of the leptomeninges, i.e., in acute virus meningoencephalitis (n = 47; M = 20.93%; SD = ±8.15%), chronic meningoencephalitis (n = 15, M = 20.42%, SD = ±10.15%), and acute attacks of multiple sclerosis (n = 21, M = 22.70%, SD = ±6.36%). A significant increase in the percentage of phagocytically positive monocytelike and macrophagelike cells was observed with the reactive alteration of the leptomeninges as a result of a fresh hemorrhage occurring less than 5 days prior to obtaining the specimen (n = 12, M = 50.25%, SD = ±8.22%) and/or an old hemorrhage occurring at least 4 weeks prior to obtaining the specimen (n = 14, M = 40.71%, SD = ±27.04%).

Three conclusions can be drawn from these investigations: (1) Phagocytizing cells were found in human CSF; (2) with the methods described here, approximately one-third of all monocytelike and macrophagelike cells in CSF demonstrated a (nonspecific) phagocytic ability after removal; and (3) the differing phagocytic behavior of the same cells in various diseases indicates the influence of external factors; no attempt was made here to investigate this matter further.

2. Cytochemical Investigations

The biochemical description of a cell can partly be used for the functional classification. This is particularly the case for demonstrating enzyme activity. The enzyme activity as

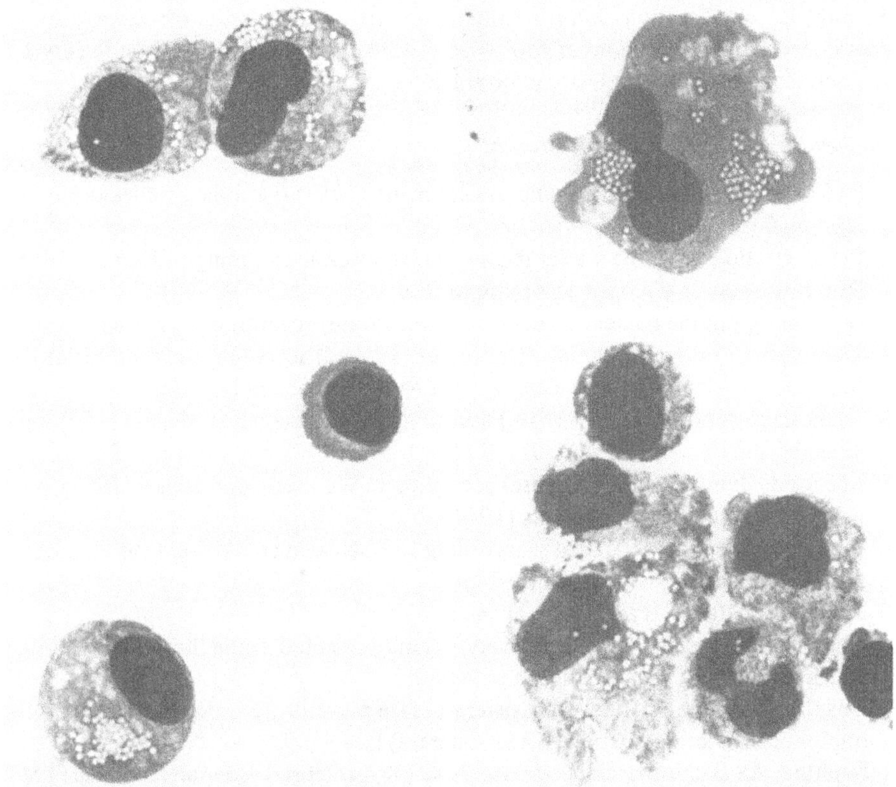

A B C D

Fig. 28 A–D. Mononuclear macrophagelike cells, which phagocytize polystyrene particles, in human CSF after in vitro administration of polystyrene suspension (Pappenheim stain; magnification: x 1200) (Fig. 28 B after Oehmichen, 1973)

well as substratchemical analysis of monocytes and macrophages was compared with the activity of resting and/or progressive microglia, of perivascular cells, of leptomeningeal macrophages, and of epiplexus cells in the following investigations.

Material and Methods

Only rabbits were used for the author's experiments. Table 4 presents the findings obtained with other species, particularly the human. [The Schaeffer and co-worker study (1970) should be consulted for additional information regarding the histochemistry of rabbit blood cells.] Blood monocytes were identified on the basis of their relatively typical morphology in normal blood smears. The smears were dried for 5–10 min and stored under airtight conditions at −70° C. Peritoneal macrophages were collected in the manner described above and spread on the slide. The slide was then dried briefly in air and stored the same as the blood smears at −70° C. After the animals had been exsanguinated, undamaged brain tissue (two rabbits) was removed as well as brain tissue obtained 4 days after a stab wound (two rabbits). The specimens were sliced into 0.5-cm-thick frontal sections and frozen in liquid nitrogen. The brain tissue was also stored under airtight conditions at -40° C and sliced at -15° C to -20° C on the cryostat. Each section was approximately 5-μ thick.

Cytochemical Methods of Demonstration

1. PAS reaction, modified according to Graumann (1953) (periodic acid leukofuchsin reaction);
2. Demonstration of fat via scarlet red and sudan black B according to Romeis (1968);
3. Demonstration of glycogen according to Best;
4. Diphosphopyridine nucleotide diaphorases (DPNase) according to Pearse (1968);
5. Triphosphopyridine nucleotide diaphorases (TPNase) according to Pearse (1968);
6. Succinic dehydrogenase (Succ.ase) according to Goebel and Puchtler (1955);
7. Adenosine triphosphatase (ATPase) according to Wachstein and Meisel (1957), modified by Ibrahim and co-workers (1974);
8. Adenosine diphosphatase (ADPase) according to Wachstein and Meisel (1957), modified by Ibrahim and co-workers (1974);
9. Uridine diphosphatase (UDPase) according to Wachstein and Meisel (1957), modified by Ibrahim and co-workers (1974);
10. Acid phosphatase (APase) (see p. 39);
11. Nonspecific esterase (refers exclusively to data presented in the literature with which no further differentiation is possible);
12. α-naphthyl acetate esterase (ANA-esterase) (see p. 39);
13. Naphthol AS acetate esterase (NASA-esterase) (see p. 39);
14. Naphthol AS-D chloroacetate esterase (NAS-DCA-esterase) according to Leder (1967), pH 7.0.

In order to obtain comparable results, each of the reactions and/or enzyme demonstrations as carried out by the same person on the same day as were the blood smears, macrophage smears, and brain sections from damaged and undamaged animals.

Only a rough, semiquantitative evaluation was carried out: O = no finding; + = identifiable, slight deposits of staining material recognizable only in isolated cells; ++ = distinct staining material deposition in most of the cells of one cell type.

Results

Table 4 presents the author's own results (cf. Fig. 29) and the results given in the literature. The following problems arose for the author in interpreting the findings.

Since the whole neuropil was diffusely stained in some of the enzyme demonstrations (e.g., APase, ANA-esterase), clear-cut identification of resting microglia was difficult. This problem was particularly serious when only a slight enzyme activity was assumed to be present in the processes of this cell type and considerably more pronounced enzyme activity, to be present in the perikaryon. Under these conditions the cell type with a positive staining reaction could no longer be identified on the basis of its morphology. The only remaining possibility was to consider perineuronal elements as resting microglia on the basis of their localization and to evaluate the corresponding deposit

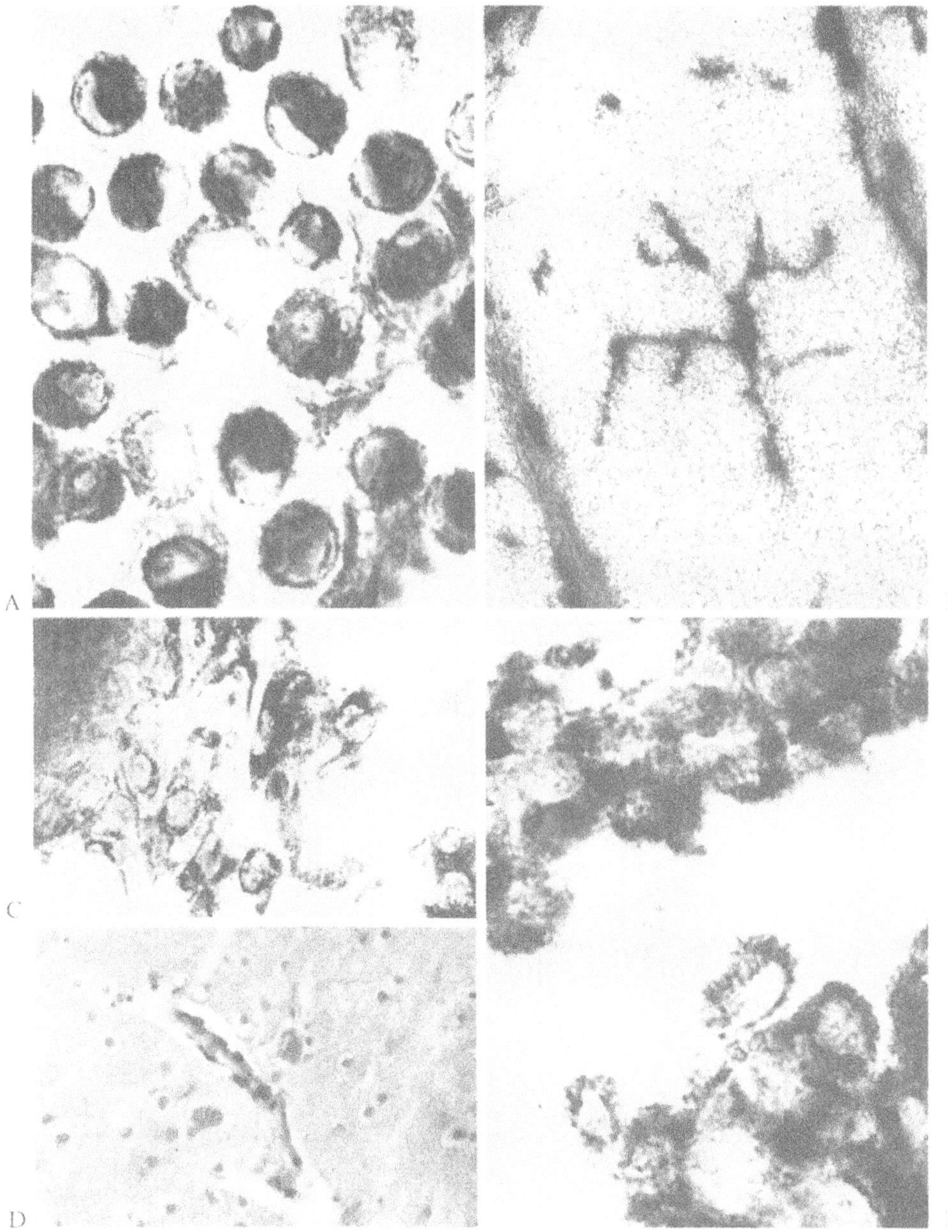

Fig. 29 A–E. Enzyme activity in various cell types. (A) Peritoneal macrophage smear, DPNase; (B) Resting microglia, ATPase; (C) Subarachnoid free cells, α-naphthyl acetate esterase; (D) Perivascular cells of intracerebral vessel, naphthyl AS-D chloroacetate esterase; (E) Epiplexus cells, TPNase [Magnification: (A–C) x 1200; (D) x 700; (E) x 500]

Table 4. Cytochemical findings in various cell types from author's investigations and from the literature

Type of cyto-chemical investigation	Blood monocyte	Peritoneal macrophage	Resting microglia	Progressive microglia	Perivascular cell	Free Sub-arachnoidal cell	Epiplexus cell
1. PAS	38 +	 +	8,16 0/+	7 +	23,38 +	16,38 +	 +
2. Fat	38 +	 ++	35,38,51 0/+	17,36,48 ++	36,38 ++	38 ++	 +
3. Glycogen	38 +	 +	 0	 0	46 0	46 +	 0
4. DPNase	6 +	49,50 +	31 0	12,27,31,42,50 +	14,24,33 +	 +	 +
5. TPNase	6 +	50 ++	24,31 +	20–22,25–27,31 42,50 ++	24,31 +	 +	 +
6. Succ.ase	6 +	 +	 0	12,21,25 +	24 +	 +	 +
7. ATPase 8. ADPase	6 +	 ++	29,30 48,49 ++	2,12,13 28,30,48,49 ++	23,24 32 +	 ++	 +
9. UDPase	 +	 ++	24 ++	 ++	24 ++	 ++	 ++
10. APase	34,43	34,37		3,4,9–12,15,17	23,29,38	41,38,45	44

	++	++	?	19,27,29,41,53 ++	45,47,51 ++	47,52 ++	++
11. Nonspecific esterase	34,38	34	30,38	30	1,18,38 39,40	38	44
12. ANA-esterase	34,38,43 ++	34 ++	38 0/+	++	38 ++	38 ++	44 ++
13. NAS-esterase	34 ++	++	?	++	++	++	+
14. NAS-DCA -esterase	34,38 +	34 ++	?	++	38 +	38 +	44 +

[a] 0 = no findings; + = slight, but identifiable deposits of staining material recognizable only in isolated cells; ++ = distinct deposits of staining material in most of the cells of one type

[b] 1. Abe et al., 1964; 2. Barron and Tuncbay, 1964; 3. Becker and Barron, 1961; 4. Bodian and Mellors, 1945; 5. Bowen and Davison, 1974; 6. Braunsteiner and Schmalzl, 1970; 7. Cammermeyer, 1967; 8. Cammermeyer, 1970b; 9. Coimbra and Tavares, 1964; 10. Colmant, 1959; 11. Colmant, 1961; 12. Colmant, 1962; 13. Colmant, 1963; 14. Duckett and Pearse, 1965; 15. Escola and Thomas, 1965; 16. Fleischhauer, 1964; 17. Friede, 1962; 18. Gomori and Chessik, 1953; 19. Hamuro, 1957; 20. Härkönen, 1964; 21. Howe and Flexner, 1947; 22. Howe and Mellors, 1945; 23. Ibrahim, 1974a; 24. Ibrahim et al., 1974; 25. Klein, 1960; 26. Kreutzberg, 1963; 27. Kreutzberg, 1966; 28. Kreutzberg, 1967; 29. Kreutzberg, 1968a; 30. Kreutzberg, 1968b; 31. Kreutzberg and Peters, 1962; 32. Landers et al., 1962; 33. Leake et al., 1964; 34. Leder, 1967; 35. Markov, 1971; 36. Markov and Dimova, 1974; 37. Nelson, 1969; 38. Oehmichen, 1973a; 39. Pearse, 1958; 40. Pepler and Pearse, 1957; 41. Robinson, 1972; 42. Rubinstein et al., 1962; 43. Schaefer et al., 1970; 44. Schwarze, 1975; 45. Shimizu, 1950; 46. Shimizu and Kumamoto, 1952; 47. Shuttleworth and Allen, 1966; 48. Sjöstrand, 1966a; 49. Sjöstrand, 1966c; 50. Smith and Rubinstein, 1962; 51. Vaughn et al., 1970; 52. Wolf et al., 1943; 53. Yanagihara et al., 1967.

of staining material. The differentiation of epiplexus cells as well as their differentiation from desquamated and detached choroidal cells presented another kind of problem. On nonfixed cryostat sections, in particular, choroidal cells also have the tendency to detach from the tissue connections. They are then extremely difficult to distinguish morphologically from epiplexus cells. Frequently, a clear-cut identification was also problematic because choroidal cells also exhibit a distinct activity with almost all of the enzymes and reactions investigated here (Oehmichen, 1973).

The following observations should be appended to the results of the investigations presented in Table 4: It was possible to demonstrate a PAS-positive reaction, fat or glycogen, in each of the investigated cell types, but the reaction was not present in all cells of the same cell type.

The most pronounced enzyme activity in the cell types examined here was that of UDPase, then ATPase, and finally ADPase. Since most of the other cells in the brain exhibited no activity in regard to the demonstration of this enzyme, it was possible to achieve an almost elective demonstration of the four investigated cell types (MP) in the CNS and resting microglia with these enzymes.

Acid phosphatase as well as the nonspecific esterases were particularly active in the perivascular cells and could be demonstrated in the free subarachnoidal cells. As a result of these demonstrations, the tissue mast cells could not always be identified with certainty. Similar activity was also found in the progressive microglia as well as in the peritoneal macrophages and in the monocytes. A slightly pronounced activity in resting microglia such as was observed in perineuronal cells could only be demonstrated in the perikaryon.

Naphthol AS-D chloroacetate esterase exhibited distinct activity in the free subarachnoidal cells, perivascular cells, epiplexus cells, and progressive microglial cells, particularly with a pH of 7.0. In each case, this activity must be differentiated from the much higher activity of perivascular mast cells. Resting microglia exhibited no activity of this enzyme.

In comparing the staining material deposition in the individual cell types examined, it was evident that resting microglia often exhibited negative or doubtful positive findings. All other cell types compared exhibited a similar cytochemical pattern; slight quantitative differences were observed.

Using oxidoreductases, particularly DPNase and TPNase, as marker enzymes to investigate the time sequence of glial activation, Hazama and Kreutzberg (1977) observed that macrophage activity increased with experimental anterograde fiber degeneration and transneuronal changes when microglial activity decreased. The number of microglial cells decreased as the number of macrophages increased.

An additional observation not included in the table should be mentioned. The blood monocytes of most laboratory animals as well as of humans contain peroxidase. No peroxidase-positive cells, however, are found in the normal neuropil. Herrlinger and coworkers (1977) were able to identify peroxidase in activated microglia of mice. Since peroxidase in extravascular monocytes (and macrophages) disappears (cf. Nichols and Bainton, 1975), this enzyme can only be demonstrated in migrated macrophages and in so-called activated microglia of laboratory animals for a very brief period of time. It can not be found in monocytic derivatives that have been located extravascularly for longer periods of time. Since peroxidase is not present in the blood monocytes of rabbits (Leder, 1967), we did not attempt to demonstrate this enzyme.

3. Investigations with Immunologic "Markers"

The investigations described below were carried out to provide information as to whether or not cells are found in the CNS which, on the basis of their immunologic reaction, can be compared either with cells of the monocyte-macrophage series or with B or T lymphocytes. The experiments were carried out in different series. The methods of examination remained basically the same; the material examined varied or was submitted to different conditions. In most of the experiments, the same immunologic labeling material was applied. The immunologic labeling methods are, therefore, dealt with first in order to describe each individual series with its special methodological presentation of the problem and the results.

Immunologic Labeling Methods

Demonstration of Fc and Complement Receptors: Sheep erythrocytes were sensitized with antibodies, using a sheep erythrocyte antibody produced in rabbit (amboceptor). The Fc fragments present on the red cell complexes can be recognized by cell types with receptors for the Fc region of IgG (Fc receptors and/or IgG receptor). Cells of the monocyte-macrophage series are, therefore, able to phagocytize this complex (LoBuglio et al., 1967; Huber et al., 1968; Shevach et al., 1973), while B lymphocytes with a Fc receptor cannot be demonstrated with these special methods (Lay and Nussenzweig, 1968; Bianco et al., 1970; Shevach et al., 1973). As far as is known at present, no other cell type exhibits a reaction type to sensitized sheep erythrocytes which is identical to that of the cells of the monocyte-macrophage series.

An antigen-antibody-complement complex is formed when the sheep erythrocyte-antibody complexes are additionally sensitized with complement. The complement bound in this way is able to react with a so-called complement receptor, independent of the Fc fragment. This receptor is present in cells of the monocyte-macrophage series and on the surface of B lymphocytes (Bentwich and Kunkel, 1973). With these experimental techniques, only the mononuclear phagocytes phagocytize the antigen-antibody complement complex; rosettes were formed by the lymphocytes through attachment.

The methods correspond to those given by Huber and Fudenberg (1968) as well as Huber and co-workers (1968). The sheep erythrocytes (*E*) were donated by Prof. R. E. Bader, Director of the Hygiene Institute, University of Tübingen. The anti-E antibody (= amboceptor and/or anti-Forssman serum) (*A*) (Behringwerke, Marburg-Lahn/FRG) was diluted with PBS (1:500, 1:2000, 1:8000, 1:32,000) and incubated with erythrocytes to obtain an *EA* complex.

The IgG and/or IgM fraction of the anti-Forssman serum was produced by the author himself according to methods described by Huber and Fudenberg (1968) or purchased (Cordis Labs. Europa, Roden/Netherlands). The fractions were also used to sensitize erythrocytes in order to produce an *EA-IgG* and/or *EA-IgM* complex.

In each case freshly removed serum from rabbits and/or humans was used as the complement (*C*). As a rule, the serum was diluted with VBS (1:80). No noticeable hemolysis occurred. After the sheep erythrocytes had been sensitized with *A* and/or *A-IgG*, they were additionally sensitized with complement; the result was an *EAC* or *EA-IgG-C* complex. After each suspension was adjusted to a 5% erythrocyte suspension, the different complexes could be utilized.

Inhibition experiments were also conducted with immunoglobulin G (*IgG*) [human IgG (Nordic Immunol. Labs., Nilburg/Netherlands); rabbit IgG (Miles Labs., Slough/England)]. In each case control experiments were conducted with washed autologous erythrocytes and *E* (sheep erythrocytes). Those mononuclear cells that had phagocytized at least one erythrocyte and/or erythrocyte complex were considered receptor positive.

Demonstration of Receptors for Sheep Erythrocytes Pretreated with Neuraminidase: Sheep erythrocytes together with a particular lymphocyte subpopulation form rosettes. The lymphocytes were T lymphocytes; the rosette test is considered specific for these cell types (Frøland, 1972; Bentwick and Kunkel, 1973). One modification of the method is the demonstration of rosette formation by T lymphocytes with *E* which were pretreated with neuraminidase (*N*) (Michlmayr et al., 1974; Gilbertsen and Metzgar, 1976; Han and Minowada, 1976). The erythrocytes pretreated in this way form a so-called *EN* complex. Those cells on which at least three erythrocytes were attached on the surface were considered positive.

Demonstration of Immunoglobulin Receptors: Determinants for immunoglobulins can be demonstrated on the surface of B lymphocytes (Raff, 1970); their demonstration is considered a specific test for this cell population (Bentwick and Kunkel, 1973). Polyvalent anti gamma globulin was applied in the experiments described here. In each case the anti gamma globulin was conjugated with fluorescein isothiocyanate: anti-human gamma globulin from goats (*AHGG*), anti-mouse gamma globulin from rabbits (*AMGG*), and anti-rabbit gamma globulin from goats (*ARGG*; Behringwerke, Marburg-Lahn/FRG). Some of the anti-sera were diluted with saline solution (1:2 and/or 1:4). After the nonfixed sections were fixed (30 s) with cold acetone (−20° C), all of the sections were incubated in a damp chamber at 4° C and/or 37° C. As a control, inhibition experiments were carried out with purified gamma globulin from humans (Behringwerke, Marburg-Lahn/FRG) and/or rabbits (Miles Labs., Slough/England). It should be noted that no specificity control was carried out and the purity grade was not checked in the authors laboratories. Before use, the free staining material was removed from the conjugated sera via a Sephadex G-25 (gel filtration). Microscopic investigations were carried out using the Zeiss photomicroscope POL. The fluorescence examination was done with a high-pressure mercury lamp HBO 200 W (exciting filter: Bg 12/4; suppression filter: 53/44).

Demonstration of Receptors for Aggregated Gamma Globulin: B lymphocytes have a receptor for aggregated gamma globulin (*AGG*, see Dickler and Kunkel, 1972; Frøland et al., 1974). Apparently, this receptor can also be demonstrated on immature B cells, which exhibit no determinants for immunoglobulin (Wernet and Kunkel, 1973). The AGG was produced according to data from Huber and co-workers (1974); conjugation with fluorescein isothiocyanate corresponded to data from Hijmans and co-workers (1969). Some of the investigations were carried out with a product made available to the author by Behringwerke (Marburg-Lahn/FRG).

Varying amounts of the immunologic markers presented here were used in five independent series of investigations.

a) Leptomeningeal Membrane Specimens

In order to obtain a fairly reliable test system, the interior surface of the leptomeninx (side nearest the brain surface) of the rabbit was first examined with immunologic markers.

Material and Methods

After cardial perfusion with warm VBS, the rabbit brain was exposed. The leptomenix was detached without damage by subarachnoidal injection of VBS. The leptomeninx was then stored in culture medium, spread out, and stretched on a plastic cover.

Membrane sections from a total of 18 rabbits were incubated together with E, EA-IgG, EAC, and EN (0.9 ml medium, 0.1 ml erythrocyte suspension for each specimen) on the vibrator at 37° C for 60 min under airtight conditions. IgG was added to some specimens for inhibition. ARGG was diluted with medium (1:2) and incubated for 60 min at 4° C. All the material was then thoroughly washed with PBS. The section of membrane was then partially fixed with formalin, stained with H&E, and spread out on a slide. After the specimen had been incubated with labeled sera, it was covered (nonfixed) and examined with the fluorescence microscope.

Results

Histologic examination primarily revealed pavementlike cells of the arachnoidea, the vessels of which are distributed. Perivascularly located clumps of cells as well as isolated cells were found only locally.

The information presented in Table 5 was provided by the immunologic tests (cf. Figs. 31 A and B p. 99). Single cells and/or cell clumps that had phagocytized EA complexes

Table 5. Results following incubation of leptomeningeal specimens with immunologic markers[a]

No. of specimens examined	Red blood cell complex	Inhibitor	Reaction
6	E		0
5	EA-IgG 1:500		+
5	EA-IgG 1:500	1 mg IgG/ml	0
5	EAC		+
5	EAC	1 mg IgG/ml	+
5	EN		0
4	ARGG		0

[a] 0 = no reaction; + = distinct reaction in the sense of red blood cell phagocytosis.

were found on the inner side. The phagocytic activity was inhibited with IgG; the inhibitory activity, counteracted by additionally sensitizing the EA complex with complement. No phagocytic process and/or rosette formation occurred after E and/or EN had been added. The investigation with ARGG yielded negative results.

No quantitative statements can be made since the number of identifiable cells varied considerably for each membrane specimen. Qualitative statements could not be made since a clear-cut classification of cells was impossible with the given preparation methods. It was established that those cells incorporated red cell complexes that were primarily located perivascularly as well as those cells appearing in large aggregation on the inner side of the leptomeninx. These aggregations were most probably the cells found in increased proportions in the sulci and/or in the cisternae between the arachnoidea and pia mater (free subarachnoidal cells and/or trabecular cells) on normal sections. No reaction was observed in the endothelial, pial, and arachnoidal cover cells. The EAC complexes exhibited a distinct tendency toward attachment and were more difficult to wash off.

b) Cells of the Subarachnoid, Ventricular, and Perivascular Spaces

Since definite classification of the cells on the exposed leptomeninx of rabbit is problematic, comparable experiments were carried out in situ. Cells could be localized in this way, thus in turn, facilitating a more exact classification of these cells.

Material and Methods

In the first series, the rabbit was perfused through the heart for 1 h with warm (37° C) VBS in order to wash the blood cells out of the cerebral (blood) vessels (cf. Fig. 30). Before the perfusion, each of the animals received heparin intraveneously. After the 1-h period had elapsed, various labeling materials such as washed sheep erythrocytes and red cell complexes (0.1 ml suspension), sometimes together with inhibitors such as dissolved IgG, were injected intrathecally, intraventricularly, and/or intracerebrally. The brains were perfused with warm VBS for an additional hour (incubation period) and then with 4% formalin for fixation. This investigation was carried out with one marker for each five rabbits (total number of animals examined: 150).

In the second series, the same injections were also undertaken with identical labeling materials in each of the five surviving animals. The animals were killed after 1 h (incubation period) by formalin perfusion through the heart.

The brains of two untreated and undamaged animals were exposed after perfusion with VBS for 10 min. The brains were cut into 0.5-cm-thick frontal slices and immediately frozen in liquid nitrogen. These blocks were then sliced on the cryostat and incubated with anti-rabbit gamma globulin.

Results

The results of the above-mentioned investigation are summarized in Table 6. The following relations were established:

No labeled cells were observed in the rabbit brain following incubation of nonfixed sections with anti gamma globulin.

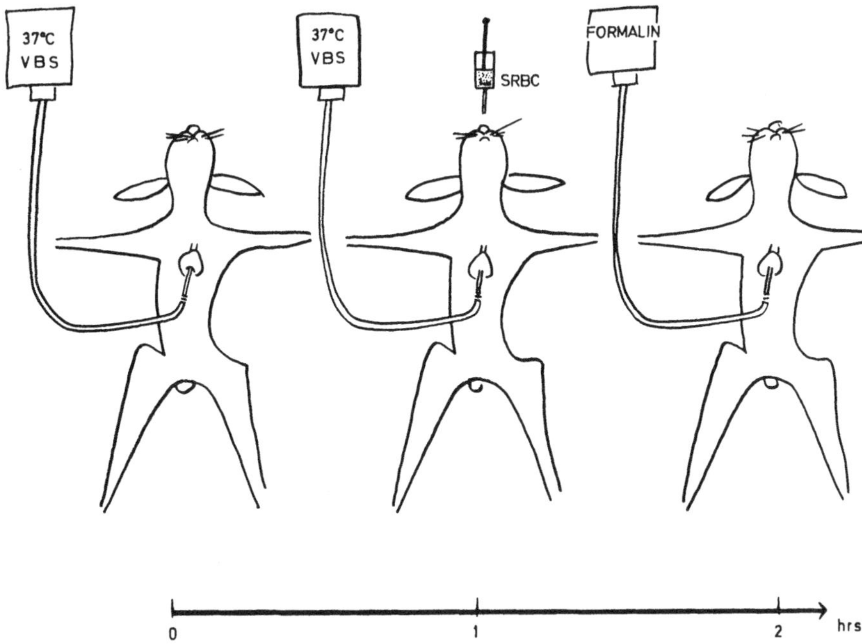

Fig. 30. Course of experimental procedure demonstrating receptor activity in different cells within the brain. Red cell complexes (SRBC) were injected intracerebrally 1 h after the brain vessels had been washed out by cardial perfusion with warm VBS. The VBS perfusion was continued for an additional hour and then formalin was perfused. The brain was removed.

Experiments involving the injection of red cell complexes into living and/or dead animals revealed slight quantitative differences. These differences were probably influenced by the circulatory movement of red cell complexes in the CSF space of living animals. In each case, the percentage of phagocytizing erythrocyte complexes was higher in living animals than in dead animals.

In both experimental series, subarachnoidal phagocytes (Figs. 31 C and D), intraventricular phagocytes (Figs. 32 A and B), and perivascular phagocytes (Figs. 32 C and D) basically exhibited the same reaction; all other cell types (cells lining the CSF space such as arachnoidal, pial, and/or ependymal or choroidal elements) did not react. The three cell types mentioned phagocytized the EA complexes in amounts directly proportional to the dosage. They did not react to washed erythrocytes; no attachment or rosette formation were observed after injection of EN complexes. Dissolved IgG inhibited the reaction with EA-IgG, even though the IgG dosage required for inhibition exceeded the physiologic level. The inhibition was distinctly reduced when EA-IgG complexes were also incubated with complement.

On the basis of these experiments, it may be concluded that subarachnoidal and perivascular cells as well as cells deposited on the choroidal plexus react in the same manner and that they exhibit the characteristics of IgG and complement receptors.

Table 6. Demonstration of receptor activity in cells from various locations inside the rabbit brain after intrathecal, intraventricular, and intracerebral injection of red cell complexes[a]

Red cell complexes	Inhibitor	Cells in the brain reacting with red cell complexes					
		Free subarachnoidal cells		Epiplexus cells		Perivascular cell of intra-cerebral vessels	
		A	B	A	B	A	B
E	–	0	0	0	0	0	0
EN		0	0	0	0	0	0
EA 1:500	–	++	+++	++	+++	+	+
EA 1:2000	–	+	++	+	++	+	+
EA 1:8000	–	0	+	0	+	0	+
EA-IgG	2 mg IgG/ml	++	+++	++	+++	+	+
EA-IgG	10 mg IgG/ml	+	++	+	++	+	+
EA-IgG	20 mg IgG/ml	+	+	0	+	0	+
EA-IgG-C	20 mg IgG/ml	++	+++	++	+++	+	+
EAC	–	++	+++	++	+++	+	+
ARGG	–	0	0	0	0	0	0

[a] A = Results after injection into brains previously perfused with VBS; B = Results after injection into brains of living animals. Note: Only a few perivascular cells exhibited receptor activity, obviously a result of the methods used; 0 = no reaction; + = slight reaction (3 red cell complexes phagocytized) of only a few cells; ++ = distinct reaction (more than 3 complexes phagocytized) of only a few cells; +++ = distinct reaction of many cells.

c) Human Cerebrospinal Fluid Cells

The above-mentioned experimental procedures were applied to cells of human CSF in order to obtain comparable results with human material.

Material and Methods

The method had to be slightly modified since, compared with the investigations carried out up to this point, receptors were to be demonstrated in cell suspension. Only those experiments were described which were necessary to establish the cells of the monocyte-macrophage series, i.e., establishing receptors for the Fc fragment and complement. The literature should be consulted for investigations regarding the quantity of B and T lymphocytes (cf. text p. 18; Oehmichen and Huber, 1978).

Demonstration via labeled antisera: Approximately 5 ml fresh cerebrospinal fluid obtained by lumbar puncture was centrifuged at 650–800 *g*/min for 5 min at room temperature. All but 1 ml sediment was discarded. In each case 0.5 ml serum labeled with fluorescein isothiocyanate was added, and the mixture was incubated for 30 and/or 60 min at 37° C and/or 4° C. The material was then washed twice by adding 5 ml physiologic saline solution each time. The supernatant was discarded again; approximately 1 ml sediment was retained. One ml medium Tc 199 was added to this sediment. The

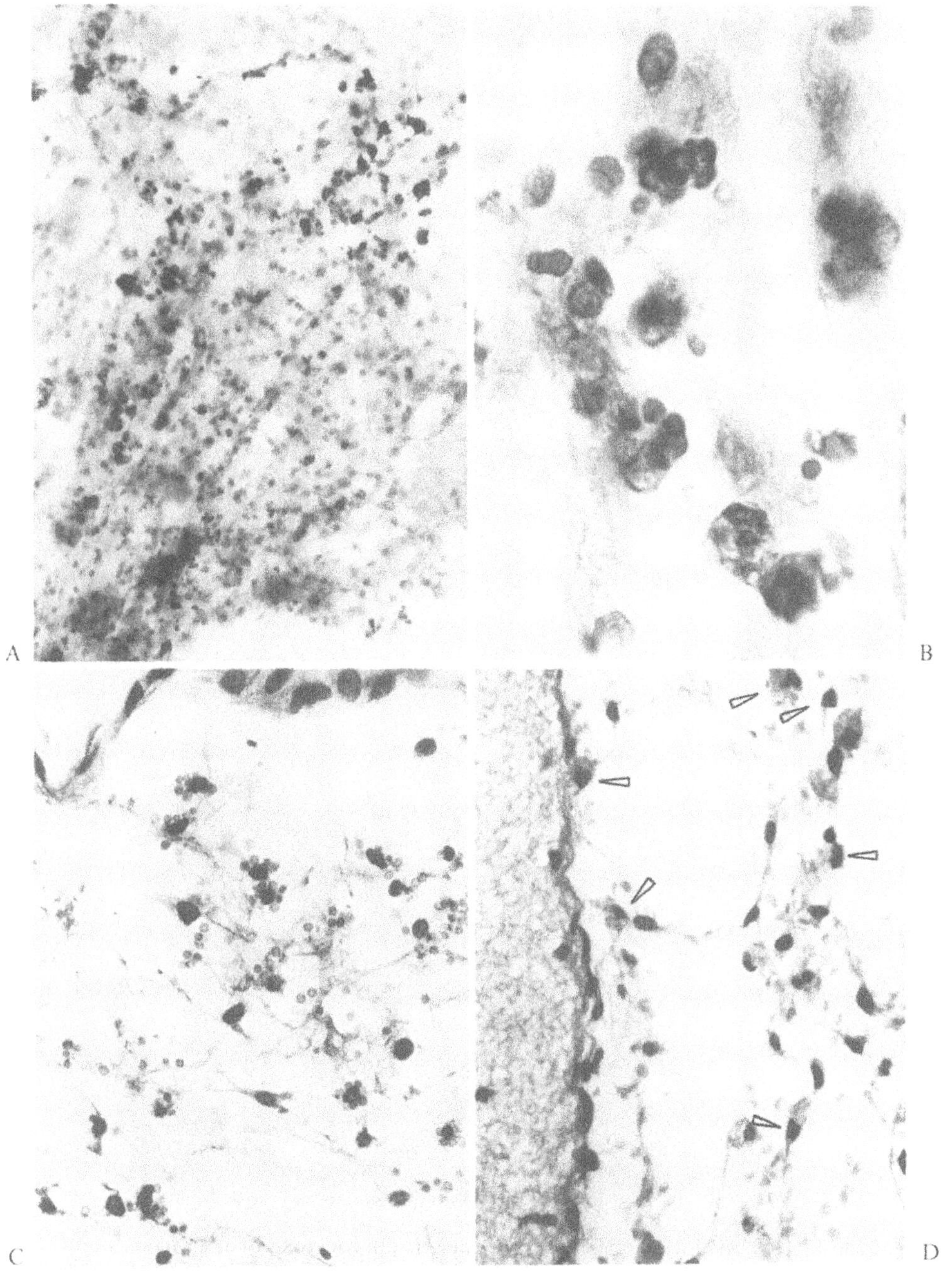

Fig. 31 A–D. Demonstration of Fc-receptor-specific phagocytosis and/or adherence of antigen-antibody complexes (sensitized red cells) with free cells in the subarachnoid space, after incubation with sensitized sheep erythrocytes. (A and B) Specimens of leptomeningeal membrane; (C and D) Section specimens following intrathecal injection of erythrocyte complexes. Arrows point to reacting mononuclear cells within the subarachnoid space. [(A–D) H&E stain; magnification: (A) x 200; (B) x 1200, (C and D) x 500] (Fig. 31 D after Oehmichen, 1976)

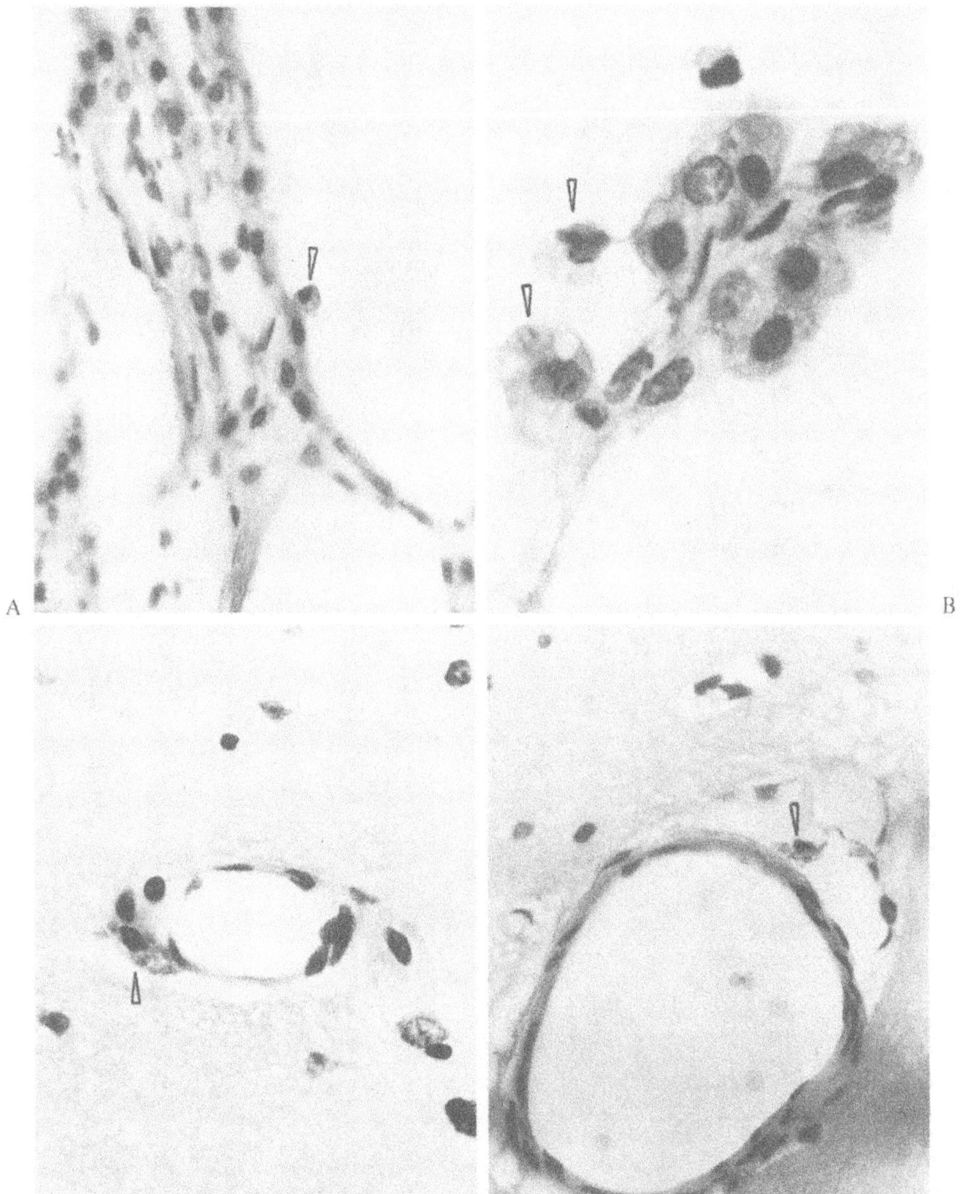

Fig. 32 A–D. Demonstration of Fc-receptor-specific phagocytosis of antigen-antibody complexes *(arrows)* with epiplexus cells, following intraventricular injection of antigen-antibody complex, i.e., sensitized sheep erythrocytes (A and B) and/or perivascular cells of intracerebral vessels (C and D), following intracerebral injection of antigen-antibody complexes . [(A–D) H&E stain; magnification: (A) x 500; (B) x 1200; (C and d) x 500] (after Oehmichen, 1976)

material was carefully mixed and allowed to settle according to Sayk (1960). The specimen was covered with glycerol (pH 7.2) and observed with the fluorescence microscope.

Demonstration via sheep erythrocytes: The demonstration of T cells by EN rosette formation was accomplished by adding 0.1 ml EN suspension adjusted for 16,000 erythrocytes/ml to 1 ml cerebrospinal fluid. This mixture was centrifuged at 800 r/min for 5 min. The supernatant was carefully removed and 1-5 drops of a 30% bovine serum albumin (Serva Feinbiochemica, Heidelberg/FRG); 2 drops of medium, and 1 drop of a 1% toluidine blue solution was added. The rosette-forming round cells were immediately counted in the Fuchs-Rosenthal chamber and again after 12 and 24 h. During this time, the CSF was refrigerated.

To demonstrate the Fc and complement receptors the CSF was washed once (or not washed at all if the cell count was extremely low) and then incubated with 1 ml 5% of an erythrocyte-complex at 37° C for 30 min. The mixture was allowed to settle (Sayk chamber) at a rate of about 30 min/ml. After sedimentation the slide was air-dried and washed; the specimen was stained according to Pappenheim.

The activity of a few enzymes was also demonstrated in the cells of human CSF. A total of 14 cerebrospinal fluid specimens taken from different patients were evaluated. Since no pathologic cell count and no chemical or serologic alterations were observed, the CSF was considered to be normal.

Results

Some of the results are summarized in Table 7 (see Fig. 33). Each mean is the result of the examination of five CSF specimens. Most of the counted mononuclear phagocytes

Table 7. Examined functional criteria from cells of human cerebrospinal fluid which exhibited no cytologic, biochemical, and serologic findings which could be interpretated as pathologic. Evaluation of 14 CSF specimens from different patients. Computation of the mean (M) and standard deviation (SD) was done after counting 100 cells from macrophagelike elements in five different specimens. Data are given in percentages of cells counted

Red cell complex	Inhibitor	Reaction with red cell complexes	
		M	SD
E	–	0.4	± 0.8
EN	–	0	0
AHGG	–	0	0
AGG	–	0	0
EA-IgG 1: 500	–	71.0	±10.9
EA-IgG 1:2000	–	36.6	± 7.1
EA-IgG 1:8000	–	14.4	± 5.4
EA-IgG 1: 500	1 mg IgG/ml	1.25	± 1.9
EA-IgG-C	1 mg IgG/ml	48.4	± 7.8
EA-IgM	–	0.6	± 0.9
EA-IgM-C	–	37.6	±11.3

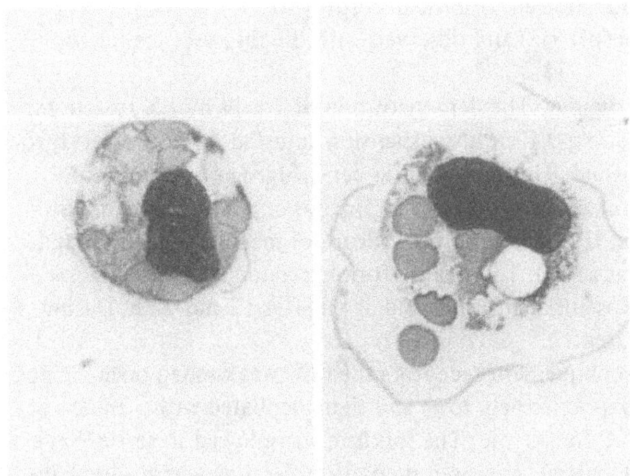

A B

Fig. 33 A and B. Demonstration of Fc-receptor-specific phagocytosis with human CSF cells. (A and B) IgG-receptor-specific phagocytosis of antigen-antibody complexes (i.e., sensitized sheep erythrocytes) with mononuclear phagocytes of human CSF. (Pappenheim stain; magnification: x 1200)

of the cerebrospinal fluid exhibited Fc and complement receptors typical for cells of the monocyte-macrophage series. The percentage of macrophagelike cells with enzyme activity for ANA esterase was M = 84,2, SD = ±9.5; for APase M = 88.0, SD = ±11.1. This enzyme content, which is identical with that of the monocyte-macrophage series, tends to support the classification as mononuclear phagocytes.

d) Glass-Induced Inflammatory Cells in the Sense of Progressive Microglia

Functional investigations with subarachnoidal phagocytes as well as mononuclear phagocytes of human CSF, epiplexus cells, and perivascular cells were carried out with the experiments described thus far. Comparable investigations with progressive microglia should be possible via the intracerebral implantation of glass. In this way, a local increase of microglial cells in the brain is possible; the cells could then adhere and grow on the glass. These glass-adhering cells were partially considered to be progressive microglia (see also Baldwin, 1975). Using phagocytosis experiments as well as the demonstration of enzyme activity and receptors for the Fc fragment and complement, the experiments take into consideration the evidence that the glass-adhering cells are actually cells of the monocyte-macrophage series. Comparable experiments with glass implantation into the skin and demonstration of surface receptors are available (Mariano et al., 1976). The remaining criteria for identification of the glass-adherent cell type (i.e., mononuclear phagocytes) were applied by other research teams in the context of other experiments (Treves et al., 1976).

Material and Methods

A sterile coverglass (maximum ϕ: 0.5 cm) was implanted in the regio precentralis agranularis of the rabbit (Rose and Rose, 1933); the opening of the lateral ventricle was avoided. After 7 days, the animals receiving an intravenous injection of heparin were killed by cardial perfusion of VBS, and the cerebral vessels were washed out. After ~1-h perfusion time, the coverglasses were removed, rinsed in culture medium, and stored. The brains were then partially fixed via formalin perfusion. Those animals for which the implanted glass was not treated with erythrocyte complexes at the end were perfused with VBS for 1 h after the glass had been removed. The erythrocyte complexes (cf. methods described above on p. 93) were then injected into these animals in the area of the brain wound produced by the glass. Only after this had been done were the animals also perfused with formalin. To exclude the possibility of an extensive hemorrhage resulting from the glass implantation, which in turn could possibly simulate nonspecific red cell phagocytosis, each brain was carefully examined histologically for hemorrhages when the respective glasses were to be used for receptor investigations. The glasses from animals receiving red cell complexes in the glass-induced wound after removal of the glass were also examined to exclude the possibility of a hemorrhage.

The following investigations were also carried out on the cells adhering to the glass: The activity of a few enzymes were demonstrated as well as the phagocytosis behavior after in vitro application of colloidal carbon (0.1 mg colloidal carbon/ml 8% suspension, incubation time: 3 h at room temperature). To demonstrate fat, a scarlet red staining was carried out on the frozen sections taken from the region of the brain wound as well as on the cells adhering to glass.

A total of 100 animals were killed in the context of this investigation. Each set of experimental results presented was based on the findings obtained from at least three identical experiments.

Results

Histologically, a large quantity of progressive microglia and isolated polynucleated giant cells were observed in the area of the glass wound on the 7th day after the implantation. A layer consisting primarily of astrocytes was found around the brain wound in the direction of the brain tissue. A few sections of wound surface were covered with a layer of fibroblasts and reticulin fibers.

Cytomophologically, three different types (Fig. 34) of glass-adhering cells should be differentiated: (1) mononuclear foam cells: some round, some spindle-shaped, some characterized by processes and frequently with vaculated cytoplasm, relatively dense (often indented) nucleus, and one or two nucleoli; (2) polynuclear giant cells with rounded nucleus: generally with several nucleoli; and (3) large spindle cells of varying diameters: frequently covered the major portion of the glass surface in a fish-scale pattern. Similar cell types were observed in cell cultures made from human brain biopsy material (see Rorke et al., 1975).

The study of the *phagocytosis activity* revealed that the mononuclear foam cells were heavily laden with carbon particles. The polynucleated giant cells also reacted in the same manner. The large spindle cells contained only a few granules in the cytoplasm. Fat could be observed only in the foam cells and polynuclear giant cells, as well as in those cells in frozen sections which were in the immediate vicinity of the brain wound and, therefore, might best be classified as progressive microglia.

The activity of the *enzymes* (NASA-esterase, ANA-esterase, APase) examined here could be easily identified in the mononuclear foam cells and in the polynuclear giant

A

B

C

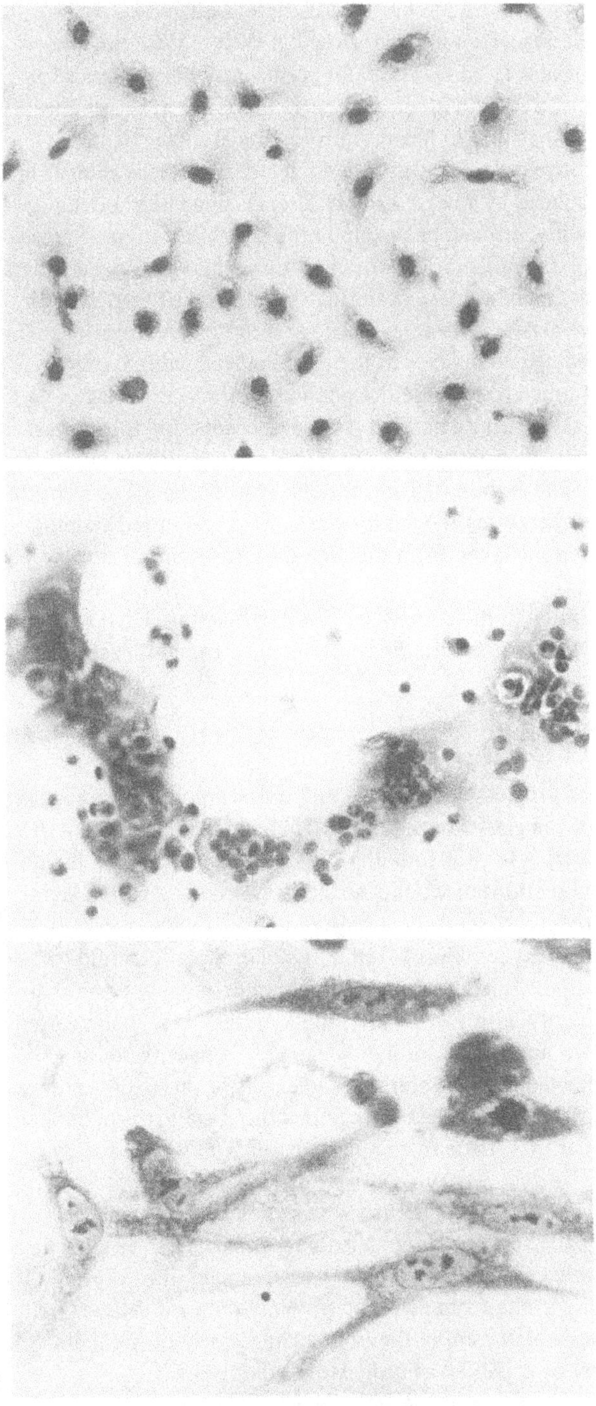

Fig. 34 A–C. Various types of glass-adhering cells following intracerebral implantation of glass
(A) Mononuclear foam cells
(B) Polynuclear giant cells
(C) Large spindle cells
[(A–C) Pappenheim stain; magnification: (A and B) x 200; (C) x 500]

cells. Isolated products of a granular reaction could also be demonstrated in the large spindle cells.

The *IgG and complement receptor activity of glass-adhering cells* is presented in Table 8 (cf. Fig. 35). Only foam cells and polynuclear giant cells phagocytized EA-IgG complexes. These reactions could be inhibited by adding dissolved IgG. The inhibition could be counteracted when the EA-IgG complex was additionally sensitized with complement. No phagocytosis was observed, however, following incubation of glasses with EA-IgM complexes. When the complex was additionally coated with complement (EAC), the same cells were able to phagocytize the red cell complexes. In these experiments, the EAC complex also exhibited an increased tendency to adhere to large spindle cells.

Table 8. Demonstration of IgG and complement receptors in glass-adhering cells following glass implantation in the brain tissue of living rabbits [a]

Red cell complexes		Inhibitor	Reaction with red cell complexes		
			Mononuclear foam cell	Polynuclear giant cell	Large spindle cell
E		–	–	–	–
ARGG		–	–	–	–
EA-IgG	1: 100	–	+++	+++	–
	1: 300	–	+++	+++	–
	1: 500	–	+++	+++	–
	1:1000	–	+++	+++	–
	1:2000	–	++	++	–
	1:8000	–	+	+	–
EA-IgG		1 mg IgG/ml	–	–	–
EA-IgM		–	–	–	–
EA-IgG-C		1 mg IgG/ml	++	++	–
EA-IgM-C		–	++	++	–

[a] 0 = no reaction; + = slight reaction (only three red cell complexes were phagocytized) of only a few cells; ++ = distinct reaction (more than three cell complexes were phagocytized) of only a few cells; +++ = distinct reaction of very many cells.

After the glass had been removed and the *EA complexes injected* in the area of the brain wound (Fig. 36), a clear-cut red cell-complex phagocytosis was observed. When the same sections were impregnated, as for microglial staining, argentophilic cells with short processes were observed which either phagocytized red cell complexes or had erythrocytes attached to their surface. The argentophilia and the morphology corresponded to that of progressive microglia.

The following evidence was provided by these experiments: A large number of cells appeared in the area of a traumatic inflammation in the brain which had been elicited by glass implantation. These cells exhibited the characteristics of cells from the monocyte-macrophage series; morphologically, they resembled the progressive microglia in the section specimens.

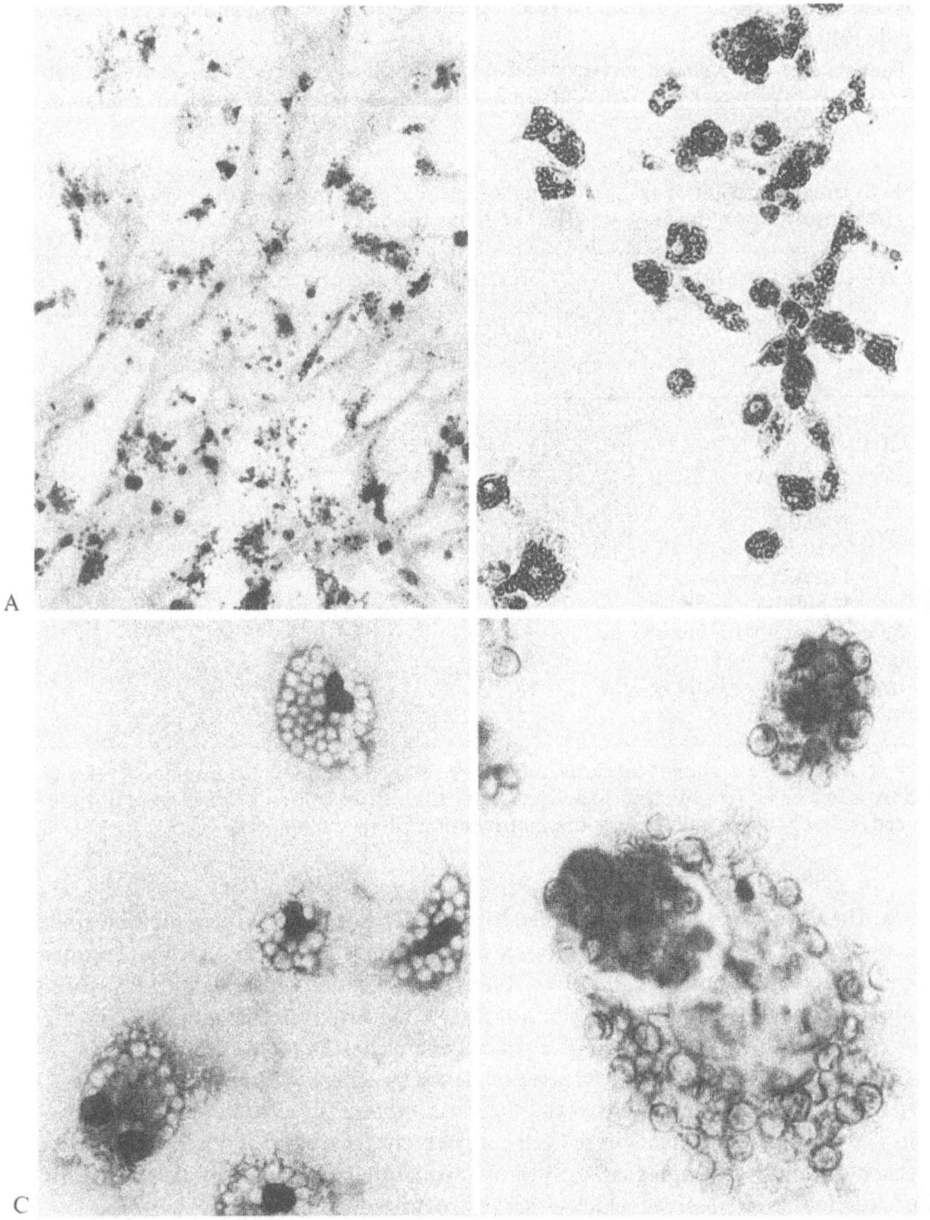

Fig. 35 A–D. Glass-adhering cells react with antibody-loaded sheep erythrocytes; indication of Fc-receptor. Pronounced phagocytosis on the part of mononuclear foam cells (A–C) and polynuclear giant cells (D). So-called large spindle cells (see shadowlike cells in the background of Fig. 35 A) show no reaction. [(A–D) Pappenheim stain; magnification: (A) x200; (B) x250; (C and D) x500]

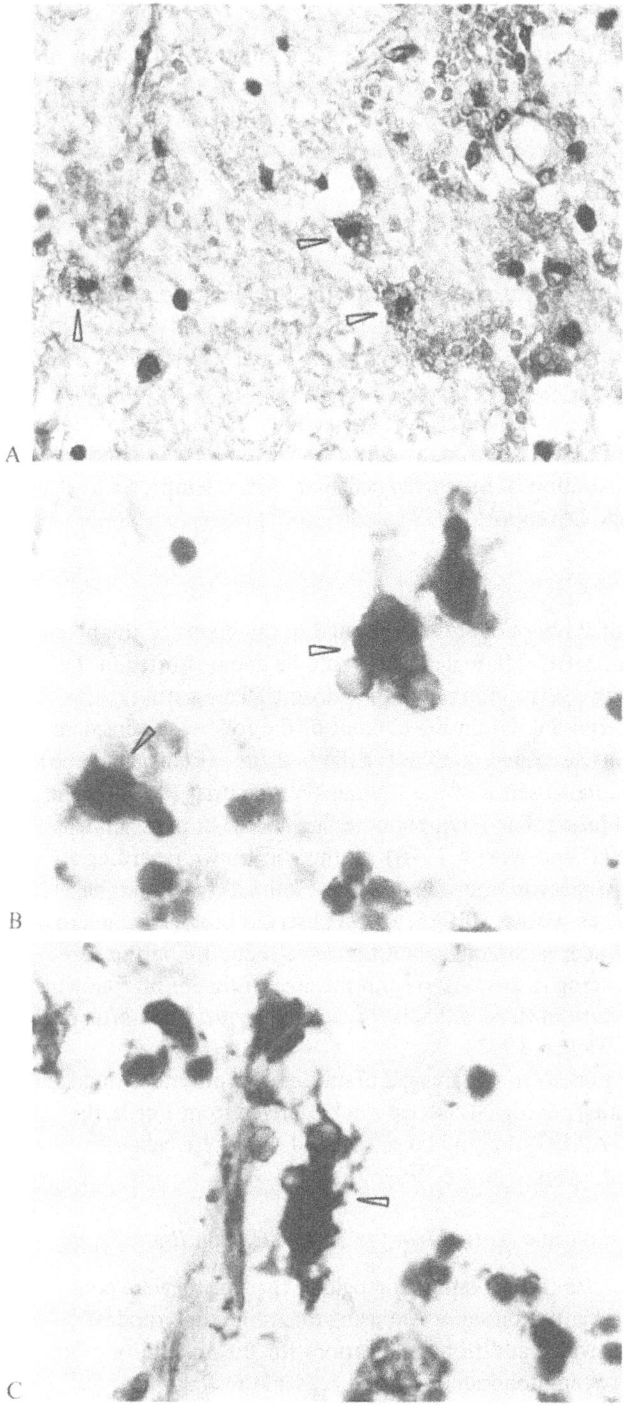

Fig. 36A–C. Demonstration of IgG receptors in cells within brain tissue in which antibody-loaded sheep erythrocytes were injected following removal of previously implanted glass
(A) Pronounced reaction of intracerebral cells in the vicinity of glass-induced brain wounds can be seen *(arrows)*
(B) Using silver impregnation method to demonstrate microglia, intracerebral cells *(arrows)* were established as argentophilic (after reacting with antigen-antibody complex) [(A) H&E stain; (B and C) Weil and Davenport; magnification: (A) x500; (B and C) x1200]

e) Brain of the Athymic or So-Called Nude Mouse

Even if the experiments described above provide eivdence for a monocytelike behavior of progressive microglia, the question has still not been answered as to whether or not resting microglia react similarly. To establish or exclude the possibility of resting microglia developing from lymphocytes, the following investigations were carried out on nude mice.

Material and Methods

The mice (breed: Han: NMRI nu/nu; Central Institute for the Breeding of Laboratory Animals, Hannover/FRG) were perfused through the heart. Three animals were perfused with VBS and three, with 4% formalin. After washing out the brain vessels with VBS, the brains were frozen in liquid nitrogen and sliced on the cryostat. The sections were incubated with anti-mouse gamma globulin (AMGG). The activity of uridine diphosphatase (UDPase) was also demonstrated. The brains fixed in formalin were sectioned with the freezing microtome. Demonstration of microglial cells was then attempted via selective silver impregnation (Weil and Davenport, 1933).

Results

No fluorescent cells indicative of B lymphocytes were found in the brains of this breed of mouse after incubation with AMGG. Microglial cells could be demonstrated in the brains of these animals via selective silver impregnation and via UDPase activity.

These findings should be interpreted within the context of the following considerations: The breed nude mouse was described in 1966 for the first time (Flanagan, 1966). It is characterized by the congenital absence of the thymus (Pantelouris, 1968). In the meantime, it has also been established that T lymphocytes are absent in these animals as well (de Sousa et al., 1969; Raff and Wortis, 1970). Nothing is known regarding alterations in the monocyte and/or macrophage values of these animals (cf. Zinkernagel and Blanden, 1975). Adachi and co-workers (1976, 1977) observed progressive microglia in the brains of nude mice under pathologic conditions. No reduction in the percentage of labeled progressive microglia was observed in the area of the lesion following a traumatic lesion of the spinal cord in those animals receiving a thymectomy after birth (Friedman et al., 1975; cf. also Walker, 1963).

If resting microglial cells are present in undamaged brain tissue of athymic animals, it may be concluded that the resting microglial cells cannot be derived from T cells. By virtue of the lack of reaction to AMGG, it could be established that these cells also cannot be derived from B lymphocytes.

f) Application of Anti-Lymphocyte and Anti-Monocyte Sera to Human Brain Tissue

To obtain additional criteria for classifying resting microglia, experiments were conducted with anti-lymphocyte and anti-monocyte sera using the immunoperoxidase technique. These experiments provided additional indications for the possibility or improbability of a relationship between mononuclear blood cells and resting microglia.

Material and Methods

The sera (anti-human-lymphocyte and anti-human-monocyte sera) were provided by Dr. M. F. Greaves (Imperial Cancer Research Laboratories, London/England). They were produced and absorbed according to the methods already published by Graeves and co-workers (1975).

The brain tissue was obtained during the course of brain surgery for tumors. The pieces of tissue (~3 mm^3) were immediately frozen in liquid nitrogen and sectioned on the cryostat. After a short fixation period (30 s) in cold acetone, parallel sections were stained to exclude the possibility of pathologic alterations, particularly tumor infiltration or inflammatory (microglial) reactions.

All sections of the tissue specimens that could be classified as normal using light-microscopic criteria were stained as follows:

1. Treated with one of the sera mentioned for 60 min at room temperature in a damp chamber: incubation with anti-human-lymphocyte serum (1:25 dilution); incubation with anti-human-monocyte serum (1:25 dilution); incubation with anti-human transferrin produced in rabbits (Behringwerke, Marburg/FRG) (1:10 dilution).
2. Washed for 15 min in PBS.
3. Incubated in a damp chamber for 60 min at room temperature with anti-rabbit serum IgG (heavy and light chains, produced in swine, peroxidase conjugated (Dako-Immunoglobulin, Copenhagen/Denmark), 1:2 dilution].
4. Washed for 15 min in PBS.
5. Diaminobenzidine reaction (Karnowsky, 1967).
6. Nuclear staining with hematoxylin.
7. Covered with DPS.

Blood smear preparations were stained in the same manner as a control for the specificity of the sera. In contrast to the brain sections prior to staining, the endogenous peroxidase of the blood cells in smears was inhibited for 60 min by 1% H_2O. Since none of the cells within the neuropil exhibited a positive (endogenous) peroxidase reaction, this enzyme was not inhibited on section specimens.

Results

Control blood smear specimens were used in which nearly all mononuclear cells had been stained with the anti-lymphocyte serum. Only monocytelike cells (~3%–5% of all cells in the blood smears) were stained when the anti-monocyte serum was applied.

Some tissue specimens showed a clear-cut reaction after the antitransferrin serum was applied. In this case, such tissue specimens were excluded from the study since obviously perifocal edema had produced excessive extravasation of plasma proteins. No positive reaction was observed in another series of tissue specimens using antitransferrin.

Since no resting microglia were stained when the various sera were applied, it must be assumed that resting microglia are not derived from mononuclear blood cells.

Conclusion

The experiments summarized and/or described regarding the functional potency of MP of the CNS yielded the following results:

1. In rabbits, a clear-cut phagocytosis activity was observed in free subarachnoidal cells, epiplexus cells, perivascular cells, in glass-adhering foam cells considered to be progressive microglia, and in polynuclear giant cells. Mononuclear phagocytes of human CSF also exhibited similar clear-cut phagocytosis.
2. Under certain conditions (e.g., following intracerebral injection of cerebrosides or glass implantation), polynuclear giant cells were present in brain tissue which should be classified as cells of the monocyte-macrophage series on the basis of cytokinetic investigations and/or on the basis of the receptor characteristics of these cells. Since the giant cells react similarly, even in their phagocytosis activity, to the other four cell types examined here, they could be described as a special type of MP in the CNS, a "transformation form."
3. The cytochemical behavior of the cell types of the brain examined here (partially also including resting microglia) is almost identical to the enzyme pattern observable with monocytes and/or macrophages.
4. Using sensitized sheep red blood to demonstrate surface receptors (Fc receptor and complement receptor), most of the mononuclear phagocytes of human cerebrospinal fluid reacted like cells of the monocyte-macrophage series. Free subarachnoidal cells, epiplexus cells, perivascular cells, and progressive microglia of rabbit also exhibited similar reactions.
5. On the basis of functional experiments using athymic nude mice, it can be assumed that resting microglia are most probably not identical to T or B lymphocytes. Cytochemically, they only react to a certain extent like cells of the monocyte-macrophage series.
6. The negative results obtained following application of anti-lymphocyte and anti-monocyte sera to sections of normal (undamaged) human brain tissue, would tend to indicate that resting microglia are not derived from mononuclear blood cells (i.e., monocytes or lymphocytes).

C. Discussion and Conclusion

An interpretation and evaluation of the described results is possible only when these findings are compared with the results from other authors. In this way, possible problems and contradictions may be clarified, at least hypothetically, or brought to our attention. Only in this way, is it possible to draw conclusions that apply generally to the mononuclear phagocyte system and/or have particular significance for the field of neuropathology.

I. Explanation of the Author's Findings

A series of experiments were conducted to provide answers to three questions: Where do the cells come from which are classified here as MP of the CNS? Can they efflux out of the cerebrum via the lymphatic system? What function and/or functional potency do they have? Here each separate group of experiments is evaluated.

1. Cytogenesis

The origin of MP in the NS was investigated in normal (undamaged) animals and in animals with experimentally inflicted damage to the NS (to increase the number of MP). This experimental increase of MP was necessary for two reasons. Under normal conditions, very few MP are found in the CNS. In order to obtain a satisfactory answer to the question posed, the results must be taken from a large number of cells. In addition, it was possible to compare normal and pathologic conditions, a comparison otherwise unobtainable.

a) Undamaged Animals

The very slight, spontaneous tendency toward cell division in undamaged brain tissue may be one reason why so few investigations are available concerning the proliferative behavior of resting microglia, leptomeningeal macrophages, perivascular cells, and epiplexus cells. With resting microglia, in particular, the additional problem of identification is present; clear-cut identification is possible only via silver impregnation or with electron microscopy. Finally, most authors discuss the theory that the above-mentioned cells, particularly microglia, are unable to divide in undamaged nerve tissue (Altman, 1962; Cammermeyer, 1965c; Mori and Leblond, 1969; Manuelidis and Manuelidis, 1971; Phillips, 1973).

A few positive results regarding the ability of local division of resting microglia under normal conditions are, however, available (cf. pp. 23–24): Adrian and Walker (1962) and Noetzel and Rox (1964) observed labeled resting microglial cells in H&E-stained autoradiographs 1 h after ^{3}H-TdR injection. They, however, did not provide any quantitatively comparable data. Adrian and Walker (1962) identified most of the labeled cells they found as microglial cells (55 of 236). Using selective impregnation methods, Hommes and Leblond (1967) demonstrated microglial cells in 20-μ-thick frozen sections and coated them with emulsion. Of 402 labeled cells found, 31% in the cerebral cortex and 10% in the corpus callosum could be considered microglia. Following application of ^{3}H-TdR, Mori and Leblond (1969) examined the corpus callosum of rats with the electron microscope. After counting a total of 3000 cells, they found 78 labeled nuclei; none of these cells could, however, be identified as microglia (cf. Skoff et al., 1976). Since Mori and Leblond only considered 4.6% of the observed cells to be microglia, ~150 microglial cells used to determine the percentage of labeled cells were observed with the electron microscope. We found three labeled microglial cells after counting 1000 elements thought to be microglia. The negative finding of Mori and Leblond (1969) could possibly have resulted from the fact that the sample of counted cells was too small.

Almost no investigations have been conducted regarding the labeling index in undamaged peripheral nerves. Here only Schwann cells are found and no microglial cells. Terry and co-workers (1974) investigated the nonmyelinized sympathetic trunk and found no labeled cells in adult animals (in contrast to the findings obtained during the developmental period, see Schupman, 1976). After counting 100 cells in the sciatic nerve, we also found no labeled cells. According to Skoff and Vaughn (1971), the percentage of labeled cells in the optic nerve was 0.1-0.2%. Since this investigation, however, involved tissue from the central nervous system, labeled astrocytes were included in the counting.

Even less data is available on the ability for division of those elements characterized as MP of the CNS. Carpenter and co-workers (1970) referred to the fact that epiplexus cells seldom exhibit mitoses. With electron-optic autoradiography, Kitamura and co-workers (1972) were able to find no labeled pericytes in the CNS following cumulative labeling, not even after traumatic damage. In their light-microscopic investigation, Skoff and Vaughn (1971) found 0.1-0.5% of the pericytes labeled. Both groups of authors limited themselves to "pericytes;" we included the whole population of the perivascular cells of intracerebral vessels. Our results correspond to the Skoff and Vaughn findings (1971). Since this investigation utilized the light microscope, it was not possible to distinguish pericytes from other types of perivascular cells. Skoff and Vaughn (1971) also investigated leptomeningeal cells concerning their proliferation (labeling index: 0.1% and/or 0.5%). No attempt was made to differentiate between the type of leptomeningeal cells (pial, arachnoidal, trabecular).

The author's results for the determination of the labeling index in undamaged animals were almost identical for the different cell types (0.2-0.3%). The negative result in counting epiplexus cells is most probably due to the fact that, in this case, only 100 cells were counted.

The labeling index for blood monocytes and/or macrophages of other organs, however, was 1-2% [mouse blood monocytes: 2.9%; mouse peritoneal macrophages: 1.3% (Van Furth and Cohn, 1968); mouse liver macrophages: 1.5% (North, 1969); mouse alveolar macrophages: 2% (Van Furth, 1970b)]. The frequency of the division of mononuclear phagocytes from other sites of the body under normal conditions was three or five times higher than that of the comparable elements in the CNS examined here. Certainly, the blood-brain barrier for thymidine, which reduced the labeling of brain cells approximately tenfold was one basic reason for the differences in the labeling indexes (Schultze et al., 1972; Mares et al., 1974).

Similar investigations with pulse labeling were evaluated only to indicate the local proliferation of the cell populations examined. Since the labeling index was extraordinarily low, the possibility could not be excluded that a cell migration might have also occurred. Our transfusion experiments with labeled cells in undamaged adult animals showed labeled cells in the neuropil of a few animals. This finding could be interpreted as an indication for such an additional migration of blood cells into the brain. Roessmann and Friede (1968) obtained the same results following injection of labeled bone marrow cells in undamaged rats. Neither these authors nor we observed labeled cells from other localizations in the brain. It could not be clarified if the migrated mononuclear blood cells were actually transformed cells such as resting microglia.

Recently, Ling (1978) observed blood-derived mononuclear cells within the undamaged brain of neonatal rats after intravenous injection of colloidal carbon. These cells were localized perivascularly, perineuronally, or were observed between the nerve fibers. Leukocytic infiltration into the brain tissue of adult animals could not be established.

b) Animals with a Lesion of the Nervous System

A considerable number of investigations can be found in the neuropathologic literature which discuss the origin of phagocytes (expecially progressive microglia) in the nervous system under pathologic conditions. Cytokinetic methods, particularly ^{3}H-thymidine autoradiography, were used. Table 9 lists the various investigations according to the mode of labeling, the various experimentally induced pathologic conditions, the applied histologic methods (light and electron microscopy), and the final conclusion regarding local proliferation and/or hematogenic migration. Different results are frequently obtained, independent of the labeling method and the type of experimentally induced disease.

Most of the cited authors assumed, however, on the basis of their results, that mononuclear cells increase following damage as a result of a migration of hematogenous elements and that these elements are also able to divide in nerve tissue after they have migrated. Various reactions, which are dependent on the type of lesion, are very probably also possible (see Stenwig, 1972; Berner et al., 1973; Torvik, 1975). On the one hand, for example, all the authors established a migration of blood cells following traumatic or inflammatory damage of the nervous system. On the other hand, most of the authors observed a proliferation of local cells in Wallerian degeneration and in retrograde degeneration; evidence for hematogenous migration was absent. It might well be that a particular response was initiated from the reacting cells by the retrograde degeneration. Since this type of damage involved a specific neuropathologic phenomenon (see especially Kreutzberg, 1967, 1968b), it cannot be compared with any other type of damage and/or any other cell reaction in the body. On the other hand, compared with inflammation and trauma, sometimes there was only a slight cell increase; negative results obtained with the methods mentioned here (particularly the cumulative labeling and transfusion of labeled cells) need not necessarily be interpreted as a definitive conclusion.

Although different and/or modified methods were applied, identical results were obtained with our investigations which, however, were not only limited to progressive microglia but were also valid for free subarachnoidal cells, perivascular cells and epiplexus cells, as well as phagocytes of the peripheral nervous system (to a limited degree). We were able to establish a migration of mononuclear blood cells in traumatic and/or inflammation-induced lesions in brain tissue; comparable experiments with orthograde and retrograde degeneration were negative. Moreover, increased local proliferation of activated MP in damaged CNS was also observed. At the same time, we were also able

Table 9. Cytokinetic investigations on the origin of mononuclear phagocytes of the nervous system (particularly of progressive microglia) in the literature (EM: electron-microscopic investigations; loc: locally proliferating; hemat: hematogenic migration)

Kinetic methods of investigation	Type of experimental lesion	Authors	Results (loc/hemat)
Pulse labeling	Trauma	Adrian and Walker, 1962	loc/hemat
		Konigsmark and Sidman, 1963	loc/hemat
		Adrian, 1968	loc/hemat
	Inflammation	Oehmichen et al., 1973	loc/hemat
	Wallerian degen.	Skoff and Vaughn, 1971	loc
	Retrograde degen.	Sjöstrand, 1965, 1966a	loc
		Kreutzberg, 1966, 1967	loc
Cumulative labeling	Trauma	Adrian and Walker, 1962	loc/hemat
		Walker, 1963	hemat
		Konigsmark and Sidman, 1963	loc/hemat
		Huntington and Terry, 1966	hemat
		Adrian, 1968	loc/hemat
		Adrian and Elliot, 1972	hemat
		Kitamura et al., 1972 (EM)	hemat
		Mori, 1972 (EM)	hemat
		(Stenwig, 1972)	hemat
		(Berner et al., 1973)	hemat
		Murray and Walker, 1973	hemat
		Adrian and Williams, 1973a,b (EM)	hemat
		Baldwin, 1975 (EM)	hemat
	Inflammation	Kosunen et al., 1963	hemat
		Sato, 1968	hemat
		Kitamura et al., 1972b (EM)	hemat
		Kitamura, 1975 (EM)	hemat
	Wallerian degen.	Olsson and Sjöstrand, 1969	hemat
		(Stenwig, 1972)	loc
		(Berner et al., 1973)	loc
		Liu, 1973, 1974 (EM)	hemat
	Retrograde degen.	Kreutzberg, 1968	loc
		Adrian and Smothermon, 1970	hemat
		Sjöstrand, 1971	loc
		(Stenwig, 1972)	loc
		(Berner et al., 1973)	loc
		Fujita and Kitamura, 1975 (EM)	hemat
		Young, 1977	hemat
Transfusion experiments	Trauma	Roessmann and Friede, 1968	hemat
		Sumner, 1974	hemat
	Inflammation	Oehmichen et al., 1973	loc/hemat
	Wallerian degen.	Roessmann and Friede, 1968	hemat
	Retrograde degen.	Roessmann and Friede, 1968	hemat
		Sumner, 1974	loc
Perinatal cumulative labeling	Trauma	Smith and Walker, 1967	hemat
		Murray and Walker, 1973	hemat
	Wallerian degen.	Asbury, 1970	hemat
X-irradiation	Trauma	Hopewell and Wright, 1967, 1970a,b	loc
	Wallerian degen.	Cavanagh, 1968a, b	loc

to observe that locally proliferating progressive microglia increased with traumatic and inflammatory brain damage; macrophagelike, DNA-synthezising cells increased with Wallerian degeneration. In contrast to other investigations, we were able to label cells with ^{3}H-DFP and exclude the possibility of tracer reutilization. With cumulative labeling and transfusion methods, reutilization was one factor casting doubt on the conclusions.

After the lesions had been inflicted, the increase in the percentage of labeled cells as a result of pulse labeling was almost the same in our two experiments (brain trauma and Wallerian degeneration). Independent of the time of investigation, the labeling index was between 1.0% and 3.4%. On the basis of these experiments, it could be assumed that a similar process had been responsible for the increase in phagocytes [compare, however, the high labeling index (18%) found by Helpap et al. (1976) after cryonecrosis of the brain]. In our transfusion experiments, the missing bits of evidence for labeled cells in orthograde and retrograde degeneration do not permit any definitive conclusions.

Quantitative data were found in the literature, particularly regarding the increase of labeled cells with pulse labeling, after cumulative labeling, as well as before various types of lesions were inflicted. A comparison is not possible because of the wide range of lesion types and/or the final evaluations and conclusions. One common factor in all the investigations was that most of the locally proliferating cells could be demonstrated between the 2nd and the 5th day after the lesion had been inflicted in retrograde degeneration (Sjöstrand, 1965; Kreutzberg, 1967, 1968; Adrian and Smothermon, 1970), in Wallerian degeneration (Friede and Johnstone, 1967; Skoff and Vaughn, 1971), and in traumatic brain damage (Konigsmark and Sidman, 1963).

Few comparable findings are available regarding perivascular cells, and those available are just as contradictory. A comparison with our findings is difficult since almost all the other investigators limited themselves to the examination of "pericytes." Mori (1972) first observed an earlier labeling of perivascular cells after the lesion and later a labeling after traumatic damage (cumulative labeling, electron microscopy). He then suggested that reactive cells migrate from the perivascular space into the neuropil. Using cryonecrosis as an experimental model for cerebral wound healing, Helpap and co-workers (1976) described an increase of labeled cells within the perivascular space (as much as 10%) even 1 h after ^{3}H-TdR application. In retrograde degeneration, Watson (1965) as well as Sjöstrand (1971) were able to observe an increase in labeled elements (pericytes and/or vascular wall cells) on the 4th and 5th day. These findings can certainly be compared to those of Cavallo and co-workers (1973): A proliferation of DNA-synthesizing pericytes was observed after tumor implantation in the skin. Skoff and Vaughn (1971), however, found no pericyte reaction at the optic nerve in their study of Wallerian degeneration, a finding that corresponds to that of the Kitamura group (Kitamura et al., 1972, 1973; Kitamura, 1973, 1975; Fujita and Kitamura, 1975, 1976). With the electron microscope, Kitamura and co-workers were unable to observe a pericyte reaction in traumatic or inflammatory retrograde and orthograde lesions following cumulative labeling. Occasionally, however, they were able to observe labeled monocytes between the perivascular basement membranes. They considered these cells to be migrated blood cells and, therefore, differentiated them from pericytes.

No investigations are available on the reaction of free subarachnoidal cells or epiplexus cells. Skoff and Vaughn (1971) mentioned leptomeningeal cells and their la-

beling index at the optic nerve in Wallerian degeneration; the index did not vary for this type of lesion. Helpap and co-workers (1976) were able to observe an increase of labeled leptomeningeal cells after cryonecrosis (as much as 25%).
Similar conclusions are possible when comparable lesions are inflicted in other areas of the body. An increase of phagocytically active cells is possible via a migration of blood cells and local proliferation; these two processes can be established independent of each other. Various labeling methods and transfusion experiments were used to obtain the findings (for survey, see Van Furth, 1970b). A direct comparison, however, is not possible with the various investigations or with the author's findings.

2. Distribution and Fate

Our results regarding the distribution and fate of intracerebral material were obtained following intracerebral injection of dyes and cells. The basic question was what happened to the injected suspensions. We observed a definite pattern of intracerebral distribution as well as an efflux of corpuscular and cellular particles into the lymphatic spaces.

a) Intracerebral Distribution

In the context of electron-optic investigations, Brightmann (1965b) observed a spreading of intracisternally applied ferritin into the preformed spaces of the leptomeninges and of the perivascular connective tissue as well as a migration through the basement membrane and a spreading from the parenchyma into the so-called intercellular spaces. The intercellular spaces were ~200 Å in diameter. This observation clarifies the findings of other authors who observed siderin in subpial astrocytes in border zone siderosis (human) following various types of subarachnoidal hemorrhages (Hughes and Oppenheimer, 1969; Koeppen and Barron, 1971). Iwanowski and Olszewski (1960), Noetzel and Ohlmeier (1963), and Blinzinger (1968) reproduced such observations in in vivo experiments following intracisternal injection of ferritin. These authors found a particularly heavy concentration of tracer in subarachnoidal phagocytes, astrocytes, and reactive microglia. Comparable findings could be obtained in in vitro experiments by incubating brain tissue cultures together with ferritin-containing medium (Kristensson and Bernstein, 1974).

Like the spontaneous appearance of border zone siderosis, all these experiments presuppose that ferritin particles are available to these cells over a period of days and weeks. Most of our investigations, however, were limited to a short incubation period (minutes and hours). The astrocytes in the injection area which are diffusely laden with ferritin can be observed via the light microscope during the short incubation periods. The process involved here is probably related to cell lesions and/or the removal of ferritin. By comparison, we felt that the iron-positive astrocytes in subpial nerve tissue after 2 months of in vivo incubation are due to the same factors that produce border zone siderosis.

It should also be noted that, in our investigations, the size of the ferritin clumps in the cytoplasm of phagocytes of the CNS were directly related to the length of the time interval between injection and examination. This finding is probably the light-microscopic equivalent of Blinzinger's electron-optic investigations (1968). Blinzinger found diffusely distributed siderin in the cells as well as in siderosomes and in intracellular structures ("giant siderosomes").

With the electron microscope, Brightman (1965 a) observed pinocytotic absorption of ferritin, particularly following intraventricular injection of ferritin in ependymal cells of rats. He also found a slight degree of absorption in the underlying neuropil. We, however, were able to observe ferritin-laden subependymally located cells in rabbits. These cells may be subependymal microglia.

The size of the particles may explain the different reaction of colloidal carbon to ferritin following intracerebral injection. As did other investigators (Field and Brierley, 1948, 1949; Woollam and Millen, 1954, 1955), we also observed this tracer within the preformed spaces as well as in cells considered to be MP of the CNS, but not in astrocytes. On the one hand, the tracer (ϕ in excess of 200 Å) was unable to penetrate the intercellular spaces and reach the astrocyte processes. On the other, phagocytosis of colloidal carbon has been considered a typical criterium for including cells in the reticuloendothelial (Biozzi et al., 1953) and/or the macrophage system (Gosselin, 1956). Apparently, other cells absorb colloidal carbon only in very small amounts.

Following intracerebral injection, the cellular elements were distributed similarly to extracellular carbon. These elements were only found in the so-called preformed spaces or in the artificial channels caused by the injection. Injected cells were found only in the damaged neuropil (particularly around the vessels) following injection of macrophages. Since these injected cells had thick processes, they could not be distinguished from progressive microglia, not even after silver impregnation of microglia.

b) Lymphatic Efflux

Although a considerable number of investigations are available on the concentration of intracerebrally injected particles, especially dyes, in the regional lymph nodes, only one publication has dealt with the problem of time sequence. Arnold and co-workers (1973) investigated the time intervals when ^{198}Au appeared in the deep cervical lymph nodes following intracisternal injection. These authors were also able to demonstrate tracer appearing after 10 min in the lymph nodes. Particles of tracer were observed 3 min after intracisternal injection of thorotrast with the electron microscope in the reticulocytes of the cervical lymph nodes. Since our investigations were carried out with the light microscope, we were able to observe measurable amounts of ferritin in the cervical lymph nodes only after 60 min. This then confirmed the extreme rapidity of lymphatic drainage observed by Arnold and co-workers (1973). The difference in the time sequences may be explained by the varying sensitivity of the investigation methods and the different animal species (guinea pig and/or rabbit) as well as by the size of the injected particle (40–50 Å and/or 120–250 Å).

Regarding cell efflux out of the CSF space, Scheid (1941), on the one hand, made a suggestion based on the experiments of Weed (1932), Wustmann (1934), and Demme (1935). He stated that cell efflux into the lymphatic space via the pacchionian granulations is as improbable as efflux via the perineurial spaces. A series of investigations on the fate of intracisternally injected erythrocytes is, however, available. Shabo and Maxwell (1968 b, see also Essick, 1920) observed phagocytosis of erythrocytes in dogs and suggested that the cells were locally destroyed. Dupont and co-workers (1961) assumed that phagocytes removed erythrocytes via the vessels (see also Klatzo et al., 1964). Adams and Prawirohardjo (1959, see also Bradford and Johnson, 1962; Usui, 1968; Alksne and Lovings, 1972; Dobrovolsky, 1974; McQueen et al., 1974) observed that some of the erythrocytes migrated directly into the vascular system. These authors assumed that the remaining erythrocytes were destroyed via phagocytotic processes. Kennady (1967), however, noted that phagocytes play little, if any, role within the first 8 h following red blood cell injection and/or spontaneous bleeding. Simmonds (1952, see also Bowsher, 1957) found additional indications for a removal of erythrocytes via the lymph tract. The findings of Dontenwill (1952) as well as Csanda (1973) can be interpreted similarly. They found siderophages in the regional lymph nodes of humans following cerebral hemorrhages.

Only one investigation is available on nucleated cells: Arnold and co-workers (1972) injected sarcoma cells intracisternally and, in the days following, were able to observe their leptomeningeal spread and growth along the nerve sheaths as far as the lymph nodes. In contrast to the author's investigations, this was a growth of cells and not an efflux of cells.

The author's investigations provided clear-cut indications for a lymphatic efflux of intracerebrally applied erythrocytes, lymphocytes, and peritoneal macrophages. These cells were, however, individual cells; only on rare occasions were groups of cells involved. Compared with the injected lymphocytes and macrophages, the number of erythrocytes appearing in the lymph nodes was relatively high. Mononuclear cells may have a greater tendency for attachment inside the connective tissue. The chance of their being washed out or removed would, therefore, be lower.

We are able to make only one observation regarding the local survival time of phagocytes. Two months after the injection we found one ^{3}H-DFP-labeled macrophage in the leptomeninges. This long survival time corresponded with Sjöstrand's observations (1971). He found labeled progressive microglial cells 3 weeks after intracisternal injection of ^{3}H-TdR. A survival period of weeks to months had also been attributed to the macrophages from other regions of the body (2 months: see Roser, 1970; Van Furth, 1970b).

Electron-microscopic investigations during the last few years have tended to indicate that the path from CSF space along the perineurial spaces to the lymph nodes is a good possibility. Communication with extracerebral tissue is possible through the open access of the perineurial space to the subarachnoid space (see above, cf. also Arnold and Ilberg, 1971). A washing out or a migration can occur through this communication. Drainage over the nerve sheaths themselves had already been described (see also Weiss et al., 1945; Field and Brierley, 1949). We were able to trace this passage along the optic nerve as far as the retro-orbital connective tissue.

It has been noted repeatedly in the literature that the washing out and removal of cells from the CSF space, even under physiologic conditions, which occurred in the reabsorption through pacchionian granulations and via drainage along the perineurial spaces was probably dependent on intracerebral pressure conditions (Gomez et al., 1973; McQueen et al., 1974; see also Bowsher, 1957; Dupont et al., 1961; Shabo and Maxwell, 1968; see to the contrary, Aklsne and Lovings, 1972, who suggested active transport processes). Authors, however, who investigated physiologic pressure conditions (among others Woollam and Millen, 1955; Arnold et al., 1972) obtained similar findings. It is, therefore, possible to compare these dye experiments with physiologic processes. The cell efflux, however, may be the result of the fact that the pressure in our experiments was not controlled. No conclusions regarding physiologic conditions can, therefore, be drawn. On the other hand, physiologic conditions are also not present with spontaneous subarachnoidal hemorrhage or meningitis. Our results, therefore, permit a conclusion to be drawn under pathologic conditions.

The possibilities of lymph drainage of the CSF space for corpuscular and cellular elements can, to a certain extent, also be compared with other regions of the body where the removal of dyes has been conclusively established. Only a few findings, however, are available on the removal of cells. At $7^1/_2$ min after the injection of chicken erythrocytes in the foot soles of guinea pigs, Litt (1967) found the erythrocytes in the regional popliteal lymph nodes. Monie and Everett (1974) conducted similar experiments; they injected labeled lymph node cells into the foot soles of their laboratory animals. Roser (1968, 1970) applied labeled peritoneal macrophages intraperitoneally and later found them in the peritoneal lymph nodes.

The final fate of corpuscular tracer and/or cellular elements, however, is still unknown. Some findings support the idea of a pulmonary removal of intraperitoneally injected cells (cf. p. 65). Recently, Bertheussen and co-workers (1978) reported evidence indicating pulmonary excretion of carbon black which was injected into the cerebral ventricles of the rat.

3. Function

The author's investigation provided evidence for the function of MP in the CNS. The results were obtained with pathocytosis experiments, by comparing the enzyme histochemistry, and by establishing a possible immunologic reaction. Even though the individual functional potencies cannot be completely separated from each other, the possibility of a differentiation between nonimmunologic and immunologic functions such as with cells of the mononuclear phagocyte system is still possible.

a) Nonimmunologic Activity

The author's findings regarding nonimmunologic activity of MP of the CNS were essentially supported by data presented in the literature. Thus far, the only functional potency of mononuclear cells of the CNS investigated here was the ability for phagocytosis. A "scavenger" function has been attributed (sometimes *expressis verbis*) to cells of the subarachnoid space [free leptomeningeal cells (Cushing, 1925; see also Essick, 1920; Kubie and Schultz, 1925)], of the ventricular space [epiplexus cells (Hosoya and Fuita, 1973; see also Kappers, 1953; Tennyson and Pappas, 1961, 1964; Carpenter et al., 1970)], of the perivascular space [perivascular cells (Kubie, 1927; Törö, 1942; Majno and Palade, 1961; Maxwell and Kruger, 1965; Cancilla et al., 1972)], and intracerebral phagocytes [progressive microglia (Penfield, 1925, 1926; Rio Hortega, 1932; von Mihalik, 1935; Dumont and Sheldon, 1965; Mori and Leblond, 1969b)]. [The difference between Fe-positive MP of the CNS and astrocytes was that MP contained considerably more ferritin in the form of coarse granules. In the astrocytes, however, small uniformly sized granules were found. The question then arises as to whether or not ferritin was actually ingested by astrocytes in the course of active phagocytosis (see Peters et al., 1976).]

R. D. Adams (1958) mentions the ability of microglial cells to form giant cells in the context of the phagocytic processes.

Only a few authors have suggested other possible functions. These suggestions were based solely on resting microglia. Glees (1958) spoke of a "consideration" when he attributed "other" tasks to microglia in addition to that of removing the products of metabolism. Even Cammermeyer's detailed survey of the functional possibilities of microglial cells (1970b) is based primarily on assertions. Cammermeyer considers the ability for ion exchange between blood vessels and neurons and/or myelin sheaths to be the most important (see also Nicholls and Wolfe, 1967; Cohn et al., 1968).

In investigations of cerebral edema, Blinzinger and Hager (1962), Klatzo and coworkers (1964, see also Klatzo and Miquel, 1960) found indications for the assimilation of material through microglia [i.e., pinocytotic process (see also Rubinstein et al., 1962; Sjöstrand, 1966)]. Blinzinger and Hager (1962) observed pinocytotic vesicles in reactive microglia; Andres (1964), in resting microglia.

The ability of ameboid mobility also appears to be unquestioned for progressive microglia cells. Such ability was first assumed on the basis of pseudopodia formation (Rio Hortega, 1932; Luse, 1968). Ibrahim and co-workers (1974) interpreted the uniformly shaped processes of staff-shaped microglia in the experimental stab wounds similarly. Mobility was directly observed in cell cultures (Marinesco and Minea, 1925, 1930; Okamoto, 1958). The distinct activity of triphosphopyridine nucleotide diaphoresis also tends to substantiate the theory of an active mobility of these cell types (Kreutzberg and Peters, 1962).

Kreutzberg's observation (1966) is also important. He suggested that the activation of perineuronal microglia in retrograde degeneration should not be interpreted as the result (i.e., first sign) of "scavenger" processes. Corresponding with the very slight phagocytic activity, only a slight activity of the oxidative (Kreutzberg, 1963; Härkönen, 1964) and the hydrolytic enzymes [e.g., acid phosphatase (Colmant, 1959; Coimbra and Tavares, 1964)] is found. According to Kreutzberg (1966), the stimulation and proliferation of microglial cells in retrograde degeneration may be triggered by a mitogenic factor initiated by irritated neurons. Since, in these experiments, microglia directly bordered on capillaries and neurons, Kreutzberg (1966) also suggested the possibility of a transport (particularly removal) of end and intermediate products of irritated nerve cells. The amount of nucleosidase activity, i.e., ATPase and ADPase, also tends to support the possibility of this type of transport process (see also Torack and Barrnett, 1963; Sjöstrand, 1966a; Kreutzberg, 1968). Enzymes are involved in this process which tend to appear particularly in connection with active membrane transport processes (Novikoff et al., 1962).

Pinocytotic processes in perivascular cells such as those in microglia (Han and Avery, 1963; Wagner et al., 1974) are postulated. The pinocytotic vesicle, which is observed with the electron microscope and sometimes appeared in connection with the cytoplasm membrane, may be involved in such transport processes between vascular wall and neuropil (Törö, 1942; Han and Avery, 1963). The cells are thought to be particularly important for maintaining the blood-brain barrier (Zimmermann, 1923; Törö, 1942; Wislocki and Leduc, 1952; Cancilla et al., 1972). The ability for ameboid mobility was observed in perivascular cells (Hama, 1961; Han and Avery, 1963; Movat and Fernando, 1964; Bergmann, 1967) in a way similar to that of microglia. Finally, a considerable ability for transformation was attributed to these cells (Begg and Garret, 1954), e.g., for reformation into smooth muscle cells or other mesenchymal cells (Rhodin, 1968; in fibroblasts: Han and Avery, 1963; in endothelial cells: Klosovskil, 1963). These cells were thought to be able to form basement membranes from capillaries and venules (Han and Avery, 1963; Rhodin, 1968).

No similar observations are available on the subarachnoidal phagocytes and epiplexus cells.

On the whole, our findings confirm the excessive ability for phagocytosis and formation of giant cells, especially for the four cell types in the CNS examined here. A comparison between these cells and elements of the monocyte-macrophage system as well as the enzyme pattern may also be possible. An identical functional potency can be demonstrated.

b) Immunologic Activity

One additional question is whether or not the cells mentioned here have some sort of function within the context of the immune response. Only a few observations in this regard are available, although it has already been established that increased numbers of MP of the CNS (particularly progressive microglia) can appear in inflammations (Rio Hortega, 1932) and tumors (Penfield, 1925, 1926; Kurobane, 1950; Imamura, 1954). Solely on the basis of morphologic similarities between microglia and cells of the reticuloendothelial system, similar modes of function have been assumed (Asua, 1927; Wells and Carmichael, 1930; Rio Hortega, 1932).

In 1934 Lebovich observed that microglial cells phagocytize bacteria (see also Costero, 1931). In the same year, Mogilnitzky and co-workers (1934) injected rats intraperitoneally with equine serum and/or caseinic acid 1–4 days prior to inflicting a mechanical lesion. They were able to obtain an accelerated microglial reaction, which they felt could only be explained immunologically. Later, proliferation inhibition of microglia with irradiation (Hopewell and Wright, 1967; Cavanagh, 1968a, b), cortisone (Foley et al., 1953; Field, 1955, 1957; Cammermeyer, 1965c; Bingham et al., 1969, 1971; Levine and Strebel, 1969), antimitotic substances (Levine and Sowinski, 1972; Pollard and Fitzpatrick, 1973), and Bordetella pertussis vaccine (Levine and Sowinski, 1972) indicated the possibility of an immunologic mode of reaction. Leibowitz (1972) finally suggested a specific macrophage-inhibiting factor (MIF) that was supposed to inhibit the migration of microglia, particularly in multiple sclerosis (cf. Meyer-Rienecker et al., 1975, 1976).

The adventitial hyperplasia and the increase of perivascular cells in brain tumors may also be interpreted similarly (Torack, 1961; see also Luse, 1960; Nystron, 1960). Transplantation experiments carried out in the skin by Cavallo and co-workers (1973) tended to indicate this type of process: The experiments showed an increase of DNA-synthesizing perivascular cells (for comparable reactions with foreign body sarcoma, see also Murad et al., 1968; Kuhn and Rosai, 1969; Johnson et al., 1973; Hahn et al., 1973). Movat and Fernando (1964) suggested that perivascular cells may possibly play a role in the counterreaction and the formation of antibodies.

Kubie and Schultz (1925) referred to the possibility of free leptomeningeal cells being involved in an immunologic reaction. They observed a proliferation of lymphocytes in the subarachnoid space in nonspecific meningeal irritation. Malloy and Low (1976) referred to the possibility of a biologic function of the free cells within the CSF cavities for maintaining asepsis. Merchant et al. (1977) were able to demonstrate cell interaction of leptomeningeal free cells in response to challenge by bacillus Calmette-Guerin.

After finding cell clumps and/or cellular fusion of epiplexus cells of cat, Carpenter and co-workers (1970) suggested that an immune reaction had taken place. The fact that lymphocytes can be repeatedly found in the ventricular space tends to support this theory (Tsusaki et al., 1952; Kappers, 1953; Schwarze, 1975).

Our findings indicate receptors for IgG and complement on the surface of all cell types referred to here as MP of the CNS within the ventricles as well as an ability for phagocytosis and giant cell formation as a result of fusion. With the methods described here, the receptor activity can be demonstrated only in cells of the monocyte-macrophage series. On the one hand, this receptor activity indicates that the cells originated in the peripheral blood. On the other, a similar behavior must be assumed for the above-mentioned cells in the context of the immune response such as that suggested for and/or established with monocytes and/or macrophages. Comparable investigations are not available.

II. Mononuclear Phagocytes of the Central Nervous System and the "Mononuclear Phagocyte System"

On the basis of the investigations described, it can be concluded that there is actually a relationship between the four types of MP of the CNS presented here and the cells of other monocyte-macrophage series. The identity of the cells will be described again briefly to show the significance of the relationship.

1. Identity

Most of those authors whose findings supported a migration of blood cells into the nervous system were unable to provide any definite data for the type of the precursor cell. Even lymphocytes were, therefore, thought to be able to transform into microglial cells (Kosunen et al., 1963; Walker, 1963; Waksman, 1965). This theory is relevant insofar as lymphocytes (or lymphocytelike elements) can be demonstrated in almost all lesions that accompany an increase of microglia (Rio Hortega, 1939; Walker, 1963; Cammermeyer, 1970b; Stensaas and Horsley, 1975). Kubie and Schultz (1925) also observed an increase of lymphocytes in the subarachnoid space following nonspecific irritation. Werdelin (1972) noted an increase of lymphocytes within the neuropil in the course of experimental allergic encephalitis. Lymphocytes were also observed in the perivascular space (Kubie, 1927) and/or next to epiplexus cells in the ventricular space (undamaged). The presence of increased numbers of microglial cells in malignant lymphomas (including also the so-called microgliomatosis) tends to support the theory of the lymphocytic derivation of phagocytes in the CNS (Lennert, 1975).

Comparative light-microscopic (Huntington and Terry, 1966; Cammermeyer, 1970b; Sjöstrand, 1971) and electron-microscopic (Blinzinger, 1965; Blackmore, 1969, 1975; Kitamura, 1975; Baldwin, 1975) investigations tend to indicate a monocytic origin. Labeled microglialike cells appearing after intravenous injection of labeled peritoneal macrophages (Sumner, 1974) tend to support the theory that this cell type is a precursor of the phagocytes in the CNS.

By intravenous injecting labeled blood monocytes and/or peritoneal macrophages, we were able to exclude the possibility of a transformation of lymphocytes into phagocytes. An identity of these labeled cells with cells of the monocyte-macrophage series was demonstrated by establishing typical monocyte enzymes in the labeled cells of the neuropil as well as of the subarachnoid, perivascular, and ventricular spaces following transfusion of labeled cells.

Ability for phagocytosis and polynuclear giant cell formation; the detailed enzyme content; the receptor activity of subarachnoidal phagocytes, perivascular cells, and epiplexus cells in undamaged brains of rabbits, in human cerebrospinal fluid cells, and following glass implantation in cells considered to be progressive microglia in rabbits–all were identical. Intracerebrally applied peritoneal macrophages also reacted morphologically and stain-wise like progressive microglia; they migrated, even if only to a slight degree, into the adjacent cervical lymph nodes via the perineurial spaces.

The cytokinetic findings as well as the various comparative investigations clearly indicated the origin and classification of the four cell types that we consider to be MP of the CNS: They must be considered to belong to the mononuclear phagocyte system. In our opinion, the four cell types are differentiated only by their localization in various compartments of the CNS, i.e., subarachnoid, perivascular, and ventricular spaces as well as the neuropil (under pathologic conditions). The different morphology and different nomenclature are determined by the location.

The role and classification of *resting microglia* remains basically unclear. In our cytokinetic investigations, little evidence was found to support a migration of cells from the blood into the (undamaged) neuropil, and this evidence was not certain. In parabiotic investigations similar to those described above, Volkman (1976) seldom found labeled (migrated) cells in nonirritated peritoneal cavities and in undamaged liver. The findings of Shands and Axelrod (1977) also yielded no evidence for a migration of monocytes into the nonirritated peritoneal cavity. These authors, therefore, postulated that, under normal conditions, the relatively slow turnover primarily results from local cell division.

Cytochemically, the resting microglia reacted only in part like monocytes and/or macrophages. In this regard, it should be mentioned that resting macrophages, particularly in tissue, exhibit another enzyme pattern than do activated cells of the same type. They contain, for example, very few lysosomes (Axline and Cohn, 1970; Robbins et al., 1971; Bar-Eli and Gallily, 1975; Kaplow, 1975). Monocytes that have migrated into the tissue contain almost no peroxisomes (Nichols and Bainton, 1975). All cited studies as well as our own research did not consider the possibility of a circadian change of enzymes such as has been observed in the last few years (von Mayersbach, 1975, 1976; Bhattacharya and von Mayersbach, 1976).

In spite of the various findings concerning resting microglia, on the one hand, and cells of the MPS, on the other, the possibility of an identity must be excluded. In our opinion these differences together with the negative findings obtained after application of extremely specific anti-monocyte seras tend not to support an identity of resting microglia and MP of the CNS and/or cells of the MPS. Our investigation did not provide information as to whether this cell type is a glial cell or a mesenchymal cell of another type.

2. Significance

The implication of the identity of the described cells with cells of the monocyte-macrophage series for the field of neuropathology is that a comparable functional behavior must be assumed in the brain as has been suggested for other regions of the body. Correspondingly, for example, *a microglia reaction must be equated with a macrophage reaction.* There are, however, two ways in which a macrophage reaction can develop:

(1) when foreign material must be removed ("scavenger" cell), and (2) when an immune reaction occurs in interaction with lymphocytes.

In both cases, the basic mode of reaction for this cell type is phagocytosis. It can be nonspecific-nonimmunologic or specific-immunologic.

On the basis of the identity of the cell types, it can also be concluded that humoral substances and medications that encourage or inhibit a macrophage reaction have the same effect and consequences in the CNS as in the rest of the body. A few experimental investigations published recently illustrate this tendency. In the subarachnoid space, Calmette-Guerin bacillus produces a threefold increase in the free cell population of the leptomeninges in 24 h and a tenfold increase in 12 days (Merchant and Low, 1977 a, b). Intracerebral implantation of silicon dioxide produces fibroblast-rich granulomas (Oehmichen and Grüninger, 1973). Infection of the CNS caused by Treponema pallidum results in a considerable increase in microglia. There, however, is evidence that virulent Treponema pallidum inhibits the migration of macrophages (Pavia et al., 1977). This may well explain the increase of microglia, possibly in the context of a delayed-type hypersensitivity.

Reduction of the microglia response in damaged brain tissue has been achieved by x-irradiation, by cortisone, by Bordetella pertussis vaccine (for literature, see above). Investigations of human CSF in which macrophage-mediating factors were found in multiple sclerosis (Meyer-Rinecker et al., 1976) and or brain tumors (Meyer-Rienecker et al., 1975) should be interpreted similarly. In various diseases, the appearance of different kinins could be interpreted as an indication of a lymphocyte-macrophage interaction (Jenssen et al., 1976).

However, relationships are present in the CNS which can be clearly differentiated from those in the rest of the body, e.g., barrier systems (Fig. 37). Barrier mechanisms are particularly important for antigens and antibodies.

The *blood-CSF and blood-brain barrier* (cf. for review of the literature see Rapoport, 1976) tend to keep the antigens from spreading. However, the spread of antibodies is inhibited. As a result, the antibody content following intravenous injection is 100–1600 times lower in the CSF than in the blood serum (Sherwin et al., 1963; cf. also Freund, 1930). Similar results were obtained by other authors who calculated a total turnover of 1 mg gamma globulin in the CSF space of the cat (Hochwald and Wallenstein, 1967 b). Even protein molecules the size of albumin [67 500 mol.wt. (compared with 150 000 to 900 000 mol.wt. of gamma globulin)] have limited passage through the blood-CSF barrier (cf. Hochwald and Wallenstein, 1976 a). Molecules with a molecular weight of 40 000 (e.g., horseradish peroxidase) are apparently able to pass more freely (Westergaard and Brightman, 1973). By osmotic opening of the blood-brain barrier with hyperosmolar solutions, it was possible to transfer larger amounts of certain antibodies into the CSF space in an experimental context (Hicks et al., 1976). In this way, an immune reaction was induced.

The biologic function of the *CSF-brain barrier* is to inhibit a spread of antigens and inflammatory reactions. For this reason, meningitis is primarily localized in the leptomeninges; encephalitis, in brain tissue; neuritis, in nerves. Apparently, the size of the protein molecule plays an important role for this barrier: The intercellular spaces within the neuropil have a diameter of ~200 Å (Brightman, 1965). Ferritin molecules (ϕ 120 Å), therefore, can pass from the CSF space into the neuropil.–It should be noted that comparable barrier mechanisms are present in the peripheral nervous system; the epineurium and the perineurium are open for intravenously injected material, while the

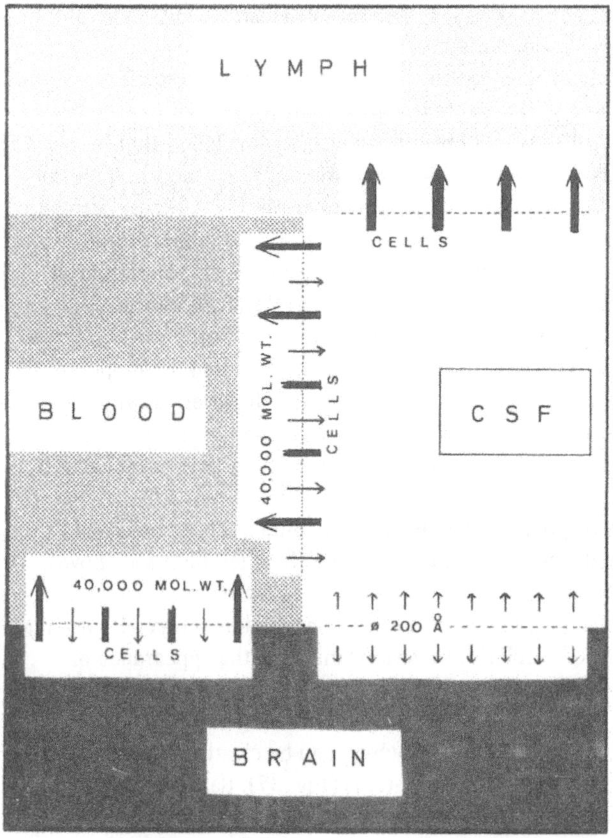

Fig. 37. Barrier system and compartments within the CNS

endoneurium forms a barrier (cf. Doinkow, 1913; Mellick and Cavanagh, 1968; Böck and Hanak, 1971; Olsson, 1971).

Compared with the above-mentioned barriers, the third barrier, the *CSF-lymph barrier,* seems to present relatively little obstruction for the passage of various sized particles. Corpuscles between 0.5 μ and 1.5 μ (Field and Brierley, 1949) as well as cells with a 20-μ diameter were found in the respective cervical lymph nodes following their intracerebral injection. The speed of this passage appears to be comparable to the speed with which the regional lymph nodes are reached in other regions of the body. It is, therefore, not amazing that antibody production following intracerebral injection of antigens occurs at about the same time as following intracutaneous injection (Jankovic et al., 1961). The efflux of gamma globulin from the CSF into the blood via similar ways have been described (Coutice and Simmonds, 1951; Bowsher, 1957). The establishment of the possibility of a migration of macrophages directly out of the CSF space into the lymph nodes tends to indicate that under certain conditions phagocytized antigen can lead to an immunologic reaction (cf. Klatzo et al., 1964). Conclusive investigations, however, are not available at present.

The *CSF-blood barrier* should also be mentioned, even though the details of this mechanism are still unclear. Apparently, erythrocytes and other components of CSF (for literature, see above) can pass through this barrier, possibly as a result of CSF pressure (Alksne and Lovings, 1972). Efflux obviously also occurs via the pacchionian villi.

In addition to the barrier mechanisms, a number of other factors may also be responsible for the fact that inflammatory reactions inside the CNS often have a different course than in the rest of the body. A few such factors are presented below.

1. Even though the qualitative composition in the CNS caused by the appearance of mononuclear phagocytes and lymphocytes is similar to that in the rest of the body, the *quantitative differences* are significant. Assuming the presence of 2000 mononuclear phagocytes and 2000 lymphocytes/ml CSF, 400000 mononuclear phagocytes and 400000 lymphocytes are then present in the CSF of an adult human (CSF: 200 ml), i.e., in the whole CNS. One ml blood, however, contains 40000 monocytes and 350000 lymphocytes.
2. The *localization* of mononuclear phagocytes as well as lymphocytes within the CNS is also conspicuous: The mononuclear phagocytes are found exclusively in CSF-containing spaces, i.e., in the ventricle as well as the perivascular and subarachnoid spaces, but not within the undamaged neuropil. This explains why all reactions of these cells arise solely from these spaces, whether via proliferation of local mononuclear phagocytes which are already present or via migration of blood monocytes.
3. *Fibrocytes* are found within the CNS only in the perivascular spaces and in the subarachnoid spaces. Chronically inflammatory reactions with fibroblast proliferation and formation of collagen fibers (occuring as a result of a macrophage reaction) are, therefore, relatively slight and always arise from the spaces mentioned.
4. Other cells also participate in the inflammatory reactions in the CNS, e.g., *astrocytes* and *oligodendrocytes.* The function of these cells in the context of inflammation is, for the most part, unknown.
5. In the presence of brain-tissue degeneration, *antibody formation against autologous brain tissue* may be induced. Antibodies against autologous brain tissue are found in cerebral infarcts and brain trauma. It must, therefore, be assumed that this process of autoaggression plays an influential role in the context of every inflammatory event.

A number of other factors should also be considered which influence the course of inflammatory reactions within the CNS, possibly also in the case of Wallerian and retrograde degeneration.

One important question pertains to the task of the so-called *resting microglia.* On the basis of this investigation, no definitive information is possible regarding the origin and classification of resting microglia. Apparently, they are not lymphocyte-derived or monocyte-derived cells. The extent to which this cell type participates in inflammatory reactions is also unknown since no definite morphologic criteria are available for the differentiation from migrated monocyte-derived cells.

In the last few years, Vaughn and co-workers (Skoff and Vaughn, 1971; for survey, see Vaughn and Skoff, 1972) as well as Fujita and Kitamura (for survey, see 1976) noted that resting microglia originated in the ectoderm. The methods applied do not appear to us convincing enough to permit this sort of definitive conclusion. For this reason, we would like to present another concept, in contrast to these concepts regarding the classification and origin of resting microglia described by the other authors mentioned as well as by Rio Hortega (for survey, see 1932) (Fig. 38). Since we were not able to offer an alternative explanation with the methods at our disposal, we would simply like to

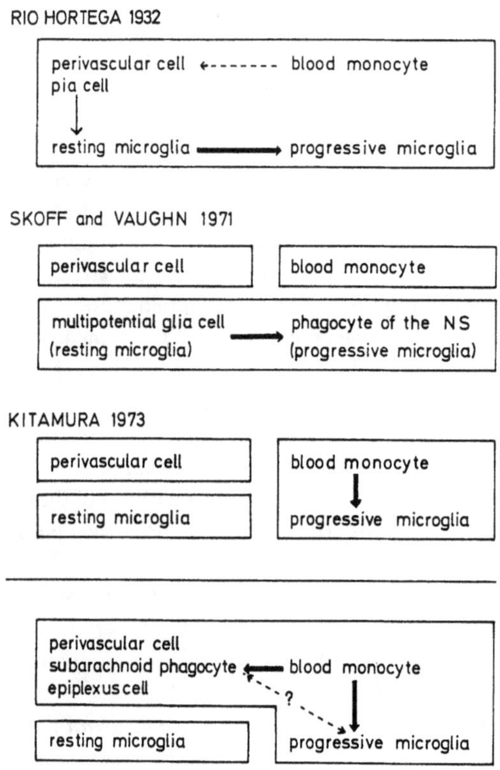

Fig. 38. Different concepts of origin and relationships of resting microglia and other cell types discussed (The concepts of Rio Hortega, Skoff and Vaughn, Kitamura, are contrary to the author's concept)

call attention to the fact that the classification of this cell type will remain unclear until convincing findings are available. One thing, however, is certain: The equation of resting microglia with the mononuclear phagocytes of the CNS mentioned here (progressive microglia, perivascular cells of intracerebral vessels, free subarachnoid cells, and epiplexus cells such as subarachnoid phagocytes) is definitely impossible on the basis of our investigation.

III. Summary of the Author's Investigations

The above investigations were conducted in order to determine if there are cells in the central (and peripheral) nervous system which belong to the "mononuclear phagocyte system," e.g., cells of the monocyte-macrophage series.

1. A survey of the literature revealed that the cells that could be included in this system were progressive microglia, free subarachnoidal cells, perivascular cells of intracerebral vessels, and epiplexus cells. At first, these cells were hypothetically considered to be mononuclear phagocytes of the central nervous system *(MP of the CNS)*. The considerable differences in considerations and findings regarding the origin and classification of these cells presented in the literature were systematically recorded.

2. The author's own investigations of proliferation and kinetics via pulse labeling with ^{3}H-thymidine (^{3}H-TdR) in undamaged rabbit brains indicated a slight, but very similar, local proliferation of the four cells types (MP in the CNS). Labeling indexes were 0.2–0.3%. Even though the indexes for the cells of the monocyte-macrophage series were very low, they were, nevertheless, ten times higher (1.5–2.5%). The blood-brain barrier for thymidine was held responsible for this difference.
3. A distinct increase of 1–2% and/or 2–3% in local proliferating cells such as MP of the CNS was established via a stab wound in the brain or, assuming identical cell populations in the peripheral nervous system, by ligation of the sciatic nerve to produce Wallerian degeneration. The increase in the labeling index corresponds with comparable experiments on the nonspecific stimulation of macrophage proliferation.
4. After labeling blood cells in a "donor" animal, labeled cells were identified in damaged brain tissue of another previously irradiated receiver animal by parabiotic experiments in rats. The brain was damaged by stab wounds, herpes meningoencephalitis, and experimental local galactocerebroside accumulation. Labeled cells were found in the typical location for cell types considered to be MP of the CNS. Labeled single nuclei in polynuclear giant cells were considered an indication of intracerebral fusion of mononuclear blood cells during giant cell formation.
5. In the transfusion experiments, radioactive labeled cells were injected intravenously into healthy and brain-damaged or nerve-damaged rabbits. The labeling was carried out in vivo on monocytes of animals with experimental monocytosis using ^{3}H-TdR, in vitro on peritoneal macrophages using ^{3}H-diisopropyl fluorophosphate (^{3}H-DFP), and in vitro on lymphocytes using ^{3}H-cytidine.
   After labeled monocyte-rich blood was injected into undamaged receiver animals, very few labeled cells were observed in the neuropil. This, however, could not be reproduced with any degree of regularity. For this reason, no definitive conclusions regarding the classification of resting microglia could be drawn on the basis of this investigation.
6. Labeled cells were found in the corresponding lesion areas of the receiver animals after damage resulting from stab wounds as well as experimental herpes virus meningoencephalitis, injection of labeled blood monocytes (^{3}H-TdR), and/or peritoneal macrophages (^{3}H-DFP). These labeled cells could sometimes be identified as monocyte derivatives via the simultaneous demonstration of nonspecific esterase. The localization corresponded to that of MP in the CNS. The transfusion of labeled blood cells into receiver animals with ligated sciatic nerve and resected facial nerve led to the appearance of labeled cells within the areas of direct traumatic damage. No labeled cells were found in the areas of Wallerian and retrograde degeneration, although the number of phagocytic cells increased.
   In experimental virus meningoencephalitis, intravenously injected labeled lymphocytes were primarily found in the leptomeninges and perivascular spaces of vessels close to the cortex. No labeled cells were found within the microglia-rich areas of brain tissue.
7. Functional investigations were carried out to control the monocyte classification of MP in the CNS. The extensive phagocytic activity of the four cell types mentioned was demonstrated by intracranial application of colloidal carbon and ferritin.

The activity of a series of enzymes was found to be identical to that of cells from the monocyte-macrophage series.

8. The receptor activity for IgG and complement was investigated by injecting sensitized sheep red blood cells into undamaged and/or traumatically damaged brain tissue of living and/or killed and perfused rabbits. In addition, human CSF cells as well as leptomeningeal membranes of rabbit and cells from rabbits which adhered to glass after intracerebral implantation of glass splinters were incubated with equal suspensions of erythrocytes. With these methods receptor activity for the Fc fragment and complement was established for MP of the CNS of rabbits as well as for phagocytes in human CSF. This receptor activity may be considered characteristic for monocytes and macrophages.
9. To classify the resting microglia, "normal" human brain tissue was incubated with anti-lymphocyte and anti-monocyte sera. The sections were stained according to the immunoperoxidase method. The resting microglia did not stain.
10. The intracerebral distribution of ferritin and colloidal carbon was described after intracranial injection. The time sequence for the efflux of tracer into the lymph paths was also observed. The tracer was found in the cervical lymph nodes no sooner than 1 h after the intracerebral injection. Light microscopy was used.
11. After intracerebral injection of radioactively labeled cells (erythrocytes: ^{51}Cr, lymphocytes: ^{3}H-cytidine, peritoneal macrophages: ^{3}H-DFP), the injected cells were distributed in the mesenchymal fissural spaces inside the brain. The macrophages within the neuropil stained like progressive microglia and had a similar feature. Isolated cells were found in the cervical lymph nodes 1–5 h after intracranial application. This finding was interpreted as indicative of lymphatic efflux and is valid for macrophages in other regions of the body.

These results, which were obtained by kinetic and comparative functional methods, were interpreted as evidence for the classification of progressive microglia, free subarachnoidal cells, perivascular cells in intracerebral vessels, and epiplexus cells in the mononuclear phagocyte system. The importance of these findings for the fields of neuropathology and neuroimmunology was discussed. The only statement that can be made in regard to the origin and importance of resting microglia is the fact that these cells are not derived from monocytes or lymphocytes.

References

Abadia-Fenoll, F.: Structure of the leptomeninx and cerebral vessels of the cat. I. The leptomeninx and its vessels. Angiology *20*, 460–482 (1969a)

Abadia-Fenoll, F.: Structure of the leptomeninx and cerebral vessels of the cat. II. Constituent elements of the intracerebral vessel wall (analogy with the meninges). Angiology *20*, 535–562 (1969b)

Abe, M., Kramer, S. P., Seligman, A. M.: The histochemical demonstration of pancreatic-like lipase and comparison with the distribution of esterase. J. Histochem. Cytochem. *12*, 364–383 (1964)

Achucarro, N.: Zur Kenntnis der pathologischen Histologie des Zentralnervensystems bei Tollwut. In: Histologische u. histopathologische Arbeiten. Nissl, F., Alzheimer, A. (eds.), Vol. III, pp. 143–199. Jena: G. Fischer 1904

Adachi, M., Volk, B. W., Amsterdam, D., Brooks, S., Tanapat, P., Broome, J. D.: Light and electron microscopic studies of "nude" mice CNS after subcutaneous administration of the E variant of the encephalomyocarditis virus. J. Neuropathol. Exp. Neurol. *35*, 318 (1976)

Adachi, M., Volk, B. W., Amsterdam, D., Brooks, S., Tanapat, P., Broome, J. D.: Light and electron microscopic studies of "nude" mice CNS after subcutaneous administration of the E variant of encephalomyocarditis (EMC) virus. Acta Neuropathol. (Berl.) *37*, 89–93 (1977)

Adams, J. E., Prawirohardjo, S.: Fate of red blood cells injected into cerebrospinal fluid pathways. Neurology (Minneap.) *9*, 561–564 (1959)

Adams, R. D.: Implications of the biology of the neuroglia and microglia cells for clinical neuropathology. In: Biology of neuroglia. Windle, W. F. (ed.), pp. 245–287. Springfield/Ill.: Ch. C. Thomas 1958

Adrian, E. K.: Cell division in injured spinal cord. Am. J. Anat. *123*, 501–520 (1968)

Adrian, E. K., Elliot, M. J.: Cell proliferation in the spinal cord following dorsal root transection. Anat. Rec. *172*, 259 (1972)

Adrian, E. K., Smothermon, R. D.: Leucocytic infiltration into the hypoglossal nucleus following injury to the hypoglossal nerve. Anat. Rec. *166*, 99–115 (1970)

Adrian, E. K., Walker, B. E.: Incorporation of thymidine-H^3 by cells in normal and injured mouse spinal cord. J. Neuropathol. Exp. Neurol. *21*, 597–609 (1962)

Adrian, E. K., Williams, M. G.: An electron microscopic study of reactive cells in the spinal cord labeled with ^{3}H-thymidine before spinal cord injury. Anat. Rec. *175*, 261–262 (1973a)

Adrian, E. K., Williams, M. G.: Cell proliferation in injured spinal cord. An electron microscopic study. J. Comp. Neurol. *151*, 1–24 (1973b)

Aguirre, C. (1971): cited by Barón u. Gallego 1972

Alksne, J. F., Lovings, E. T.: The role of the arachnoid villus in the removal of red blood cells from the subarachnoid space. An electron microscope study in the dog. J. Neurosurg. *36*, 192–200 (1972)

Allen, D. J.: Scanning electron microscopy of epiplexus macrophages (Kolmer cells) in the dog. J. Comp. Neurol. *161*, 197–213 (1975)

Allen, D. J., Didio, L. J. A.: Scanning and transmission electron microscopy of the encephalic meninges in dogs. J. Submicr. Cytol. *9*, 1-22 (1977)

Allen, D. J., Low, F. N.: Scanning electron microscopy of the subarachnoid space in the dog. III. Cranial levels. J. Comp. Neurol. *161*, 515-539 (1975)

Allen, J. C., Sheremata, W., Cosgrove, J. B., Osterland, K.: Cerebrospinal fluid T and B lymphocyte kinetics related to exacerbation of multiple sclerosis. Neurology (Minneap.) *25*, 352 (1975)

Allen, J. C., Sheremata, W., Cosgrove, J. B. R., Osterland, K., Shea, M.: Cerebrospinal fluid T and B lymphocyte kinetics related to exacerbation of multiple sclerosis. Neurology (Minneap.) *26*, 579-583 (1976)

Altman, J.: Autoradiographic study of degeneration and regenerative proliferation of neuroglia cells with tritiated thymidine. Exp. Neurol. *5*, 302-318 (1962)

Alzheimer, A.: Histologische Studien zur Differentialdiagnose der progressiven Paralyse. In: Histologische u. histopathologische Arbeiten. Nissl, F., Alzheimer, A. (Hsg.), Vol. I, S. 18-314. Jena: G. Fischer 1904

Alzheimer, A.: Einige Methoden zur Fixierung der zelligen Elemente der Cerebrospinalflüssigkeit. Cbl. Nervenheilk. Psychiatr. *30*, 449-451 (1907)

Andernach, L.: Beiträge zur Untersuchung des Liquor cerebrospinalis mit besonderer Berücksichtigung der zelligen Elemente. Arch. Psychiatr. *47*, 806-818 (1910)

Andersen, H., Matthiessen, M. E.: The histiocyte in human foetal tissues. Its morphology, cytochemistry, origin, function, and fate. Z. Zellforsch. *72*, 193-211 (1966)

Anderson, D. R.: Ultrastructure of meningeal sheaths. Arch. Ophthalmol. *82*, 659-674 (1969)

Andres, K. H.: Mikropinozytose im Zentralnervensystem. Z. Zellforsch. *64*, 63-73 (1964)

Andrew, W.: Phagocytic activity of the oligodendroglia and amphicytes in the brain, spinal cord and semilunar ganglion of the mouse during inanition. Am. J. Pathol. *17*, 421-436 (1941)

Anker, R. L.: Leucocyte as a marker of experimental neural degeneration in perinatal cats. Exp. Neurol. *49*, 601-605 (1975)

Anzil, A. P., Blinzinger, K., Mehraein, P., Dorn, G., Neuhäuser, G.: Cytoplasmic inclusions in a child affected with Krabbe's disease (globoid leucodystrophy) and in the rabbit injected with galactocerebroside. J. Neuropathol. Exp. Neurol. *31*, 370-388 (1972)

Arnold, W., Ilberg, C., von: Verbindungswege zwischen Liquor und Perilymphraum. Arch. Ohren Nasen Kehlkopfheilkd. *198*, 247-261 (1971)

Arnold, W., Ritter, R., Nitze, H. R., Wagner, W.: Morphologische und kinetische Studien zum Lymphabfluß des Liquor cerebrospinalis. Arch. Klin. Exp. Ohren Nasen Kehlkopfheilkd. *202*, 389-394 (1972)

Arnold, W., Ritter, R., Wagner, W. H.: Quantitative studies on the drainage of the cerebrospinal fluid into the lymphatic system. Acta Otolaryngol. (Stockh.) *76*, 156-161 (1973)

Arnvig, J.: Cerebrospinalvaeskens produktion og resorption. Inaug. Diss. Kopenhagen 1948

Asbury, A. K.: The histogenesis of phagocytosis during Wallerian degeneration. Radioautographic observations. In: VIth Internat. Congr. Neuropathol, pp. 666-682. Paris: Masson et Cie. Editeurs 1970

Aschoff, L.: Das retikuloendotheliale System. Ergeb. Inn. Med. Kinderheilkd. *26*, 2-118 (1924)

Aschoff, L., Kiyono, K.: Zur Frage der großen Mononukleären. Folia Haematol. (Leipz.) *15*, 383-390 (1913)

Ashton, N.: Oxygen and the growth and development of retinal vessels. Am. J. Ophathalmol. *62*, 412-435 (1966)

Aström, K. E., Webster, H. de F., Arnason, B. G.: The initial lesion in experimental allergic neuritis. J. Exp. Med. *128*, 469-496 (1968)

Asua, F. J. de: Die Mikroglia (Hortegasche Zellen) und das retikulo-endotheliale System. Z. Gesamte Neurol. Psychiatr. *109*, 354-379 (1927)

Athens, J. W., Mauer, A. M., Ashenbrucker, H., Cartwright, G. E., Wintrobe, M. M.: A method for labeling leukocytes with radioactive diisopropy fluorophosphate (DFP^{32}). Ann. N.Y. Acad. Sci. *77*, 773–776 (1959)

Austin, J. H., Lehfeldt, D.: Studies in globoid (Krabbe) leukodystrophy. III. Significance of experimentally–produced globoid–like elements in rat white matter and spleen. J. Neuropathol. Exp. Neurol. *24*, 265–289 (1965)

Axline, S. G., Cohn, Z. A.: In vitro induction of lysosomal enzymes by phagocytosis. J. Exp. Med. *131*, 1239–1260 (1970)

Ayer, J. B.: A pathological study of experimental meningitis from subarachnoid inoculation. Monogr. Rockefeller Inst. Med. Res. *12*, 26–44 (1920)

Baggenstoss, A. H., Kernohan, J. W., Drapiewski, J. F.: The healing process in wounds of the brain. Am. J. Clin. Pathol. *13*, 333–348 (1943)

Bagley, C.: Blood in the cerebrospinal fluid. Resultant functional and organic alterations in the central nervous system. A. Experimental data. Arch. Surg. *17*, 18–81 (1928)

Baker, R. N., Cancilla, P. A., Pollock, P. S., Frommes, S. P.: The movement of exogenous protein in experimental cerebral edema. J. Neuropathol. Exp. Neurol. *30*, 668–679 (1971)

Baldwin, F.: The origin of macrophages in a simple cerebral lesion. In: Mononuclear phagocytes in immunity, infection and pathology. Furth, V. R., Van (ed.), pp. 241–257. Oxford, London, Edinburgh, Melbourne: Blackwell Sci. Publ. 1975

Baldwin, F., Wendell-Smith, C. P., Blunt, J. J.: The nature of microglia. J. Anat. *104*, 401 (1969)

Bannwarth, A.: Die Zellen der Cerebrospinalflüssigkeit. Arch. Psychiatr. *100*, 533–573 (1933)

Bannwarth, A.: Zur Klinik und Pathogenese der „chronischen lymphocytären Meningitis". I. Mitteilung. Arch. Psychiatr. *117*, 161–185 (1944a)

Bannwarth, A.: Zur Klinik und Pathogenese der „chronischen lymphocytären Meningitis". II. Mitteilung. Arch. Psychiatr. *117*, 682–717 (1944b)

Bar-Eli, M., Gallily, R.: The effect of macrophage hydrolytic enzyme levels on the uptake and degradation of antigen and immune complexes. J. Reticuloendothel. Soc. *18*, 317–328 (1975)

Bargmann, W.: Histologie und mikroskopische Anatomie des Menschen, 6th ed. Stuttgart: G. Thieme 1967

Barka, T., Anderson, P. J.: Histochemical methods for acid phosphatase using hexazonium pararosanilin as coupler. J. Histochem. Cytochem. *10*, 741–753 (1962)

Barón, M., Gallego, A.: The relation of the microglia with the pericytes in the cat cerebral cortex. Z. Zellforsch. *128*, 42–57 (1972)

Barron, K. D., Tuncbay, T. O.: Phosphatase histochemistry of feline cervical spinal cord after brachial plexectomy. Hydrolysis of beta-glycerophosphate thiamine pyrophosphate and nucleoside diphosphates. J. Neuropathol. Exp. Neurol. *23*, 368–386 (1964)

Bauer, K. Fr., Vester, G.: Das elektronenmikroskopische Bild der Hirnkapillaren menschlicher Feten. Fortschr. Neurol. Psychiatr. *38*, 269–318 (1970)

Becker, N. H., Barron, K. D.: The cytochemistry of anoxic and anoxic ischemic encephalopathy in rats. I. Alterations in neuronal lysosomes identified by acid phosphatase activity. Am. J. Pathol. *38*, 161–175 (1961)

Begg, C. G., Garret, R.: Hemangiopericytoma occuring in the meninges. Cancer *7*, 602–606 (1954)

Belezky, W. K.: Über die Histiogenese der Mesoglia. Virchows Arch. [Pathol. Anat.] *284*, 295–311 (1932)

Beletzky, W., Garwaki, N.: Die Mesogliazellen und die hämatoencephalitische Schranke. Z. Gesamte Neurol. Psychiatr. *132*, 474–483 (1931)

Benested, H. B., Iversen, J. G., Rolstad, B.: Macrophage proliferation in leukocyte populations from rat blood and lymph during immune responses. Scand. J. Haematol. *8*, 44–52 (1971)

Bennet, H. S., Luft, J. H., Hampton, J. C.: Morphological classifications of vertebrate blood capillaries. Am. J. Physiol. *196*, 381–390 (1959)

Bennet, W. E., Cohn, Z. A.: The isolation and selected properties of blood monocytes. J. Exp. Med. *123*, 145-160 (1966)
Benninghoff, A.: Über die Formenreihe der glatten Muskulatur und die Bedeutung der Rouget'schen Zellen an den Kapillaren. Z. Zellforsch. *4*, 125-170 (1926)
Benninghoff, A.: Die Capillaren. In: Handbuch der mikroskopischen Anatomie des Menschen. Möllendorf, W., von (Hrsg.), Vol. II, S. 18-49. Berlin: J. Springer 1930
Bensley, R. R., Vimtrup, B.: On the nature of the Rouget cells of capilaries. Anat. Rec. *39*, 37-55 (1928)
Bentwich, Z., Kunkel, H. G.: Specific properties of human B and T lymphocytes and alteration in disease. Transplant. Rev. *16*, 29-50 (1973)
Berner, A., Torvik, A., Stenwig, E. A.: Origin of macrophages in traumatic lesions and Wallerian degeneration in peripheral nerves. Acta Neuropathol. (Berl.) *25*, 228-236 (1973)
Bertheussen, K. J., Diemer, N. H., Proestholm, J., Klinken, L.: Pulmonary excretion of carbon black injected into the cerebral ventricles of the rat. Acta pathol. microbiol. scand. *86*, 90-92 (1978)
Besta, C.: Dati sul reticulo periferico della cellula nervosa, sulla rete interstiziale diffusa e sulla loro probabile derivazione da particolari elementi cellulari. Boll. Soc. Ital. Biol Sper. *3*, 966-973 (1929)
Bhattacharya, R., Mayersbach, H., von: Histochemistry of circadian changes of some lysosomal enzymes in rat liver. Acta Histochem. (Jena) Suppl. *16*, 109-115 (1976)
Bianco, C., Patrick, R., Nussenzweig, V.: A population of lymphocytes bearing a membrane receptor for antigen-antibody-complement complexes. I. Separation and characterization. J. Exp. Med. *132*, 702-720 (1970)
Bignami, A., Ralston, H. J.: The cellular reaction to Wallerian degeneration in the central nervous system of the cat. Brain Res. *13*, 444-461 (1969)
Bingham, W. G., Paul, S. E., Sastry, K. S.: Effects of cold injury on six enzymes in rat brain. Arch. Neurol. *21*, 649-660 (1969)
Bingham, W. G., Paul, S. E., Sastry, K. S.: Effects of steroid on enzyme response to cold injury in rat brain. Neurology (Minneap.) *21*, 111-121 (1971)
Binswanger, O., Berger, H.: Beiträge zur Kenntnis der Lymphzirkulation in der Großhirnrinde. Virchows Arch. [Pathol. Anat. Physiol.] *152*, 525-544 (1898)
Bintliff, S. J., Walker, B. E.: Radioautographic studies of skeletal muscle regeneration. Am. J. Anat. *106*, 233-250 (1960)
Biondi, G.: Zur Histopathologie des menschlichen Plexus chorioideus und des Ependyms. Arch. Psychiatr. Nervenkr. *101*, 666-728 (1934)
Biozzi, G., Benacerraf, B., Halpern, B. N.: Quantitative study of the granulopectic activity of the reticulo-endothelial system. II. A study of the kinetics of the granulopectic activity of the R.E.S. in relation to the dose of carbon injected. Relationship between the wheight of the organs and their activity. Br. J. Exp. Pathol. *34*, 441-457 (1953)
Blakemore, W. F.: The ultrastructure of the subependymal plate of the rat. J. Anat. *104*, 423-433 (1969)
Blakemore, W. F.: Observations on oligodendrocyte degeneration, the resolution of status spongiosus and remyelination in cuprizone intoxication in mice. J. Neurocytol. *1*, 423-426 (1972)
Blakemore, W. F.: The ultrastructure of normal and reactive microglia. Acta Neuropathol. (Berl.) Suppl. *4*, 273-278 (1975)
Blakemore, W. F., Jolly, R. D.: The subependymal plate and associated ependyma in the dog. An ultrastructural study. J. Neurocytol. *1*, 69-84 (1972)
Bleier, R.: The relations of ependyma to neurons and capillaries in the hypothalamus. A Golgi-Cox study. J. Comp. Neurol. *142*, 439-463 (1971)
Bleier, R.: Structural relationship of ependymal cells and their processes within the hypothalamus. In: Brain-endocrine interaction. Median eminence: structure and function. Knigge, K. M., Scott, D. E., Weindl, A. (eds.), pp. 306-318. Basel: Karger 1972

Bleier, R.: Surface fine structure of supraependymal elements and ependyma of hypothalamic third ventricle of mouse. J. Comp. Neurol. *161*, 555-567 (1975)
Bleier, R., Albrecht, R., Cruce, J. A. F.: Supraependymal cells of hypothalamic third ventricle: Identification as resident phagocytes of the brain. Science *189*, 299-301 (1975)
Blinzinger, K. H.: Das submikroskopische Bild der experimentellen Coli-Meningitis und seine durch Streptomycin bewirkte Abwandlung. In: Neuropathology. Lüthy, F., Bischoff, A. (eds.), pp. 270-286. International Congress Series, No. 100. Amsterdam: Excerpta Medica 1965
Blinzinger, K. H.: Untersuchungen über die feinere Morphologie und Verteilung von Eisenablagerungen im zentralnervösen Gewebe bei einer experimentell erzeugten Randzonensiderose. Verh. Dtsch. Ges. Pathol. *52*, 269-274 (1968a)
Blinzinger, K. H.: Elektronenmikroskopische Beobachtungen bei experimentell erzeugter Randzonensiderose des Kaninchengehirns. Acta Neuropathol. (Berl.) Suppl. *4*, 146-157 (1968b)
Blinzinger, K. H., Hager, H.: Elektronenmikroskopische Untersuchungen über die Feinstruktur ruhender und progressiver Mikrogliazellen im Säugetiergehirn. Beitr. Pathol. Anat. *127*, 173-192 (1962)
Blinzinger, K. H., Hager, H.: Elektronenmikroskopische Untersuchungen zur Feinstruktur ruhender und progressiver Mikrogliazellen im ZNS des Goldhamsters. Prog. Brain Res. *6*, 99-111 (1964)
Blinzinger, K. H., Kreuzberg, G.: Displacement of synaptic terminals from regenerating motoneurons by microglial cells. Z. Zellforsch. *85*, 145-157 (1968)
Bodian, D.: An electron-microscopic study of the monkey spinal cord. Johns Hopkins Med. J. *114*, 13-119 (1964)
Bodian, D., Mellors, R. C.: The regenerative cycle of motoneurons with special reference to phosphatase activity. J. Exp. Med. *81*, 496-488 (1945)
Böck, P., Hanak, H.: Die Verteilung exogener Peroxydase im Endoneuralraum. Histochemie *25*, 361-371 (1971)
Bolsi, D.: Le transformazioni patologiche della microglia studiate con un nuovo metodo d'impregnazioni all'argento ridotto (Cellule a bastoncello e corpi granuloadiposi). Riv. Pat. Nerv. Ment. *32*, 907-947 (1928)
Borst, M.: Neue Experimente zur Frage nach der Regenerationsfähigkeit des Gehirns. Zieglers Beitr. Pathol. Anat. *36*, 1-87 (1904)
Bowen, D. M., Davison, A. N.: Macrophages and cathepsin A activity in multiple sclerosis brain. J. Neurol. Sci. *21*, 227-231 (1974)
Bowsher, D.: Pathways of absorption of protein from the cerebrospinal fluid: an autoradiographic study in the cat. Anat. Rec. *28*, 23-39 (1957)
Boya, J.: An ultrastructural study of the relationship between pericytes and cerebral macrophages. Acta Anat. (Basel) *95*, 598-608 (1976)
Bradford, F. K., Johnson, P. C.: Passage of intact iron labelled erythrocytes from subarachnoid space to systemic circulation in dogs. J. Neurosurg. *19*, 332 (1962)
Bradley, W. G., Asbury, A.: Duration of synthesis phase in neurilemma cells in mouse sciatic nerve during degeneration. Exp. Neurol. *26*, 275-282 (1970)
Bratiano, S., Llombart, A.: Système réticulo-endothélial local de l'encéphale. Rôle de la pie-mêre profonde et superficielle. Rôle de la mesoglie. C.R. Soc. Biol. (Paris) *101*, 905-907 (1929a)
Bratiano, S., Llombart, A.: La mésoglie (microglie) dans la maladie de Borna. C.R. Soc. Biol. (Paris) *101*, 792-794 (1929b)
Braunsteiner, H., Schmalzi, F.: Cytochemistry of monocytes and macrophages. In: Mononuclear phagocytes. Furth, R., Van (ed.), pp. 62-81. Oxford, Edinburgh: Blackwell Sci. Publ. 1970
Bremer, K., Fliedner, T. M.: RNA metabolism of circulating-lymphocytes studied in man after autotransfusions and in vitro ^{3}H-cytidin labeling. Acta Haematol. (Basel) *45*, 181-191 (1971)

Brichova, H.: Contribution to the question of the existence and function of microglia cells in the rat CNS. Folia Morphol. (Praha) *20*, 85-87 (1972)

Brierley, J. B.: Die Doppelherkunft der Fettkörnchenzellen in ischämischen Läsionen des Primatengehirns. Zbl. Gesamte Neurol. Psychiatr. *205*, 182 (1972)

Brightman, M. W.: The distribution within the brain of ferritin injected into cerebrospinal fluid compartments. I. Ependymal distribution. J. Cell Biol. *26*, 99-123 (1965a)

Brightman, M. W.: The distribution within the brain of ferritin injected into cerebrospinal fluid compartments. II. Parenchymal distribution. Am. J. Anat. *117*, 193-219 (1965b)

Brownson, R. H.: Perineuronal satellite cells in the motor cortex of aging brains. J. Neuropathol. Exp. Neurol. *15*, 190-195 (1956)

Bunge, M. B., Bunge, R. P., Pappas, G. D.: Electron microscopic demonstration of connections between glia and myelin sheaths in the developing mammalian central nervous system. J. Cell. Biol. *12*, 448-453 (1962)

Cajal, S. R.: Sobre un nuevo proceder de impregnacion de la neuroglia y sus resultados en los centros nerviosos del hombre y animales. Trab. Lab. Invest. Biol. Univ. Madrid *11*, 219-252 (1913a)

Cajal, S. R.: Contribución al conocimiento de la neuroglia del cerebro humano. Trab. Lab. Invest. Biol. Univ. Madrid *11*, 255-315 (1913b)

Cajal, S. R.: Algunas consideraciones sobre la mesoglia de Robertson y Rio Hortega. Trab. Lab. Invest. Biol. Univ. Madrid *18*, 109-127 (1920)

Cajal, S. R.: Contribution al la connaissance de la névroglie cérébrale et cérébelleuse dans la paralysie générale progressive. Avec quelques indications techniques sur l'imprégnation argentique du tissu nerveux pathologique. Trav. Lab. Rech. Biol. Univ. Madrid *23*, 157-216 (1925)

Caley, D. W., Maxwell, D. S.: An electron microscopic study of the neuroglia during postnatal development of the rat cerebrum. J. Comp. Neurol. *133*, 45-70 (1968)

Camazine, S. M., Ryan, G. B., Unanue, E. R., Karnovsky, M. J.: Isolation of phagocytic cells from the rat renal glomerulus. Lab. Invest. *35*, 315-326 (1976)

Cammermeyer, J.: Differences in shape and size of neuroglial nuclei in the spinal cord due to individual, regional, and technical variations. Acta Anat. (Basel) *40*, 149-177 (1960)

Cammermeyer, J.: Juxtavascular karyokinesis and microglia cell proliferation during retrograde reaction in the mouse facial nucleus. Ergeb. Anat. Entwicklungsgesch. *38*, 1-22 (1965a)

Cammermeyer, J.: Endothelial and intramural karyokinesis during retrograde reaction in the facial nucleus of rabbits of varying age. Ergeb. Anat. Entwicklungsgesch. *38*, 23-45 (1965b)

Cammermeyer, J.: Histiocytes, juxtavascular mitotic cells and microglia cells during retrograde changes in the facial nucleus of rabbits of varying age. Ergeb. Anat. Entwicklungsgesch. *38*, 195-229 (1965c)

Cammermeyer, J.: The hypependymal microglia cell. Z. Anat. Entwicklungsgesch. *124*, 543-561 (1965d)

Cammermeyer, J.: The association between microglia and myelin in silver-impregnated sections. Z. Anat. Entwicklungsgesch. *125*, 367-377 (1966)

Cammermeyer, J.: Microglia cells in diffuse and granulomatous encephalitis in the rabbit. Acta Neuropathol. (Berl.) *7*, 261-274 (1967)

Cammermeyer, J.: A light microscopic study of microglial cells: mitosis, development, and proliferation. In: VIth Internat. Congr. Neuropathol., pp. 424-436. Paris: Masson et Cie., Editeurs 1970a

Cammermeyer, J.: The life history of the microglia cell: A light microscopic study. In: Neuroscience research. Ehrenpreis, S., Solnitsky, O. Z. (eds.), Vol. III, pp. 43-129. New York Academic Press 1970b

Cancilla, P. A., Pollock, P. S., Baker, R. N., Andrews, J. M.: The fate of exogenous protein in experimental cerebral edema. In: VIth Internat. Congr. Neuropathol., pp. 1033–1034. Paris: Masson et Cie. Editeurs 1970

Cancilla, P. A., Baker, R. N., Pollok, P. S., Frommes, S. P.: The reaction of pericytes of the central nervous system to exogenous protein. Lab. Invest. *26*, 376–383 (1972)

Capobianco, F.: Della participiazione mesodermica nella genesi della neuroglia cerebrale. Arch. Ital. Biol. *37*, 152–155 (1901)

Cappell, D. F.: Intravitam and supravital staining. II. Blood and organs. J. Pathol. Bacteriol. *32*, 629–675 (1929)

Carmichael, A. E.: Microglia: An experimental study in rabbits after intracerebral injection of blood. J. Neurol. Psychopathol. *9*, 209–216 (1929)

Carmichael, F. A., Kernohan, J. W., Adson, A. W.: Histopathogenesis of cerebral abscess. Arch. Neurol. Psychiatr. (Chic.) *42*, 1001–1029 (1939)

Carpenter, S. J.: An electron microscopic study of the choroid plexus of Necturnus maculosus. J. Comp. Neurol. *127*, 413 (1966)

Carpenter, S. J., McCarthy, L. E., Borison, H. L.: Morphologic and functional effects of intracerebroventricular administration of autologous blood in cats. Neurology (Minneap.) *17*, 993–1002 (1967)

Carpenter, S. J., McCarthy, L. E., Borison, H. L.: Electron microscopic study on the epiplexus (Kolmer) cells of the rat choroid plexus. Z. Zellforsch. *110*, 471–486 (1970)

Carr, I.: The macrophage. A review of ultrastructure and function. London, New York: Academic Press 1973

Cavallo, T., Sade, R., Folkman, J., Cotran, R. S.: Ultrastructural autoradiographic studies of the early vasoproliferative response in tumor angiogenesis. Am. J. Pathol. *70*, 345–362 (1973)

Cavanagh, J. B.: Effects of X-irradiation on the proliferation of cells in peripheral nerve during Wallerian degeneration in the rat. Br. J. Radiol. *41*, 275–281 (1968a)

Cavanagh, J. B.: Prior X-irradiation and the cellular response to nerve crush: Duration of effect. Exp. Neurol. *22*, 253–258 (1968b)

Cerletti, U.: Die Gefäßvermehrung im Zentralnervensystem. In: Histologische u. histopathologische Arbeiten. Nissl, F., Alzheimer, A. (Hrsg.), Vol. IV, S. 11–168. Jena: G. Fischer 1910

Cervos-Navarro, J.: Elektronenmikroskopische Befunde an den Kapillaren der Hirnrinde. Arch. Psychiatr. Nervenkr. *204*, 484 (1963)

Cervos-Navarro, J.: Elektronenmikroskopie der Hämangioblastome des ZNS und der angioblastischen Meningiome. Acta Neuropathol. (Berl.) *19*, 184–207 (1971)

Chamberlain, J. G.: Scanning electron microscopy of epiplexus cells (macrophages) in the fetal rat brain. Am. J. Anat. *139*, 443–446 (1974)

Ciaccio: cited by Cammermeyer (1970b)

Clark, E. R., Clark, E. L.: The development of adventitial (Rouget-)cells on the blood capillaries of amphibian larvae. Am. J. Anat. *35*, 239–264, 265–282 (1925)

Cliff, W. J.: Observations on healing tissue: a combined light and electron microscopic investigation. Philos. Trans. R. Soc. Lond. (Biol. Sci.) *246*, 305–325 (1963)

Cloyd, M. W., Low, F. N.: Scanning electron microscopy of the subarachnoid space in the dog. I. Spinal cord levels. J. Comp. Neurol. *153*, 325–367 (1974)

Coates, P. W.: Scanning electron microscopic studies of third ventricle from infant monkey brains disclose supraependymal cells. J. Cell. Biol. *55*, 47a (1972)

Coates, P. W.: Supraependymal cells: light and transmission electron microscopy extends scanning electron microscopic demonstration. Brain Res. *57*, 501–507 (1973a)

Coates, P. W.: Supraependymal cells in recesses of the monkey third ventricle. Am. J. Anat. *136*, 533–539 (1973b)

Coates, P. W.: Scanning electron microscopy of a second type of supraependymal cell in the monkey third ventricle. Anat. Rec. *182*, 275–288 (1975)

Cohen, M. W., Gerschenfeld, H. M., Kuffler, S. W.: Ionic environment of neurones and glial cells in the brain of an amphibian. J. Physiol. (Lond.) *197*, 363–380 (1968)

Cohn, Z. A.: Lysosomes in mononuclear phagocytes. In: Mononuclear Phagocytes. Furth, R., Van (ed.), pp. 50–58. Oxford, Edinburgh: Blackwell Sci. Publ. 1970

Coimbra, A., Tavares, A. S.: Deoxiribonuclease II, acid ribonuclease, and acid phosphatase activities in normal and chromatolytic neurons. Histochemical and photometric study. Histochemie *3*, 509–520 (1964)

Colmant, H. J.: Aktivitätsschwankungen der sauren Phosphatase im Rückenmark und den Spinalganglien der Ratte nach Durchschneidung des Nervus ischiadicus. Arch. Psychiatr. Nervenkr. *199*, 60–71 (1959)

Colmant, H. J.: Ergebnisse der Enzymhistochemie am zentralen und peripheren Nervensystem. Fortschr. Neurol. Psychiatr. *29*, 61–124 (1961)

Colmant, H. J.: Enzymhistochemische Befunde an der elektiven Parenchymnekrose des Rattenhirns. In: IV. Internat. Congr. Neuropathol. München 1961. Jacobi, H. (ed.), Vol. I, pp. 89–95. Stuttgart: G. Thieme 1962

Colmant, G. W.: Zerebrale Hypoxie. Stuttgart: G. Thieme 1963

Colmant, H. J.: Allgemeine Histopathologie der Glia. Acta Neuropathol. (Berl.) Suppl. *4*, 61–76 (1968)

Comini, A.: Ricerche istologiche sui plessi coroidei dei pesei. Pubbl. Staz. Zool. Napoli *9*, 213–235 (1929)

Cone, W.: Acute pathologic changes in neuroglia and in microglia. Arch. Neurol. Psychiatr. (Chic.) *20*, 34–68 (1928)

Conradi, S.: Ultrastructure and its distribution of neuronal and glial elements on the motoneuron surface in the lumbosacral spinal cord of the adult cat. Acta Physiol. Scand. Suppl. *332*, 5–48 (1969)

Cook, R. D., Wisniewski, H. M.: The role of oligodendrocytes in Wallerian degeneration. J. Neuropathol. Exp. Neurol. *32*, 160 (1973)

Corria, C. M. R.: Réaction de la microglie dans la méningoencephalite tuberculeuse. Compt. Rend. Soc. Biol. *96*, 902–903 (1927)

Costero, I.: Studien an Mikrogliazellen (sogen. Hortegazellen) in Gewebskulturen von Gehirn. Arb. Staatsinst. Exp. Ther. *23*, 27–37 (1930)

Costero, I.: Experimenteller Nachweis der morphologischen und funktionellen Eigenschaften und des mesodermischen Charakters der Mikroglia. Z. Gesamte Neurol. Psychiatr. *132*, 372–406 (1931)

Coulter, H. D.: Electron microscopic identification of glial cells in the central nervous system of adult mice and rats after perfusion fixation. Anat. Rec. *148*, 273 (1964)

Courtice, F. C., Simmonds, W. J.: The removal of protein from the subarachnoid space. Aust. J. Exp. Biol. Med. Sci. *29*, 255–263 (1951)

Cravioto, H.: Wallerian degeneration: Ultrastructural and histochemical studies. Bull. Los Angeles Neurol. Soc. *34*, 233–253 (1969)

Creutzfeld, H. G., Metz, A.: Über Gestalt und Tätigkeit der Hortegazellen bei pathologischen Vorgängen. Z. Gesamte Neurol. Psychiatr. *106*, 18–53 (1926)

Cronkite, E. P., Fliedner, T. M., Bond, V. P., Rubini, J. R., Brecher, G., Quastler, H.: Dynamics of hemopoietic proliferation in man and mice studied by H^3-thymidine incorporation into DNA. Ann. N.Y. Acad. Sci. *77*, 803–820 (1959)

Csanda, E.: Schrankenmechanismen im zentralen Nervensystem. Vortrag: 18. Tagung der Vereinigung deutscher Neuropathologen u. Neuroanatomen, Hamburg 1973

Cserr, H. F., Ostrach, L. H.: Bulk flow of interstitial fluid after intracranial injection of blue dextran 2000. Exp. Neurol. *45*, 50–60 (1974)

Cushing, M.: Studies in intracranial physiology and surgery. Edinburgh: Cameron Lect. 1925

Daems, W. T., Brederoo, P.: The fine structure of mononuclear phagocytes as revealed by freeze-etching. In: Mononuclear phagocytes. Furth, R., Van (ed.), pp. 29–42. Oxford, Edinburgh: Blackwell Sci. Publ. 1970

Das, G. D.: Resting and reactive macrophages in the developing cerebellum. An experimental ultrastructural study. Virchows Arch. [Zellpathol.] *20*, 287–298 (1976a)

Das, G. D.: Gitter cells and their relationship to macrophages in the developing cerebellum. An electron microscopic study. Virchows Arch. [Zellpathol.] *20*, 299-305 (1976b)

Das, G. D., Pfaffenroth, M. J.: A further note on the presence of the endogenous macrophages in the developing cerebellum. Virchows Arch. [Zellpathol.] *22*, 299-304 (1976)

Davidoff, M.: Über die Glia im Hypoglossuskern der Ratte nach Axotomie. Z. Zellforsch. *141*, 427-442 (1973)

Davson, H.: Physiology of the cerebrospinal fluid. London: Churchill 1967

Demme, H.: Die Liquordiagnostik in Klinik und Praxis. München: J. F. Lehmann 1935

De Robertis, E., Gerschenfeld, H. M.: Submicroscopic morphology and function of glial cells. Int. Rev. Neurobiol. *3*, 1-65 (1961)

De Sousa, M. A. B., Parrott, D. M. V., Pantelouris, E. M.: The lymphoid tissues in mice with congenital aplasia of the thymus. Clin. Exp. Immunol. *4*, 637-644 (1969)

Devaux, A.: Étude histologique de foyers de nécrose de l'écorce cérébrale. In: Histologische u. histopathologische Arbeiten. Nissl, F. (Hrsg.), Vol. II, S. 115-144. Jena: G. Fischer 1908

Dewulf, A.: La microglie normal chez le singe (Macacus rhesus). J. Belge Neurol. Psychiatr. *37*, 341-365 (1937)

Dickler, H. B., Kunkel, H. G.: Interaction of aggregated globulin with lymphocytes. J. Exp. Med. *136*, 191-196 (1972)

Dimova, R. N.: Donnees ultrastructurales sur la proliferation des astrocytes et de la microglie. Arch. Biol. (Liege) *87*, 303-314 (1976)

Dimova, R. N., Markov, D. V.: cited by Markov and Dimova, 1974

Dobrovolsky, G. F.: Significance of the ulstrastructure of the arachnoid membrane of the human brain in removing erythrocytes of the subarachnoidally effused blood (electron microscopic investigation). Vopr. Neirokhir. *38*, 32-37 (1974)

Dodson, R. F., Tagashira, Y., Chu, L. W.-F.: Acute pericytic response to cerebral ischemia. J. Neurol. Sci. *29*, 9-16 (1976)

Doinkow, B.: Histologische und histopathologische Untersuchungen am peripheren Nervensystem mittels vitaler Färbung. Folia Neuro-Biol. *7*, 731 (1913)

Donahue, S., Pappas, G. D.: The fine structure of capillaries in the cerebral cortex of the rat at various stages of development. Am. J. Anat. *108*, 331-347 (1962)

Dontenwill, W.: Beitrag zur Genese des Hydrocephalus bzw. der beginnenden Hydranencephalie und zur Frage der Liquorabflußwege. Frankf. Z. Pathol. *63*, 493-503 (1952)

Dougherty, T. F.: Studies on the cytogenesis of microglia and their relation to cells of the reticulo-endothelial system. Am. J. Anat. *74*, 61-89 (1944)

Dublin, W. B.: Histogenesis of compound granular corpuscles in response to cerebral trauma. Am. J. Clin. Pathol. *15*, 228-229 (1945)

Duckett, S., Pearse, A. G. E.: A pericapillary cell in the central nervous system of the human embryo and adult. Acta Neuropathol. (Berl.) *4*, 442-445 (1965)

Dumont, A., Sehldon, H.: Changes in the fine structure of macrophages in experimentally produced tubercoulous granulomas in hamsters. Lab. Invest. *14*, 2034-2055 (1965)

Dunning, H. S., Furth, J.: Studies on the relation between microglia, histiocytes, and monocytes. Am. J. Pathol. *11*, 895-911 (1935)

Dunning, H. S., Stevenson, L.: Microglia-like cells and their reaction following injury to the liver, spleen, and kidney. Am. J. Pathol. *10*, 343-348 (1934)

Dupont, J.-R., Wart, Ch. Van, Kraintz, L.: The clearance of major components of whole blood from cerebrospinal fluid following simulated subarachnoid hemorrhage. J. Neuropathol. Exp. Neurol. *20*, 450-455 (1961)

Eager, R. P., Eager, P. R.: Glial responses to degenerating cerebellar cortico-nuclear pathways in the cat. Science *153*, 553-555 (1966)

Ebaugh, F. G., Emerson, C. P., Ross, J. F.: The use of radioactive chromium 51 as an erythrocyte tagging agent for the determination of red cell surviva in vivo. J. Clin. Invest. *32*, 1260-1276 (1953)

Eberth (1871): cited by Han and Avery, 1963
Eichhorst, H.: Über die Entwicklung des menschlichen Rückenmarks und seiner Formelemente. Virchows Arch. [Pathol. Anat. Physiol.] *64*, 425–475 (1875)
Eliot, C.: The origin of phagocytic cells in the rabbit. Bull. J. Hopkins Hosp. *39*, 149–157 (1926)
Escola, J., Thomas, E.: Elektronenmikroskopische Untersuchungen über die Lokalisation der sauren Phosphatase im Reaktionsbereich experimentell erzeugter Hirngewebsnekrosen. Acta Neuropathol. (Berl.) *4*, 380–391 (1965)
Essick, C. R.: Formation of macrophages by the cells lining the subarachnoid cavity in response to the stimulus of particulate matter. Contr. Embryol. Carneg. Inst. No. 42, *9*, 377–388 (1920)
Eyre, J., Rosen, P. J., Perry, S.: Relative labeling of leukocytes, erythrocytes and platelets in human blood by ^{51}Cromium. Blood *36*, 250–253 (1970)
Farquhar, M. G., Hartmann, J. F.: Electron microscopy of cerebral capillaries. J. Neuropathol. Exp. Neurol. *16*, 18–39 (1956)
Farrar, C. B.: On the phenomena of repair in the cerebral cortex. In: Histologische u. histopathologische Arbeiten. Nissl, F. (Hrsg.), Vol. II, S. 1–70. Jena: G. Fischer 1908
Feigin, I.: Mesenchymal tissues of the nervous system. The indigenous origin of brain macrophages in hypoxic states and in multiple sclerosis. J. Neuropathol. Exp. Neurol. *28*, 6–24 (1969)
Feinendegen, L. E.: Tritium-labeled molecules in biology and medicine. New York, London: Academic Press 1967
Fernando, D. A.: A third glial cell seen in retrograde degeneration of the hypoglossal nerve. Brain Res. *27*, 365–368 (1971)
Fernando, D. A.: An electron microscopic study of the neuroglial reaction in the hypoglossal nucleus after transsection of the hypoglossal nerve. Acta Anat. (Basel) *86*, 1–14 (1973a)
Fernando, D. A.: An electron microscopic study of the neuroglial reaction in Wallerian degeneration of the corticospinal tract. Acta Anat. (Basel) *86*, 459–473 (1973b)
Ferner, H., Kautzky, R.: Angewandte Anatomie des Gehirns und seiner Hüllen. In: Handbuch der Neurochirurgie. Olivercrona, H., Tönnis, W. (Hrsg.), Vol. I/1, S. 2–90. Berlin, Göttingen, Heidelberg: Springer 1959
Ferraro, A., Davidoff, L. M.: The reaction of the oligodendroglia to injury of the brain. Arch. Pathol. *6*, 1030–1053 (1928)
Field, E. J.: Observations on the development of microglia together with a note on the influence of cortisone. J. Anat. *89*, 201–208 (1955)
Field, E. J.: Histogenesis of compound granular corpuscles in the mouse brain after trauma and a note on the influence of cortisone. J. Neuropathol. Exp. Neurol. *16*, 48–56 (1957)
Field, E. J., Brierley, J. B.: The lymphatic connections of the subarachnoid space. An experimental study of the dispersion of particulate matter in the cerebrospinal fluid, with special reference to the pathogenesis of poliomyelitis. Br. Med. J. *1948/I*, 1167–1171
Field, E. J., Brierley, J. B.: The retroorbital tissue as a site of outflow of cerebrospinal fluid. Proc. R. Soc. Med. *42*, 447–450 (1949)
Fink, M. (ed.): The macrophage, its role in tumour immunology. New York, San Francisco, London: Academic Press 1976
Fink, M. A. (ed.): Macrophages in neoplasia. New York: Academic Press 1976
Fischer, O.: Die anatomische Grundlage der cerebrospinalen Pleocytose. Monatsschr. Psychiatr. Neurol. *27*, 512–530 (1910)
Flanagan, S. P.: "Nude," a new hairless gene with pleiotropic effects in the mouse. Genet. Res. (Camb.) *8*, 295–309 (1966)
Fleischhauer, K.: Über die Fluoreszenz perivasculärer Zellen im Gehirn der Katze. Z. Zellforsch. *64*, 140–152 (1964)

Flexner, L. B.: The development of the meninges in amphibia: A study of normal and experimental animals. Contr. Embryol. *20*, 31-49 (1929)
Földi, M.: Physiologie und Pathophysiologie des Lymphgefäßsystems. In: Handbuch der allgemeinen Pathologie. Meessen, H. (Hrsg.) Bd. III/6, S. 239-310. Berlin, Heidelberg, New York: Springer 1972
Foley, J. M., Chambers, R. A., Adams, R. D.: The effect of cortisone on the early repair of brain wounds in guinea pigs. J. Neuropathol. Exp. Neurol. *12*, 101-104 (1953)
Foot, N. C.: The endothelial phagocyte. A critical review. Anat. Rec. *30*, 15-51 (1925)
Forberg, S., Odeblad, E., Söremark, R., Ulleberg, S.: Autoradiography with isotopes emitting internal conversion electrons and Auger electrons. Acta Radiol. [Ther.] (Stockh.) *2*, 241-262 (1964)
Forbes, I. J.: Mitosis in mouse peritoneal macrophages. J. Immunol. *96*, 734-743 (1966)
Forster, E.: Experimentelle Beträge zur Lehre der Phagocytose der Hirnrindenelemente. In: Histologische u. histopathologische Arbeiten. Nissl, F. (Hrsg.), Bd. 2, S. 173-192. Jena: G. Fischer 1908
Freund, J.: Accumulation of antibodies in the central nervous system. J. Exp. Med. *51*, 889-902 (1930)
Fraher, J. P., McDougall, R. D.: Macrophages related to leptomeninges and ventral nerve roots. An ultrastructural study. J. Anat. *120*, 537-549 (1975)
Frederickson, R. G., Haller, F. R.: The subarachnoid space interpretated as a special portion of the connective tissue space. Proc. N.Y. Acad. Sci. *24*, 142-159 (1971)
Frederickson, R. G., Low, F. N.: Blood vessels and tissue space associated with the brain of the rat. Am. J. Anat. *125*, 123-146 (1969)
Friede, R. L.: An enzyme histochemical study of cerebral arteriosclerosis. Acta Neuropathol. (Berl.) *2*, 58-72 (1962)
Friede, R. L., Johnstone, M. A.: Responses of thymidine labeling of nuclei in gray matter and nerve following sciatic transection. Acta Neuropathol. (Berl.) *7*, 218-231 (1967)
Friedman, H. M., Gilden, D. H., Roosa, R. A., Nathanson, N.: The effect of neonatal thymectomy on Tamiami virus induced central nervous system disease. J. Neuropathol. Exp. Neurol. *34*, 159-166 (1975)
Friedmann, M.: Studien zur pathologischen Anatomie der acuten Encephalitis. Arch. Psychiatr. *21*, 836-862 (1890)
Frøland, S. S.: Binding of sheep erythrocytes to human lymphocytes. A probable marker of T lymphocytes. Scand. J. Immunol. *1*, 269-280 (1972)
Frøland, S. S., Natvig, J. B., Michaelsen, T. E.: Binding of aggregated IgG by human B lymphocytes independent of Fc receptors. Scand. J. Immunol. *3*, 375-380 (1974)
Fujita, S.: An autographic study on the origin and fate of the sub-pial glioblast in the embryonic chick spinal cord. J. Comp. Neurol. *124*, 51-60 (1965)
Fujita, S., Kitamura, T.: Origin of brain macrophages and the nature of the so-called microglia. Acta Neuropathol. (Berl.) Suppl. *4*, 291-296 (1975)
Fujita, S., Kitamura, T.: Origin of brain macrophages and the nature of the microglia. In: Progr. neuropathol. Zimmerman, H. M. (ed.), Vol. III, pp. 1-50. New York, San Francisco, London: Grune & Stratton 1976
Furth, R.,Van: The origin and turnover of promonocytes, monocytes, and macrophages in normal mice. In: Mononuclear phagocytes. Furth, R. Van (ed.), pp. 151-165. Oxford, Edinburgh: Blackwell Sci. Publ. 1970a
Furth, R., Van: Origin and kinetics of monocytes and macrophages. Semin. Hematol. *7*, 125-141 (1970b)
Furth, R., Van (ed.): Mononuclear phagocytes. Oxford, Edinburgh: Blackwell Sci. Publ. 1970c
Furth, R., Van (ed.): Mononuclear phagocytes in immunity, infection, and pathology. Oxford, London, Edinburgh, Melbourne: Blackwell Sci. Publ. 1975
Furth, R., Van: Origin and kinetics of mononuclear phagocytes. Ann. N.Y. Acad. Sci. USA *278*, 161-175 (1976)
Furth, R., Van, Cohn, Z. A.: The origin and kinetics of mononuclear phagocytes. J. Exp. Med. *128*, 415-435 (1968)

Furth, R., Van, Cohn, Z. A., Hirsch, J. G., Spector, W. G., Langevoort, H. L.: The mononuclear phagocyte system: a new classification of macrophages, monocytes, and their precursor cells. Bull. W.H.O. *46*, 845–852 (1972)

Furth, R., Van, Langevoort, H. L., Schaberg, A.: Mononuclear phagocytes in human pathology. Proposal for an approach to improved classification. In: Mononuclear phagocytes in immunity, infection, and pathology. Furth, R. Van (ed.), pp. 1–15. Oxford, London, Edinburgh, Melbourne: Blackwell Sci. Pub. 1975

Gall, J. G., Johnson, W. W.: Is there "metabolic" DNA in the mouse seminal vesicle? J. Biophys. Biochem. Cytol. *7*, 657–665 (1960)

Gelderen, C., Van: Über die Entwicklung der Hirnhäute bei Teleostiern. Anat. Anz. *60*, 48–57 (1926)

Genser, B. M., Howard, J. G.: The isolation of lymphocytes and macrophages. In: Handbook of experimental immunology. Weir, D. M. (ed.), pp. 1009–1033. Oxford: Blackwell Sci. Publ. 1967

Gerecke, D., Gross, R.: Autoradiographic evidence for reutilization of DNA catabolites by granulopoiesis in the rat. Scand. J. Haematol. *17*, 132–142 (1976)

Gilbertsen, R. B., Metzgar, R. S.: Human T and B lymphocyte rosette tests: Effect of enzymatic modification of sheep erythrocytes (E) and the specificity of neuraminidase treated E. Cell. Immunol. *24*, 97–108 (1976)

Gillette, R. W., Lance, E. M.: Kinetic studies of macrophages. I. Distributional characteristics of radiolabeled peritoneal cells. J. Reticuloendothel. Soc. *10*, 223–237 (1971)

Glees, P.: Neuroglia, morphology and function. Springfield: Ch. C. Thomas 1955

Glees, P.: The biology of the neuroglia: A summary. In: Biology of neuroglia. Windle, W. F. (ed.), pp. 134–142. Springfield/Ill.: Ch. C. Thomas 1958

Gluge, G.: Experimente über Encephalitis. Abh. Physiol. Pathol. (Jena) *2*, 13–47 (1841)

Go, K. G., Stokroos, I., Blaauw, E. H., Zuiderveen, F., Molenaar, I.: Changes of ventricular ependyma and choroid plexus in experimental hydrocephalus, as observed by scanning electron microscopy. Acta Neuropathol. (Berl.) *34*, 55–64 (1976)

Goasguen, J., Sabouraud, O.: Rosettes mouton sur lymphocytes de liquide cephalorachidien. Nouv. Presse Med. *3*, 2266 (1974)

Goebel, A., Puchtler, H.: Untersuchungen zur Methodik der Darstellung der Succinodehydrogenase im histologischen Schnitt. Virchows Arch. [Pathol. Anat.] *326*, 312–331 (1955)

Goldmann, E.: Vitalfärbungen im Zentralnervensystem. Beitrag zur Physio-Pathologie des Plexus chorioideus und der Hirnhäute. Abh. Klg. Preuß. Akad. Wiss.-Physik.-Mathemat. Cl. *1*, 1–60 (1913)

Goldstein, M. N.: Formation of giant cells from human monocytes cultivated on cellophane. Anat. Rec. *118*, 577–591 (1959)

Gomez, D. G., Potts, D. G., Deonarine, V., Reilly, K. F.: Effects of pressure gradient changes on the morphology of arachnoid villi and granulations of the monkey. Lab. Invest *28*, 648–657 (1973)

Gomori, G., Chessick, R. D.: Esterases and phosphatases of the brain. A histochemical study. J. Neuropathol. Exp. Neurol. *12*, 387–396 (1953)

Gonatas, N. K., Levine, S., Shoulson, R.: Phagocytosis and regeneration of myelin in an experimental leukoencephalopathy. Am. J. Pathol. *44*, 565–583 (1964)

Gosselin, R. S.: The uptake of radiocolloids by macrophages in vitro. J. Gen. Physiol. *39*, 625–635 (1956)

Gozzano, M.: L'istogenesi della microglia. Riv. Neurol. *4*, 225–265 (1931)

Graumann, W.: Zur Standardisierung des Schiffschen Reagens. Z. Wiss. Mikrosk. *61*, 225–226 (1953)

Gray, E. G.: Ultrastructure of synapses of the cerebral cortex and of certain specializations of the neuroglial membranes. In: Electron Microscopy in Anatomy. Boyd, J. D., Johnson, F. R., Lever, J. D. (eds.), pp. 54–73. London: Edward Arnold 1961

Gray, E. G.: Tissues of the central nervous system. In: Electron microscopy in anatomy. Kurtz, S. M. (ed.), pp. 369–417. New York: Academic Press 1964

Greaves, M. F., Falk, J. A., Falk, R. E.: A surface antigen marker for human monocytes. Scand. J. Immunol. *4*, 555–562 (1975)

Grüninger, H., Oehmichen, M.: Modifikation der Parabiosetechnik. Exp. Pathol. *6*, 343–345 (1972)

Guseo, A.: Über die Makrophagen des Liquor cerebrospinalis. Z. Neurol. *200*, 136–147 (1971)

Guseo, A.: Morphological signs as indications of function of cells in the cerebrospinal fluid. J. Neurol. *212*, 159–170 (1976)

Guth, L.: Regeneration in the mammalian peripheral nervous system. Physiol. Rev. *36*, 441–478 (1956)

Hackenberg, P.: Kritische Erwägungen zur Frage der „maskierten Makrophagen" im Liquorzellsediment. Dtsch. Z. Nervenheilkd. *192*, 124–138 (1967)

Hager, H.: Elektronenmikroskopische Befunde zur Feinstruktur der Hirngefäße und der perivaskulären Räume im Säugetiergehirn. Ein Betrag zur Kenntnis des morphologischen Substrates der sogenannten Bluthirnschranke. Acta Neuropathol. (Berl.) *1*, 9–33 (1961)

Hager, H.: Die feinere Cytologie und Cytopathologie des Nervensystems. Stuttgart: G. Fischer 1964

Hager, H.: Pathologie der Makro- und Mikroglia im elektronenmikroskopischen Bild. Acta Neuropathol. (Berl.) Suppl. *4*, 86–97 (1968)

Hager, H.: EM findings on the source of reactive microglia on the mammalian brain. Acta Neuropathol. (Berl.) Suppl. *6*, 279–283 (1975)

Hahn, M. J., Dawson, R., Esterly, J. A., Joseph, D. J.: Hemangiopericytoma. An ultrastructural study. Cancer *31*, 255–261 (1973)

Hain, R. F.: Discussion of the lecture of Königsmark a. Sidman (1963a). J. Neuropath. Exp. Neurol. *22*, 327–328 (1963)

Haller, F. R., Low, F. N.: The fine structure of the peripheral nerve root sheat in the rat and other laboratory animals. Am. J. Anat. *131*, 1–20 (1971)

Haller, F. R., Haller, A. C., Low, F. N.: The fine structure of cellular layers and connective tissue space at spinal nerve root attachments in the rat. Am. J. Anat. *133*, 109–124 (1972)

Hama, K.: On the existence of filamentous structures in endothelial cells of the amphibian capillary. Anat. Rec. *139*, 437–441 (1961)

Hamuro, Y.: Histochemical studies on glycogen and certain other enzymes in the recovery of the brains injury. II. Histochemical studies on certain enzymes (phosphatases, succinic dehydrogenase, cytochrome oxidase, 5-nucleotidase, and phosphorylase) in recovery of brain injuries. Arch. Histol. Jap. *13*, 69–87 (1957)

Han, S. S., Avery, J. K.: The ultrastructure of capillaries and arterioles of the hamster dental pulp. Anat. Rec. *145*, 549–571 (1963)

Han, T., Minowada, J.: Enhanced E- and EAC-rosette formation by neuraminidase. J. Immunol. Methods *12*, 253–260 (1976)

Härkönen, M.: Carboxylic esterases, oxidative enzymes and catecholamines in the superior cervical ganglion of the rat and the effect of pre- and post-ganglionic nerve division. Acta Physiol. Scand. *63*, Suppl. 237 (1964)

Harvey, S., Burr, H.: Development of the meninges. Arch. Neurol. Psychiatr. (Chic.) *15*, 545–567 (1926)

Harvey, S., Burr, H., Campenhout, E., Van: Development of the meninges. Further experiments. Arch. Neurol. Psychiatr. (Chic.) *29*, 683–690 (1933)

Hasenjäger, T., Stroescin, G.: Über den Zusammenhang zwischen Meningitis und über die Morphogenese der Ependymitis granularis. Arch. Psychiatr. Nervenkr. *109*, 46–81 (1939)

Hasselt, U. E., Van: Zur Zytokinetik der Blutmonozyten beim Menschen. Inaug.-Diss. Ulm/Donau 1970

Hatai, S.: On the origin of neuroglia tissue from mesoblast. J. Comp. Neurol. *12*, 291-296 (1902)

Hauw, J. J., Berger, B., Escourolle, R.: Electron microscopic study of the developing capillaries of human brain. Acta Neuropathol. (Berl.) *31*, 229-242 (1975)

Hazama, F., Kreutzberg, G. W.: Histochemical study of anterograde fiber degeneration and transneuronal changes in the optic system of the rabbit. Acta Histochem. Cytochem. Jap. *10*, 337-349 (1977)

Heil, S.: Zur Genese und Reifung der sog. konzentrischen Körperchen der menschlichen Arachnoidea. Anat. Anz. *130*, 326-374 (1972)

Held, H.: Über die Neuroglia marginalis der menschlichen Großhirnrinde. Monatsschr. Psychiatr. *26*, 360-416 (1909)

Helpap, B., Cremer, H., Grouls, V.: Reutilisation von markierten DNS-Bausteinen bei der Wundheilung. Naturwissenschaften *58*, 574-575 (1971)

Helpap, B., Breining, H., Cappel, S., Sturm, K. W., Lymberopoulos, S.: Wound healing of the brain of rats after cryonecrosis. Autoradiographic investigations with ^{3}H-thymidine. Virchows Arch. [Zellpathol.] *22*, 151-161 (1976)

Herndon, R. M.: The fine structure of the rat cerebellum. II. The stellate neurons, granule cells and glia. J. Cell. Biol. *23*, 277-293 (1964)

Herndon, R. M.: Thiophen induced granular cell necrosis in the rat cerebellum: An electron microscopic study. Exp. Brain Res. *6*, 49-68 (1968)

Herndon, R. M.: The electron microscopic study of cerebrospinal fluid sediment. J. Neuropathol. Exp. Neurol. *28*, 128 (1969)

Herndon, R. M., Johnson, M.: A method for the electron microscopic study of cerebrospinal fluid sediment. J. Neuropathol. Exp. Neurol. *29*, 320-330 (1970)

Herrlinger, H., Blinzinger, K., Luh, S., Anzil, A. P.: Der cytochemische Nachweis von endogener peroxydatischer Aktivität als Markierungsmethode für Untersuchungen über die Herkunft reaktiver mononukleärer Zellelemente im zentralnervösen Gewebe. Report given on the 22nd Meeting of the German Society for Neuropathology and Neuroanatomy, Tübingen 1977

Hicks, J. T., Albrecht, P., Rapoport, S. I.: Entry of neutralizing antibody to measles into brain and cerebrospinal fluid of immunized monkeys after osmotic opening of the blood-brain barrier. Exp. Neurol. *53*, 768-779 (1976)

Hijmans, W., Schuit, H. R. E., Klein, F.: An immuno fluorescence procedure for the detection of intracellular immunoglobulins. Clin. Exp. Immunol. *4*, 457-472 (1969)

Hills, C. P.: Ultrastructural changes in the capillary bed of the rat cerebra cortex in anoxic-ischemic brain lesions. Am. J. Pathol. *44*, 531-551 (1964)

Himango, W. A., Low, F. N.: The fine structure of a lateral recess of the subarachnoid space in the rat. Anat. Rec. *171*, 1-20 (1971)

Hirano, A., Zimmerman, H. M., Levine, S.: Reaction of ependyma to cryptococcal polysaccharide implantation. J. Neuropathol. Exp. Neurol. *25*, 152 (1966)

Hirano, A., Cervos-Navarro, J., Ohsugi, T.: Capillaries in the subarachnoid space. Acta Neuropathol. (Berl.) *34*, 81-85 (1976)

Hirsch, J. G., Fedorko, M. E.: Morphology of mouse mononuclear phagocytes. In: Mononuclear phagocytes. Furth, R. Van (ed.), pp. 7-28. Oxford, Edinburgh: Blackwell Sci. Publ. 1970

His, W.: Über ein perivasculäres Canalsystem in den nervösen Centralorganen und über dessen Beziehungen zum Lymphsystem. Z. Wiss. Zool. *15*, 127-141 (1865)

His, W.: Die Neuroblasten und deren Entstehung im embryonalen Mark. Arch. Anat. Physiol. 249-300 (1889)

Hochwald, G. M., Wallenstein, M.: Exchange of albumin between blood, cerebrospinal fluid, and brain in the cat. Am. J. Physiol. *212*, 1199-1204 (1967a)

Hochwald, G. M., Wallenstein, M. C.: Exchange of γ-globulin between blood, cerebrospinal fluid and brain in the cat. Exp. Neurol. *19*, 115-126 (1967b)

Holländer, H., Brodal, P., Walberg, F.: Electron microscopic observations on the struc-

ture of the pontine nuclei and the mode of termination of the corticopontine fibres. An experimental study in the cat. Exp. Brain Res. *7*, 95–110 (1969)
Holtzman, E., Novikoff, A. B.: Lysosomes in the rat sciatic nerve following crush. J. Cell Biol. *27*, 651–669 (1965)
Hommes, O. R., Leblond, C. P.: Mitotic division of neuroglia in the normal rat. J. Comp. Neurol. *129*, 296–278 (1967)
Hopewell, J. W., Wright, E. A.: Effects of previous X-irradiation on the response of brain to injury. Nature (Lond.) *215*, 1405–1406 (1967)
Hopewell, J. W., Wright, E. A.: The nature of latent cerebral irradiation damage and its modification by hypertension. Br. J. Radiol. *43*, 161–167 (1970a)
Hopewell, J. W., Wright, E. A.: Modification of subsequent freezing damage by previous local brain irradiation. Exp. Neurol. *26*, 160–172 (1970b)
Hörstadius, S.: The neural crest: Its properties and derivatives in the light of experimental research. London: Oxford University Press 1950
Horvat, B., Pena, C., Fisher, E. R.: Primary reticulum cell sarcoma (microglioma) of brain. An electron microscopy study. Arch. Pathol. *87*, 609–619 (1969)
Hosoya, Y., Fujita, T.: Scanning electron microscope observation of intraventricular macrophages (Kolmer cells) in the rat brain. Arch. Histol. Jap. *35*, 133–140 (1973)
Howarth, F., Cooper, E. R. A.: The fate of certain foreign colloids and crystalloids after subarachnoid injection. Acta Anat. (Basel) *25*, 112–140 (1955)
Howe, H. A., Flexner, J. B.: Succinic dehydrogenase in regeratin neurons. J. Biol. Chem. *167*, 663–671 (1947)
Howe, H. A., Mellors, R. C.: Cytochrome oxidase in normal and regeneration neurons. J. Exp. Med. *81*, 489–500 (1945)
Huber, C., Dworzak, E., Fink, U., Michlmayr, G., Braunsteiner, H., Huber, H.: Receptor sites for aggregated gammaglobulin (AGG) on lymphocytes in lymphoproliferative disease. Br. J. Haematol. *27*, 643–654 (1974)
Huber, H., Fudenberg, H. H.: Receptor sites of human monocytes for IgG. Int. Arch. Allergy Appl. Immunol. *34*, 18–31 (1968)
Huber, H., Holm, G.: Surface receptors of mononuclear phagocytes: effect of immune complexes on in vitro function in humam monocytes. In: Mononuclear phagocytes in immunity, infection, and pathology. Furth, R., Van (ed.), pp. 291–301. Oxford, London, Edinburgh, Melbourne: Blackwell Sci. Publ. 1975
Huber, H., Polley, M. J., Linscott, W. D., Fudenberg, H. H., Müller-Eberhard, H. J.: Human monocytes: distinct receptor sites for the third component of complement and for immunoglobulin G. Science *162*, 1281–1283 (1968)
Huber, H., Michlmayr, G., Müller-Eberhard, J. G., Fudenberg, H. H.: Rezeptoren an menschlichen Monozyten für IgG und Komplement. Schweiz. Med. Wochenschr. *100*, 344–347 (1970)
Huber, H., Douglas, S., Nusbacher, J., Kochwa, S., Rosenfield, R. E.: IgG subclass specificity of human monocyte receptor sites. Nature (Lond.) *229*, 419–420 (1971)
Huebschmann, P.: Die Leukozyten bei der Leptomeningitis tuberculosa und die Cohnheimsche Lehre. Münch. Med. Wochenschr. *98*, 1497–1498 (1956)
Hughes, J. T., Oppenheimer, D. R.: Superficial siderosis of the central nervous system. Acta Neuropathol. (Berl.) *13*, 56–74 (1969)
Hughes, W. L., Bond, V. P., Brecher, G., Cronkite, E. P., Painter, R. B., Quastler, H., Sherman, F. G.: Cellular proliferation in the mouse as revealed by autoradiography with triated thymidine. Proc. Natl. Acad. Sci. USA *44*, 476–483 (1958)
Humphrey, J H., White, R. G.: Immunology for students of medicine, 3rd. ed. Oxford, Edinburgh: Blackwell Sci. Publ. 1970
Huntington, H. W., Terry, R. D.: The origin of the reactive cells in cerebral stab wounds. J. Neuropathol. Exp. Neurol. *25*, 643–653 (1966)
Ibrahim, M. Z. M.: The mast cells of the mammalian central nervous system. Part 1. Morphology, distribution, and histochemistry. J. Neurol. Sci. *21*, 431–478 (1974a)

Ibrahim, M. Z. M.: The mast cells of the mammalian central nervous system. Part 2. The effect of proton irradiation in the monkey. J. Neurol. Sci. *21*, 479–499 (1974b)
Ibrahim, M. Z. M., Call, N., Noden, P.: Modifications of the Hortega silver carbonate method adapted for celloidinembedded and frozen sections. Acta Neuropathol. (Berl.) *10*, 258–260 (1968)
Ibrahim, M. Z. M., Khreis, Y., Koshayan, D. S.: The histochemical identification of microglia. J. Neurol. Sci. *22*, 211–233 (1974)
Iida, T.: Elektronenmikroskopische Untersuchungen an oberflächlichen Anteilen des Gehirns bei Hund und Katze. Arch. Histol. Jap. *27*, 267–285 (1966)
Imamura, S.: Microglia in gliomas. Folia Psychiatr. Neurol. Jap. *8*, 99–126 (1954)
Ishikawa, K.: On the genesis of Hortega cells. Folia Anat. Jap. *10*, 229–248 (1932)
Iwanowski, L., Olszewski, J.: Experimental hemochromatosis of the central nervous system. J. Neuropathol. Exp. Neurol. *19*, 175 (1960)
Izumi, S., Penrose, J. M., More, D. G., Nelson, D. S.: Further observations on the immunological induction of DNA synthesis in mouse peritoneal macrophages. Role of products of activated lymphocytes. Int. Arch. Allergy Appl. Immunol. *49*, 573–584 (1975)
Jakob, A.: Normale und pathologische Anatomie und Histologie des Großhirns. In: Handbuch der Psychiatrie. Aschaffenburg, G. (Hrsg.), Abt. 1, Teil 1. Leipzig, Wien: F. Deuticke 1927 und 1929
Jankovic, B. D., Draskoci, M., Isakovic, K.: Antibody response in rabbits following injection of sheep erythrocytes into lateral ventricle of brain. Nature (Lond.) *191*, 288–289 (1961)
Janzen, W.: The relationship between the perivascular and the subarachnoidal space. Psychiatr. Neurol. Neurochir. *64*, 37–45 (1961)
Jellinger, K.: Spezielle Pathologie des zentralen und peripheren Nervensystems sowie der neuromuskulären Peripherie. In: Spezielle Pathologie. Holzner, J. H. (Hrsg.), Bd. 4. München, Berlin, Wien: Urban & Schwarzenberg 1976
Jenssen, H. L., Meyer-Rienecker, H. J., Werner, H.: Nachweis eines Faktors mit elektrophoretischer Zellmobilitätshemmung im Liquor cerebrospinalis bei Multipler Sklerose. J. Neurol. *214*, 45–59 (1976)
Johnson, K. H., Ghobrial, H. K. G., Buoen, L. C., Brand, I., Brand, K.: Nonfibroblastic origin of foreign body sarcomas implicated by histological and electron microscopic studies. Cancer Res. *33*, 3139–3154 (1973)
Jones, E. G.: On the mode of entry of blood vessels into the cerebral cortex. J. Anat. *106*, 507–520 (1970)
Joos, F., Roos, B., Bürki, H., Bürki, K., Laissue, J.: Umsatz, Proliferation und Phagozytosefähigkeit der freien Zellen im Peritonealraum der Maus nach Injektion von Polystyren-Partikeln. Z. Zellforsch. *95*, 68–85 (1969)
Juba, A.: Untersuchungen über die Entwicklung der Hortegaschen Mikroglia des Menschen. Arch. Psychiatr. *101*, 577–592 (1934a)
Juba, A.: Das erste Erscheinen und die Urformen der Hortegaschen Mikroglia im Zentralnervensystem. Arch. Psychiatr. *102*, 225–232 (1934b)
Kaplan, G.: Differences in the mode of phagocytosis with Fc and C3 receptors in macrophages. Scand. J. Immunol. *6*, 797–807 (1977)
Kaplow, L. S.: Cytochemical heterogeneity of human circulating monocytes. Acta Cytol. (Baltimore) *19*, 358–365 (1975)
Kappers, J. Ariens: Beitrag zur experimentellen Untersuchung von Funktion und Herkunft der Kolmerschen Zellen des Plexus choroideus beim Axolotl und Meerschweinchen. Z. Anat. Entwicklungsgesch. *117*, 1–19 (1953)
Kappers, J. Ariens: Structural and functional changes in the telencephalic choroid plexus during human ontogenesis. In: Ciba Foundation Symposium on the Cerebrospinal Fluid Production, Circulation, and Absorption. Wolstenholme, G. E. W., O'Connor, C. M. (eds.), pp. 3–25. London: J. a. A. Churchill 1958
Karnowsky, M. J.: Ultrastructural basis of capillary permeability studied with peroxidas

as a tracer. J. Cell Biol. *35*, 213-236 (1967)
Kaufmann, E.: Lehrbuch der speziellen pathologischen Anatomie. Berlin: Georg Reimer 1904
Kennady, J. C.: Investigation of the early fate and removal of subarachnoid blood. Pacific Med. Surg. *75*, 163-168 (1967)
Kerns, J. M., Hinsman, E. J.: Neuroglial response to sciatic neurectomy. I. Light microscopy and autoradiography. J. Comp. Neurol. *151*, 237-254 (1973a)
Kerns, J. M., Hinsman, E. J.: Neuroglial response to sciatic neurectomy. II. Electron microscopy. J. Comp. Neurol. *151*, 255-280 (1973b)
Kershman, J.: Genesis of microglia in the human brain. Arch. Neurol. Psychiatr. (Chic.) *41*, 24-50 (1939)
Key, A., Retzius, G.: Studien in der Anatomie des Nervensystems und des Bindegewebes. Stockholm: Samson u. Wallin 1875
King, J. S.: A light and electron microscopic study of perineuronal glial cells and processes in the rabbit neocortex. Anat. Rec. *161*, 111-124 (1968)
King, J. S., Schwyn, R. C.: The fine structure of neuroglial cells and pericytes in the primate red nucleus and substantia nigra. Z. Zellforsch. *106*, 309-321 (1970)
Kirkpatrick, J. B.: Chromatolysis in the hypoglossal nucleus of the rat: An electron microscopic analysis. J. Comp. Neurol. *132*, 189-212 (1968)
Kitamura, T.: The origin of brain macrophages. Some considerations on the microglia theory of Del Rio Hortega. Acta Pathol. Jap. *23*, 11-26 (1973)
Kitamura, T.: Hematogenous cells in experimental Japanese encephalitis. Acta Neuropathol. (Berl.) *32*, 341-346 (1975)
Kitamura, T., Fujita, S.: The role of hematogenous cells in alteration of mouse brains following stab wounding, inoculation of Japanese encephalitis virus and retrograde degeneration of facial nerve. In: Proceedings of the VIIth International Congress of Neuropathology in Budapest, 1974. Környey, S., Tariska, S., Gosztonyi, G. (eds.), Vol. I, pp. 37-40. Amsterdam, Budapest: Excerpta Medica-Akademia Kiado 1975
Kitamura, T., Hattori, H., Fujita, S.: Autoradiographic studies on histogenesis of brain macrophages in the mouse. J. Neuropathol. Exp. Neurol. *31*, 502-518 (1972)
Kitamura, T., Hattori, H., Fujita, S.: EM-autoradiographic studies on the inflammatory cells in the experimental Japanese encephalitis (Japan.). J. Electron. Microsc. (Tokyo) *21*, 315-322 (1973)
Kitamura, T., Tsuchihashi, Y., Tatebe, A., Fujita, S.: Electron microscopic features of the resting microglia in the rabbit hippocampus, identified by silver carbonate staining. Acta Neuropathol. (Berl.) *38*, 195-202 (1977)
Kiyono, K.: Die vitale Karminspeicherung. Ein Beitrag zur Lehre von der vitalen Färbung mit besonderer Berücksichtigung der Zelldifferenzierungen im entzündeten Gewebe. Jena: G. Fischer 1914
Klatzo, I., Miquel, J.: Observations on pinocytosis in nervous tissue. J. Neuropathol. Exp. Neurol. *19*, 475-487 (1960)
Klatzo, I., Miquel, J., Tobias, C., Haymaker, W.: Effect of alpha particle radiation on the rat brain including vascular permeability and glycogen studies. J. Neuropathol. Exp. Neurol. *20*, 459-483 (1961)
Klatzo, I., Miquel, J., Otenasek, R.: The application of fluorescein labelled serum proteins (FLSP) to the study of vascular permeability in the brain. Acta Neuropathol. (Berl.) *2*, 144-160 (1962)
Klatzo, I., Miquel, J., Ferris, P. J., Prokop, J. D., Smith, D. E.: Observations on the passage of the fluorescein labeled serum proteins (FLSP) from the cerebrospinal fluid. J. Neuropathol. Exp. Neurol. *23*, 18-35 (1964)
Klatzo, I., Wisniewski, H., Smith, D. E.: Observations on penetration of serum proteins into the central nervous system. In: Biology of neuroglia. Robertis, E. D. P., de, Carrera, R. (eds.), pp. 73-88. Prog. Brain Res., Vol. XV. Amsterdam, New York: Elsevier 1965

Klein, H.: Der Nachweis einer oxydativen Stoffwechselsteigerung in der „primär gereizten" Spinalganglienzelle am Verhalten der Bernsteinsäuredehydrogenase. Arch. Psychiatr. Nervenkr. *201*, 81–96 (1960)
Klika, E.: The ultrastructure of meninges in vertebrates. Acta Univ. Carol. [Med.] (Praha) *13*, 53–71 (1967)
Klima, R., Beyreder, J.: Über monozytäre Reaktionen in Ergüssen seröser Körperhöhlen und in entzündlich veränderten Körperflüssigkeiten und Geweben. Folia Haematol. (Leipz.) *69*, 250–263 (1950)
Klosovskii, B. N.: Fundamental facts concerning the stages and principles of development of the brain and its response to noxious agents. In: The development of the brain and its disturbance by harmful factors. Klosovskii, B. N. (ed.), pp. 12–15. Oxford, London: Pergamon Press 1963
Koburg, E., Maurer, W.: Autoradiographische Untersuchungen mit (H-3) Thymidin über die Dauer der Desoxyribonukleinsäure-Synthese und ihren zeitlichen Verlauf bei den Darmepithelien und anderen Zelltypen der Maus. Biochem. Biophys. Acta *61*, 229–242 (1962)
Koelliker, A.: Entwicklungsgeschichte des Menschen und der höheren Tiere, 2nd ed. Leipzig: Engelmann 1879
Koenig, H., Bunge, M. B., Bunge, R. P.: Nucleic acid and protein metabolism in white matter. Arch. Neurol. *6*, 177–193 (1962)
Koeppen, A. H. W., Barron, K. D.: Superficial siderosis of the central nervous system; a histological, hostochemical, and chemical study. J. Neuropathol. Exp. Neurol. *30*, 448–469 (1971)
Kolbe, C. F.: Zur Kenntnis der embolischen Gehirnerweichung. Inaug.-Diss. Marburg 1889
Kolmer, W.: Über eine eigenartige Beziehung von Wanderzellen zu den Chorioidalplexus des Gehirns der Wirbeltiere. Anat. Anz. *54*, 15–19 (1921)
Komiya, E., Katsunuma, H., Shibamoto, G., Kawakubo, R., Noda, M., Sugimoto, T., Sato, S., Hoshi, K., Kawashimo, N.: Extraktion der neurohumoralen blutregulierenden Wirkstoffe. 2. Mitteilung: Extraktion von Monopoetin, Thrombopoetin und Erythropoetin. Folia Haematol. N.F. *5*, 328–348 (1961)
Konigsmark, B. W.: Discussion of the paper of Feigin, 1969
Konigsmark, B. W., Sidman, R. L.: Origin of gitter cells in the mouse brain. J. Neuropathol. Exp. Neurol. *22*, 327–328 (1963a)
Konigsmark, B. W., Sidman, R. L.: Origin of brain macrophages in the mouse. J. Neuropathol. Exp. Neurol. *22*, 643–676 (1963b)
Konigsmark, B. W., Sidman, R. L.: Responses of astrocytes to brain injury. J. Neuropathol. Exp. Neurol. *24*, 142 (1964)
Kopriwa, B., Leblond, C. P.: Improvements in the coating technique of radioautography. J. Histochem. Cytochem. *10*, 269–284 (1962)
Kosunen, T. U., Waksman, B. H., Samuelsson, I. H.: Radioautographic study of cellular mechanisms in delayed hypersensitivity. II. Experimental allergic encephalitis in the rat. J. Neuropathol. Exp. Neurol. *22*, 367–380 (1963)
Kozma, M., Zoltan, O. T., Csillik, B.: Die anatomischen Grundlagen des prälymphatischen Systems im Gehirn. Acta Anat. (Basel) *81*, 409–420 (1972)
Kreutzberg, G. W.: Changes of coenzyme (TPN) diaphorase and TPN-linked dehydrogenase during axonal reaction of nerve cell. Nature (Lond.) *199*, 393–394 (1963)
Kreutzberg, G. W.: Autoradiographische Untersuchung über die Beteiligung von Gliazellen an der axonalen Reaktion im Facialiskern der Ratte. Acta Neuropathol. (Berl.) *7*, 149–161 (1966)
Kreutzberg, G. W.: DNA metabolism in glial cells during retrograd changes. Proc. Internat. Sympos. Metabol. Nucleic Acids Proteins and Funct. Neurons. Praha 1967
Kreutzberg, G. W.: Autoradiographie am Nervensystem bei gleichzeitiger histochemischer Enzymreaktion. Acta Histochem. (Jena) Suppl. *8*, 299–303 (1968a)
Kreutzberg, G. W.: Über perineuronale Mikrogliazellen (autoradiographische Untersuchung). Acta Neuropathol. (Berl.) Suppl. *4*, 141–145 (1968b)

Kreutzberg, G. W., Peters, G.: Enzymhistochemische Beobachtungen beim experimentellen Hirntrauma der Ratte. In: Livre Jubilaire Dr. Ludo van Bogaert, pp. 454-464. Bruxelles: Les Editions "Acta medica belgica" 1962

Kristensson, K., Bornstein, M. B.: Effects of iron-containing substance on nervous system in vitro. Acta Neuropathol. (Berl.) *28*, 281-292 (1974)

Krogh, A., Vimtrup, B.: The capillaries. In: Special cytology. cowdr, E. V. (ed.), 2nd ed., pp. 477-503. New York: Hoeber 1932

Kruger, L., Hamori, J.: An electron microscopic study of dendritic degeneration in the cerebral cortex resulting from laminar lesions. Exp. Brain Res. *10*, 1-16 (1970)

Kruger, L., Maxwell, D. S.: Electron microscopy of oligodendrocytes in normal rat cerebrum. Am. J. Anat. *118*, 411-436 (1966)

Kruger, L., Maxwell, D. S.: Wallerian degeneration in the optic nerve of a reptile: An electron microscopic study. Am. J. Anat. *125*, 247-270 (1969)

Kubie, L. S.: A study of the perivascular tissues of the central nervous system with the supravital technique. J. Exp. Med. *46*, 615-626 (1927)

Kubie, L. S., Schultz, G. M.: Vital and supravital studies of the cells of the cerebrospinal fluid and of the meninges in the cat. Bull. Johns Hopkins Hosp. *37/2*, 91-129 (1925)

Kuhn, C., Rosal, J.: Tumors arising from pericytes. Ultrastructure and organ culture of a case. Arch. Pathol. *88*, 653-663 (1969)

Kurobane, T.: Microglia in gliomas; a contribution to the study of microglia. Folia Psychiatr. Neurol. Jap. *4*, 123-131 (1950)

Lafarga, M., Palacios, G.: Ultrastructural study of pericytes in the rat supraoptic nucleus. J. Anat. *120*, 433-438 (1975)

Lampert, P. W.: Mechanism of demyelination in experimental allergic neuritis. Electron microscopic studies. Lab. Invest. *20*, 127-138 (1969)

Lampert, P. W., Carpenter, S.: Electron microscopic studies on the vascular permeability and the mechanism of demyelination in experimental allergic encephalomyelitis. J. Neuropathol. Exp. Neurol. *24*, 11-24 (1965)

Landers, J. W., Chason, J. L., Gonzalez, J. E., Polutke, W.: Morphology and enzymatic activity of rat cerebral capillaries. Lab. Invest. *11*, 1253-1259 (1962)

Langevoort, H. L., Cohn, Z. A., Hirsch, J. G., Humphrey, J. H., Spector, W. G., Furth, R. Van: The nomenclature of mononuclear phagocytic cells. Proposal for a new classification. In: Mononuclear Phagocytes. Furth, R. Van (ed.), pp. 1-6. Oxford, Edinburgh: Blackwell Scientific Publications 1970

Langhammer, H., Büll, U., Pfeiffer, K. J., Hör, G., Pabst, H. W.: Experimental studies on lymphatic drainage of the peritoneal cavity using ^{198}Au-colloid. Lymphology *6*, 149-157 (1973)

Laskin, A. I., Lechevalier, H. (eds.): Macrophages and cellular immunity. Cleveland/Ohio: CRC Press 1972

Lay, W. H., Nussenzweig, V.: Receptors for complement on leukocytes. J. Exp. Med. *128*, 991-1007 (1968)

Leake, E. S., Gonzales-Ojeda, D., Myrvik, Q. N.: Enzymatic differences between normal alveolar macrophages and oil-induced peritoneal macrophages obtained from rabbits. Exp. Cell. Res. *33*, 553-560 (1964)

LeBeaux, Y. J., Willemot, J.: Actin- and myosin-like filaments in rat brain pericytes. Anat. Rec. *190*, 811-826 (1978)

Lebowich, R. J.: Phagocytic behavior of interstitial cells of brain parenchyma of adult rabbit toward colloidal solutions and bacteria. Arch. Pathol. *18*, 50-71 (1934)

Leder, L. D.: Über die selektive fermentcytochemische Darstellung von neutrophilen myeloischen Zellen und Gewebsmastzellen im Paraffinschnitt. Klin. Wochenschr. *42*, 553 (1964)

Leder, L. D.: Der Blutmonocyt. Berlin, Heidelberg, New York: Springer 1967

Lee, J. C., Olszewski, J.: Penetration of radioactive bovine albumin from cerebrospinal fluid into brain tissue. Neurology (Minneap.) *10*, 814-822 (1960)

Leibowitz, S.: Immunology of multiple sclerosis. In: Research on multiple sclerosis.

Adams, C. W., Leibowitz, S. (eds.), pp. 149–168. Springfield: Ch. C. Thomas 1972
Lennert, K.: Morphology and classification of malignant lymphomas and so-called reticuloses. Acta Neuropathol. (Berl.) Suppl. *4*, 1–16 (1975)
Leonhardt, H.: Über ependymale Tanycyten des III. Ventrikels beim Kaninchen in elektronenmikroskopischen Betrachtungen. Z. Zellforsch. *74*, 1–11 (1966)
Levine, S., Sowinski, R.: Inhibition of macrophage response to brain injury. Am. J. Pathol. *67*, 349–360 (1972)
Levine, S., Strebel, R.: Allergic encephalomyelitis: Inhibition of cellular passive transfer by exogenous and endogenous steroids. Experientia *25*, 189–190 (1969)
Levine, S., Hirano, A., Zimmermann, H. M.: Hyperacute encephalomyelitis. Am. J. Pathol. *47*, 209–221 (1965)
Levinson, A. I., Lisak, R. P., Zweiman, B.: Immunologic characterization of cerebrospinal fluid lymphocytes: Preliminary report. Neurology (Minneap.) *26*, 693–695 (1976)
Lewandowski, M.: Zur Lehre von der Cerebrospinalflüssigkeit. Z. Klin. Med. *40*, 480–494 (1910)
Lewis, P. D.: The fate of the subependymal cell in the adult rat brain, with a note on the origin of microglia. Brain *91*, 721–736 (1968)
Lilien, D. L., Spivak, J. L., Goldman, I. D.: Chromate transport in human leukocytes. J. Clin. Invest. *49*, 1551–1551–1557 (1970)
Ling, E. A.: Some aspects of amoeboid microglia in the corpus callosum and neighbouring regions of neonatal rats. J. Anat. *121*, 29–45 (1976)
Ling, E. A.: Brain macrophages in rats following intravenous labelling of mononuclear leucocytes with colloidal carbon. J. Anat. *125*, 101–106 (1978)
Ling, E. A., Paterson, J. A., Privat, A., Mori, S., Leblond, C. P.: Investigation of glial cells in semithin sections. I. Identification of glial cells in the brain of young rats. J. Comp. Neurol. *149*, 43–72 (1973)
Litt, M.: Studies of the latent period. I. Primary antibody in guinea pig lymph nodes 7 1/2 minutes after introduction of chicken erythrocytes. Cold Spring Harbor Symp. Quant. Biol. *32*, 477–492 (1967)
Liu, H. M.: Schwann cell properties: I. Origin of Schwann cell during peripheral nerve regeneration. J. Neuropathol. Exp. Neurol. *32*, 458–473 (1973)
Liu, H. M.: Schwann cell properties. II. The identity of phagocytes in the degenerating nerve. Am. J. Pathol. *75*, 395–406 (1974)
LoBuglio, A. F., Cotran, R. S., Jandl, J. H.: Red cells coated with immunoglobulin G: binding and sphering by mononuclear cells in man. Science *158*, 1582–1585 (1967)
Löffler, H.: Cytochemischer Nachweis von unspezifischer Esterase in Ausstrichen. Klin. Wochenschr. *39*, 1220–1227 (1961)
Löffler, H., Berghoff, W.: Eine Methode zum Nachweis von saurer Phosphatase in Ausstrichen. Klin. Wochenschr. *40*, 363–364 (1962)
Logan, W. J.: Amino acid transport by two glial cell lines and by proliferating glia. Exp. Neurol. *53*, 431–443 (1976)
Lopes, C. A. S., Mair, W. G. P.: Ultrastructure of the outer cortex and pia mater in man. Acta Neuropathol. (Berl.) *28*, 79–86 (1974a)
Lopes, C. A. S., Mair, W. G. P.: Ultrastructure of the arachnoid membrane in man. Acta Neuropathol. (Berl.) *28*, 167–173 (1974b)
Luk, S. C., Simon, G. T.: Phagocytosis of colloidal carbon and heterologous red blood cells in the bone marrow of rats and rabbits. Am. J. Pathol. *77*, 423–430 (1974)
Luse, S. A.: Electron microscopic observations of the central nervous system. J. Biophys. Biochem. Cytol. *2*, 531–542 (1956)
Luse, S. A.: Electron microscopic studies of brain tumor. Neurology (Minneap.) *10*, 881–905 (1960)
Luse, S. A.: Microglia. In: Pathology of the nervous system. Minckler, J. (ed.), Vol. I, pp. 531–538. New York, Toronto, Sydney, London: McGraw-Hill Book Co. 1968
Macklin, C. C., Macklin, M. T.: A study of brain repair in the rat by the use of trypan

blue, with special reference to the vital staining of the macrophages. Arch. Neurol. Psychiatr. (Chic.) *3*, 353–393 (1920)
Magari, S., Akashi, Y., Asano, S.: Über die feinstrukturellen Veränderungen im Ependym des III. Ventrikels des Kaninchens bei experimenteller Blokade des zervikalen Lymphsystems. Acta Anat. (Basel) *85*, 232–247 (1973)
Majno, G.: Ultrastructure of the vascular membrane. In: Handbook of physiology, Sect. 2: Circulation. Hamilton, W. F., Dow, P. (eds.), Vol. III, p. 2293. Washington/DC: American Physiological Society 1965
Majno, G., Palade, G. E.: Studies on inflammation. I. The effect of histamine and serotonin on vascular permeability: an electron microscic study. J. Biophys. Biochem. Cytol. *11*, 571–605 (1961)
Malloy, J. J., Low, F. N.: Scanning electron microscopy of the subarachnoid space in the dog. IV. Subarachnoid macrophages. J. Comp. Neurol. *167*, 257–283 (1976)
Malmfors, T.: Electron microscopic description of the glial cells in the nervous opticus in mice. J. Ultrastruct. Res. *8*, 193 (1963)
Mandelstamm, M., Krylow, L.: Vergleichende Untersuchungen über die Farbspeicherung im Zentralnervensystem bei Injektion von Farbe ins Blut und in den Liquor cerebrospinalis. II. Mitteilung. Z. Gesamte Exp. Med. *60*, 63–85 (1928)
Mantovani, B., Rabinovitch, M., Nussenzweig, V.: Phagocytosis of immune complexes by macrophages. Different roles of the macrophage receptor sites for complement (C3) and for immunoglobulin (IgG). J. Exp. Med. *135*, 780–792 (1972)
Manuelidis, L., Manuelidis, E. E.: An autoradiographic study of the proliferation and differentiation of glial cells in vitro. Acta Neuropathol. (Berl.) *18*, 193–213 (1971)
Marchand, F.: Über die bei Entzündung in der Peritonealhöhle auftretenden Zellformen. Verh. Dtsch. Ges. Pathol. *1*, 63–81 (1898)
Marchand, F.: Untersuchungen über die Herkunft der Körnchenzellen des Zentralnervensystems. Beitr. Pathol. Anat. *45*, 161–196 (1909)
Marchand, F.: Die örtlichen reaktiven Vorgänge (Lehre von der Entzündung). In: Handbuch der allgemeinen Pathologie. Krehl, L., Marchand, F. (Hrsg.), Band 4. Leipzig: Hirzel 1924a
Marchand, F.: Ältere und neuere Beobachtungen zur Histologie des Omentum. Haematologica (Messina) *5*, 304–348 (1924b)
Mares, V., Schultze, B., Maurer, W.: Stability of the DNA in Purkinje cell nuclei of the mouse. An autoradiographic study. J. Cell Biol. *63*, 665–674 (1974)
Mariano, M., Spector, W. G.: The formation and properties of macrophage polykaryons (inflammatory giant cells). J. Pathol. *113*, 1–19 (1974)
Mariano, M., Nikitin, T., Malucelli, B. E.: Immunological and nonimmunological phagocytosis by inflammatory macrophages, epitheloid cells and macrophage polykaryons from foreign body granulomata. J. Pathol. *120*, 151–159 (1976)
Marinesco, G., Minea, I.: Die Kultur des Gliagewebes der Großhirnrinde in vitro. Angaben zur Bildung und Funktion der amöboiden Zellen. (Rumän.) Spitalul *45*, 9–11 (1925)
Marinesco, G., Minea, I.: Contribution à l'etude de la culture in vitro de la névroglie et de la microglie. Rev. Neurol. (Paris) *1*, 994–999 (1930)
Markov, D.: Ultrastructure of microglia. In: The spinal cord. Galabov, G. (ed.), Vol. II, pp. 79–95. Sofia: Publishing House of Bulgarian Acad. Sci. 1971
Markov, D. V., Dimova, R. N.: Ultrastructural alterations of rat brain microglial cells and pericytes after chronic lead poisoning. Acta Neuropathol. (Berl.) *28*, 25–35 (1974)
Marshall, A. H. E.: Histiocytic medullary reticulosis. J. Pathol. Bacteriol. *71*, 61–71 (1956)
Mathé, G., Florentin, I., Simmler, M. C. (eds.): Lymphocytes, macrophages and cancer. Berlin, Heidelberg, New York: Springer 1976
Matsumoto, H.: Ultrastructural studies of the meninx. Acta Pathol. Jap. *25*, 663–679 (1975)

Matsuyama, H., Komatsu, N., Senda, R.: Origin of macrophage in the telencephalic wall of the rat fetus. An observation based on methylazoxymethanol and radiation induced lesions. Acta Pathol. Jap. *25*, 691–706 (1975)

Matthews, M. A.: Microglia and reactive "M" cells of degenerating central nervous system: Does similar morphology and function imply a common origin? Cell Tissue Res. *148*, 477–491 (1974)

Matthews, M. A., Kruger, L.: Electron microscopy of non-neuronal cellular changes accompanying neural degeneration in thalamic nuclei of the rabbit. I. Reactive hematogeneous and perivascular elements within the basal lamina. J. Comp. Neurol. *148*, 285–311 (1973a)

Matthews, M. A., Kruger, L.: Electron microscopy of non-neuronal cellular changes accompanying neural degeneration in thalamic nuclei of the rabbit. II. Reactive elements within the neuropil. J. Comp. Neurol. *148*, 313–346 (1973b)

Maximow, A.: Bindegewebige und blutbildende Gewebe. In: Handbuch der mikroskopischen Anatomie des Menschen. Möllendorf, W., v. (Hrsg.), Bd. I/1, S. 232–583. Berlin: Springer 1927

Maximow, A.: The macrophages or histiocytes. In: Special cytology. Cowdry, E. V. (ed.), pp. 427–484. New York: Paul B. Hoeber, Inc. 1928

Maxwell, D. S., Kruger, L.: Small blood vessels and the origin of phagocytes in the rat cerebral cortex following heavy paricle irradiation. Exp. Neurol. *12*, 33–54 (1965)

Maxwell, D. S., Kruger, L.: The reactive oligodendrocyte. An electron microscopic study of cerebral cortex following alpha particle irradiation. Am. J. Anat. *118*, 437–460 (1966)

Mayersbach, H., von: Die Zeit, ein Schlüssel zur Standardisierung der Zytochemie und Zellbiologie? Acta Histochem. (Jena) Suppl. *14*, 207–220 (1975)

Mayersbach, H., von: Time – a key in experimental and practical medicine. Arch. Toxicol. *36*, 185–216 (1976)

Maynard, E. A., Schultz, R. L., Pease, D. C.: Electron microscopy of the vascular bed of rat cerebral cortex. Am. J. Anat. *100*, 409–433 (1957)

McCabe, J. S., Low, F. N.: The subarachnoid angle: An area of transition in peripheral nerve. Anat. Rec. *164*, 15–34 (1969)

McDonald, T. F.: The formation of phagocytes from perivascular cells in the irradiated cerebral cortex of the rat as seen in the electron microscope. Anat. Rec. *142*, 257 (1962)

McQueen, J. D., Northrup, B. E., Leibrock, L. G.: Arachnoid clearance of red blood cells. Neurol. Neurosurg. Psychiatr. *37*, 1316–1321 (1974)

Mellick, R., Cavanagh, J. B.: The function of the perineurium and its relation to the flow phenomen within the endoneural spaces. Proc. Aust. Assoc. Neurol. *5*, 521–525 (1968)

Merchant, R. E.: A non-hematogenous origin of subarachnoid macrophages in response to secondary challenge by bacillus Clmette-Guerin (BCG). Anatom. Rec. (in press – 1978)

Merchant, R. E., Low, F. N.: Scanning electron microscopy of the subarachnoid space in the dog. V. Macrophages challenged by bacillus Calmette-Guerin. J. Comp. Neurol. *172*, 381–408 (1977a)

Merchant, R. E., Low, F. N.: Identification of challenged subarachnoid free cells. Am. J. Anat. *148*, 143–148 (1977b)

Merchant, R. E., Olson, G. E., Low, F. N.: Scanning and transmission electron microscopy of leptomeningeal free cells: cell interactions in response to challenge by bacillus Calmette-Guerin. J. Reticuloendothel. Soc. *22*, 199–207 (1977)

Merker, G.: Einige Feinstrukturbefunde an den Plexus chorioidei von Affen. Z. Zellforsch. *134*, 565–584 (1972)

Merzbacher, L.: Ergebnisse der Untersuchung des Liquor cerebrospinalis. Neurol. Cbl. *23*, 548–559 (1904)

Merzbacher, L.: Untersuchungen über die Morphologie und Biologie der Abräumzellen im Zentralnervensystem. In: Histologische u. histopathologische Arbeiten. Nissl, F. (Hrsg.), Bd. 3, S. 1-142. Jena: G. Fischer 1910

Mestres, P., Breipohl, W.: Morphology and distribution of supraependymal cells in the third ventricle of the albino rat. Cell Tissue Res. *168*, 303-314 (1976)

Metschnikoff, E.: Lectures on the comparative pathology of inflammation (1891). Reprinted, New York: Dove Publ. 1968

Metschnikoff, E.: Die Lehre von den Phagocyten und deren experimenteller Grundlage. In: Handbuch der pathogenen Mikroorganismen. Kolle, W., Wassermann, A., von (Hrsg.), Bd. 2, S. 655-731. Jena: G. Fischer 1913

Metz, A.: Über die Bewegungsfähigkeit der Hortegazellen (Mikroglia). Zbl. Gesamte Neurol. Psychiatr. *43*, 8 (1926)

Metz, A., Spatz, H.: Die Hortegaschen Zellen (= das sogenannte „dritte Elemente") und über ihre funktionelle Bedeutung. Z. Gesamte Neurol. Psychiatr. *89*, 138-170 (1924)

Meuret, G.: Disorders of the mononuclear phagocyte system. An analytical review. Blut *34*, 317-328 (1977)

Meuret, G., Hoffmann, G.: Monocyte kinetic studies in normal and disease states. Br. J. Haematol. *24*, 275-285 (1973)

Meyer-Rienecker, H., Jenssen, H. L., Köhler, H., Günther, J. K.: Zur Bedeutung des Makrophagen-Elektrophores-Mobilitätstests für die Diagnostik der Geschwülste des Zentralnervensystems. Dtsch. Med. Wochenschr. *100*, 538-543 (1975)

Meyer-Rienecker, H., Jenssen, H. L., Köhler, H., Günther, J. K.: Der Makrophagen-Elektrophorese-Mobilitäts-LAD-Test als diagnostisches Verfahren für die multiple Sklerose. J. Neurol. *211*, 229-240 (1976)

Michlmayr, G., Huber, Ch., Fink, U., Falkensamer, M., Huber, H.: T-Lymphozyten in peripherem Blut und Lymphknoten bei lymphatischen Systemerkrankungen. Schweiz. Med. Wochenschr. *104*, 815-820 (1974)

Mihalik, P., von: Über die Nervengewebekulturen, mit besonderer Berücksichtigung der Neuronenlehre und der Mikrogliafrage. Arch. Exp. Zellforsch. *17*, 119-176 (1935)

Millen, J. W., Woollam, D. H. M.: Observation on the nature of the pia mater. Brain *84*, 514 (1961)

Millen, J. W., Woollam, D. H. M.: The anatomy of the cerebrospinals fluid. London: Oxford University Press 1962

Minor, L.: Traumatische Erkrankungen des Rückenmarks (Rückenmarkquetschung, Hämatolmyelie, Nekrose etc.). In: Handbuch der pathologischen Anatomie des Nervensystems. Flatau, E., Jacobsohn, L., Minor, L. (Hrsg.), Bd. 2, S. 1008-1058. Berlin: S. Karger 1904

Miyagawa, R.: Study of Hortega's cells (Japan.). Mitt. Med. Akad. Kioto *11*, 99-147 (1934)

Mogilnitzky, B. N., Marcuse, K., Schdanow, I.: Die Einwirkungen der Sensibilisierung auf die Mesoglia und das reticuloendotheliale System. Frankf. Z. Pathol. *46*, 210-217 (1934)

Monie, H. J., Everett, N. B.: The popliteal node assay for graft-versus-host interaction in mice. II. Location and proliferation of donor and host cells within the popliteal node. Anat. Rec. *179*, 19-25 (1974)

More, D. G., Penrose, J. M., Keanney, R., Nelson, D. S.: Immunological induction of DNA synthesis in mouse peritoneal macrophages. An expression of cell-mediated-immunity. Int. Arch. Allergy Appl. Immunol. *44*, 611-630 (1973)

Morgan, H., Martinez, A. J., Kapp, J. P., Robertson, J. T., Astruc, J.: Aseptic meningitis due to atheromatous material in the subarachnoid space. Acta Neuropathol. (Berl.) *30*, 145-154 (1974)

Mori, S.: Cytological features and mitotic ability of microglia in the injured rat brain. Proc. VII. Internat. Congr. Electron Microscopy, pp. 57-80. Grenoble 1970

Mori, S.: Uptake of (^{3}H) thymidine by corpus callosum cells in rats following a stab wound of the brain. Brain Res. *46*, 177-186 (1972)

Mori, S., Leblond, C. P.: Identification of microglia in light and electron microscopy. J. Comp. Neurol. *135*, 57-79 (1969)
Morris, J. H., Hudson, A. R., Weddel, G.: A study of degeneration and regeneration in divided rat sciatic nerve based on electron microscopy. I. The traumatic degeneration of myelin in the proximal stump of the divided nerve. Z. Zellforsch. *124*, 76-102 (1972)
Morse, D. E., Low, F. N.: Regional variations in the fine structure of the pia mater of the rat. Anat. Rec. *169*, 467 (1971)
Morse, D. E., Low, F. N.: The fine structure of the pia mater of the rat. Am. J. Anat. *133*, 349-368 (1972a)
Morse, D. E., Low, F. N.: The fine structure of subarachnoid macrophages in the rat. Anat. Rec. *174*, 469-475 (1972b)
Moser, R. P., Robinson, J. A., Prostko, E. R.: Lymphocyte subpopulations in human cerebrospinal fluid. Neurology (Minneap.) *26*, 726-728 (1976)
Movat, H. Z., Fernando, N. V. P.: The fine structure of the terminal vascular bed. IV. The venules and their perivascular cells (pericytes, adventitial cells). Exp. Mol. Pathol. *3*, 98-114 (1964)
Mugnaini, E., Walberg, F.: Ultrastructure of neuroglia. Ergeb. Anat. Entwicklungsgesch. *37*, 194-236 (1964)
Mugnaini, E., Walberg, F.: "Dark cells" in electron micrographs from the central nervous system of vertebrates. J. Ultrastruct. Res. *12*, 235-236 (1965)
Mugnaini, E., Walberg, F., Brodal, A.: Mode of termination of primary vestibular fibres in the lateral vestibular nucleus. An experimental electron microscopical study in the cat. J. Comp. Neurol. *4*, 187-211 (1967a)
Mugnaini, E., Walberg, F., Hauglie-Hanssen, E.: Observations on the fine structure of the lateral vestibular nucleus (Deiter's nucleus) in the cat. J. Comp. Neurol. *4*, 146-186 (1967b)
Murad, T. M., Haam, E., von, Murthy, M. S. N.: Ultrastructure of a hemangiopericytoma and a glomus tumor. Cancer *22*, 1239-1249 (1968)
Murray, H. M., Walker, B. E.: Comparative study of astrocytes and mononuclear leukocytes reacting to brain trauma in mice. Exp. Neurol. *41*, 290-302 (1973)
Myers, D. K., Feinendegen, L. E.: Double labeling with (^{3}H) thymidine and (^{125}I) iododeoxyuridine as a method for determining the fate of injected DNA and cells in vivo. J. Cell Biol. *67*, 484-488 (1975)
Nabeshima, S.: Morphological basis of meningeal barriers to peroxidase. Anat. Rec. *169*, 384 (1971)
Nabeshima, S., Reese, T. S., Landis, D. M. D., Brightman, M. W.: Junctions in the meninges and marginal glia. J. Comp. Neurol. *164*, 127-169 (1975)
Nachlas, M. M., Seligman, A. M.: The histochemical demonstration of esterase. Cancer Inst. *9*, 415-425 (1949)
Naess, A.: Demonstration of T lymphocytes in cerebrospinal fluid. Scand. J. Immunol. *5*, 165-168 (1976)
Naoumenko, J., Feigin, I.: A modification for paraffin sections of silver carbonate impregnation for microglia. Acta Neuropathol. (Berl.) *2*, 402-406 (1963)
Nelson, D. S.: Macrophages and immunity. Amsterdam, London: North-Holland Publ. Co. 1969
Nelson, D. S. (ed.): Immunobiology of the macrophage. New York, San Francisco, London: Academic Press 1976
Nelson, E., Blinzinger, K. H., Hager, H.: Ultrastructural observations on phagocytosis of bacteria in experimental (E. coli) meningitis. J. Neuropathol. Exp. Neurol. *21*, 155-169 (1962a)
Nelson, E., Blinzinger, K. H., Hager, H.: Electron microscopic observations on subarachnoid and perivascular spaces of the Syrian hamster brain. Neurology (Minneap.) *11*, 285-295 (1962b)
Nelson, E., Blinzinger, K. H., Hager, H.: An electron-microscopic study of bacterial men-

ingitis. Arch. Neurol. *6*, 390-403 (1962c)
Netsky, M. G., Shuangshoti, S.: Studies on the choroid plexus. In: Neurosciences research. Ehrenpreis, S., Solnitzky, O. (eds.), Vol. III, pp. 131-178. New York, London: Academic Press 1970
Nichols, B. A., Bainton, D. F.: Ultrastructure and cytochemistry of mononuclear phagocytes. In: Mononuclear phagocytes in immunity, infection, and pathology. Furth, R., Van (ed.), pp. 17-55. Oxford, London, Edinburgh, Melbourne: Blackwell Scientific Publications 1975
Nicholls, J. G., Wolfe, D. E.: Distribution of ^{14}C-labeled sucrose, inulin, and dextran in extracellular spaces and in cells of the leech central nervous system. J. Neurophysiol. *30*, 1574-1592 (1967)
Nicol, T., Bilbey, D. L. J.: Elimination of macrophage cells of the reticulo-endothelial system by way of the bronchial tree. Nature (Lond.) *182*, 192-193 (1958)
Niessing, K.: Zellformen und Zellreaktionen der Mikroglia des Mäusehirns. Morphol. Jahrb. *92*, 102-122 (1952)
Niessing, K.: Zellreaktionen der Hortegaglia bei Anwendung pharmakologischer und hormoneller Reize. Anat. Anz. Suppl. *100*, 266-271 (1954)
Nissl, F.: Über einige Beziehungen zwischen Nervenzellenerkrankungen und gliösen Erscheinungen bei verschiedenen Psychosen. Arch. Psychiatr. *32*, 656-676 (1899)
Nissl, F.: Kritische Bemerkungen zu H. Schmaus: Vorlesungen über die pathologische Anatomie des Rückenmarks. Zentralbl. Nervenheilkd. Psychiatr. N.S. *14*, 88-107 (1903)
Nissl, F.: Zur Histopathologie der paralytischen Rindenerkrankung. In: Histologische u. histopathologische Arbeiten. Nissl, F., Alzheimer, A. (Hrsg.), Bd. 1, S. 315-494. Jena: G. Fischer 1904
Noetzel, H., Ohlmeier, R.: Zur Frage der Randzonensiderose des Zentralnervensystem. Tierexperimentelle Untersuchungen. Acta Neuropathol. (Berl.) *3*, 164-183 (1963)
Noetzel, H., Rox, J.: Autoradiographische Untersuchungen über Zellteilung und Zellentwicklung im Gehirn der erwachsenen Maus und des erwachsenen Rhesus-Affen nach Injektion von radioaktivem Thymidin. Acta Neuropathol. (Berl.) *3*, 326-342 (1964)
North, R. J.: The mitotic potential of fixed phagocytes in the liver as revealed during the development of cellular immunity. J. Exp. Med. *130*, 315-326 (1969)
Novikoff, A. B., Essner, E., Goldfischer, S., Heus, M.: Nucleosidephosphatase activities of cytomembranes. In: The interpretation of ultrastructure. Symposia of the International Society for Cell Biology. Harris, R. J. C. (ed.), Vol. I, pp. 149-192. New York, London: Academic Press 1962
Nutschnikoff: cited by Cammermeyer, 1970b
Nystrom, S.: Pathological changes in blood vessels of human glioblastoma multiforme. Acta Pathol. Microbiol. Scand. *49*, Suppl. 137, 1-71 (1960)
O'Daly, J. A., Imaeda, T.: Electron microscopic study of Wallerian degeneration in cutaneous nerves caused by mechanical injury. Lab. Invest. *17*, 744-766 (1967)
Oehmichen, M.: Kombinierte autoradiographisch-enzymhistochemische Untersuchungen an Blutzellen. Beschreibung einer Methode. Klin. Wochenschr. *49*, 282-284 (1971)
Oehmichen, M.: Substrathistochemische und enzymhistochemische Untersuchungen an Mesenchymzellen – einschließlich Mikroglia – des normalen Kaninchengehirns. Acta Histochem. (Jena) *47*, 289-304 (1973a)
Oehmichen, M.: Enzymatic activity of intravasal neutrophils and monocytes of rabbits at different age levels; first results by application of a combined cytochemical-autoradiographical method. Microscopica Acta *75*, 117-129 (1973b)
Oehmichen, M.: Histochemische Untersuchungen zum Fettgehalt und Fettstoffwechsel des Plexus choroideus des Kaninchens. Z. Zellforsch. *142*, 387-397 (1973c)
Oehmichen, M.: IgG- und Komplement-Rezeptoren an mononukleären Phagozyten des menschlichen Liquor cerebrospinalis. In: Proc. VII. Int. Congr. Neuropathol. Budapest. Környey, S., Tariska, S., Gosztonyi, G. (eds.), pp. 83-86. Amsterdam, Budapest: Excerpta medica - Akademiai Kiado 1975

Oehmichen, M.: Recent experimental methods for demonstrating blood derived cells in nervous tissue. Neuropathol. Appl. Neurobiol. *2*, 160-161 (1976a)

Oehmichen, M.: Receptor activity on some mesenchymal cells in CNS of normal rabbits. Indications of the monocytic origin of intracerebral perivascular cells, epiplexus cells and mononuclear phagocytes in the subarachnoid space. Acta Neuropathol. (Berl.) *35*, 205-218 (1976b)

Oehmichen, M.: Characterization of mononuclear phagocytes of human CSF using membrane markers. Acta Cytol. *20*, 548-552 (1976c)

Oehmichen, M.: Cerebrospinal fluid cytology. Stuttgart: G. Thieme 1976d

Oehmichen, M.: Differenzierung mononukleärer Zellen des Liquor cerebrospinalis mit immunologischen und zytochemischen Methoden. In: Pathologie der Liquorräume. Mertens, H. G., Dommasch, D. (Hrsg.). Stuttgart: G. Thieme (in press)

Oehmichen, M., Grüninger, H.: Parabioseversuche zur Herkunft der Fibroblasten im ZNS. Autoradiographische Untersuchungen am Granulationsgewebe nach Kieselsäure-Implantation. Virchows Arch. (Zellpathol.) *13*, 351-356 (1973)

Oehmichen, M., Grüninger, H.: Cytokinetic studies on the origin of cells of the cerebrospinal fluid, with a contribution to the cytogenesis of the leptomeningeal mesenchym. J. Neurol. Sci. *22*, 165-176 (1974a)

Oehmichen, M., Grüninger, H.: Zur Entstehung von mehrkernigen Riesenzellen bei der experimentell-induzierten und spontanen Krabbeschen Krankheit (Globoid Cell Leukodystrophy). Beitr. Pathol. *153*, 111-132 (1974b)

Oehmichen, M., Huber, H.: Reactive microglia with membrane features of mononuclear phagocytes. J. Neuropathol. Exp. Neurol. *35*, 30-39 (1976)

Oehmichen, M., Huber, H.: Supplementary cytodiagnostic analyses of cerebrospinal fluid cells: Differentiation of mononuclear cells of cerebrospinal fluid using cytologic markers. J. Neurol. *218*, 187-196 (1978)

Oehmichen, M., Saebisch, R.: Zur Problematik histochemischer Färbungen und autoradiographische Technik. Acta Histochem. (Jena) *41*, 353-364 (1971)

Oehmichen, M., Torvik, A.: The origin of reactive cells in retrograde and Wallerian degeneration. Cell Tissue Res. *173*, 343-348 (1976)

Oehmichen, M., Treff, W. M.: Unterschiedliches postpunktionelles Phagocytoseverhalten von Liquorzellen. Verh. Dtsch. Ges. Pathol. *57*, 268-271 (1973)

Oehmichen, M., Saebisch, R., Grüninger, H.: Intravasale Cytokinetik der Leukocyten beim Kaninchen. Virchows Arch. [Zellpathol.] *9*, 28-44 (1971)

Oehmichen, M., Grüninger, H., Saebisch, R., Maas, B.: Die Monozyten bei carmininduzierter Monozytose. Enzymhistochemische und autoradiographische Untersuchungen an Blutzellen des Kaninchens. Folia Haematol. (Leipz.) *98*, 271-287 (1972)

Oehmichen, M., Grüninger, H., Saebisch, R., Narita, Y.: Mikroglia und Pericyten als Transformationsformen der Blut-Monocyten mit erhaltener Proliferationsfähigkeit. Experimentelle autoradiographische und enzymhistochemische Untersuchungen am normalen und geschädigten Kaninchen- und Rattengehirn. Acta Neuropathol. (Berl.) *23*, 200-218 (1973).

Oehmichen, M., Grüninger, H., Gencic, M.: Experimental studies on kinetics and functions of mononuclear phagocytes of the central nervous system. Acta Neuropathol. (Berl.) Suppl. *6*, 285-290 (1975)

Oehmichen, M., Wiethölter, H., Greaves, M. F.: Immunological analysis of human microglia: Lack of monocytic and lymphoid membrane differentiation antigens. J. Neuropathol. exp. Neurol. (in press–1978)

Ohno, F.: Beiträge zur Frage der neurophysiologischen Entzündungslehre. Beitr. Pathol. Anat. *72*, 722-759 (1924)

Okamoto, M.: Observations on neurons and neuroglia from the area of the reticular formation in tissue culture. Z. Zellforsch. *47*, 269-287 (1958)

Oksche, A.: Die Bedeutung des Ependyms für den Stoffaustausch zwischen Liquor und Gehirn. Anat. Anz. Suppl. *103*, 162-172 (1956)

Olsson, Y.: Studies on vascular permeability in peripheral nerves. IV. Distribution of intravenously injected protein tracers in the peripheral nervous system of various species. Acta Neuropathol. (Berl.) *17*, 114-126 (1971)

Olsson, Y., Sjöstrand, J.: Origin of macrophages in Wallerian degeneration of peripheral nerves demonstrated autoradiographically. Exp. Neurol. *23*, 102-112 (1969)

Onishi, N.: Study on reticulo-endothelial system in the central nervous system. Folia Psychiatr. Neurol. Jap. *5*, 263-282 (1952)

Page, R. C., Davies, P., Allison, A. C.: Participation of mononuclear phagocytes in chronic inflammatory diseases. J. Reticuloendothel. Soc. *15*, 413-438 (1974)

Palay, S. L.: An electron microscopical study of neuroglia. In: Biology of neuroglia. Windle, W. F. (ed.), pp. 24-38. Springfield/Ill.: Ch. C. Thomas 1958

Palmer, E., Rees, R. J. W., Weddell, G.: The phagocytic activity of Schwann cells. In: Proceedings of the anatomical society of Great Britain and Ireland, pp. 49-52. London: Taylor and Francis 1961

Pantelouris, E. M.: Absence of thymus in a mouse mutant. Nature (Lond.) *217*, 370-371 (1968)

Papadimitriou, J. M., Sforsina, D., Papaellias, L.: Kinetics of multinucleate giant cell formation and their modification by various agents in foreign body reactions. Am. J. Pathol. *73*, 349-361 (1973)

Patek, P. R.: The perivascular space of the mammalian brain. Anat. Rec. *88*, 1-24 (1944)

Paterson, J. A., Privat, A., Ling, E. A., Leblond, C. P.: Investigation of glial cells in semithin sections. III. Transformation of subependymal cells into glial cells, as shown by radioautography after ^{3}H-thymidine injection into the lateral ventricle of the brain of young rats. J. Comp. Neurol. *149*, 83-102 (1973)

Pearse, A. G. E.: Esterases of the hypothalamus and neurohypophysis and their functional significance. Proc. Int. Congr. Neuropath., pp. 329-335. Milano 1958

Pearse, A. G. E.: Histochemistry, theoretical, and applied. London: J. a. A. Churchill Ltd. 1968

Pease, D. C., Schultz, R. L.: Electron microscopy of rat cranial meninges. Am. J. Anat. *102*, 301-321 (1958)

Penfield, W.: Microglia and the process of phagocytosis in gliomas. Am. J. Pathol. *1*, 77-89 (1925)

Penfield, W.: Phagocytic activity of microglia in the central nervous system. Zentralbl. Gesamte Neurol. Psychiatr. *43*, 9-10 (1926)

Penfield, W.: Neuroglia and microglia. The interstitial tissue of the central nervous system. In: Special cytology. Cowdry, E. V. (ed.), Vol. II, pp. 1032-1068. New York: Paul B. Hoeber 1928

Pepler, W. J., Pearse, A. G. E.: The histochemistry of the esterases of rat brain with special reference to those of the hypothalamic nuclei. J. Neurochem. *1*, 193-202 (1957)

Persson, L.: Cellular reactions to small cerebral stab wounds in the rat frontal lobe. Virchows Arch. [Zellpathol.] *22*, 21-37 (1976)

Pestalozzi, H.: Über Aneurismata spuria der kleinen Gehirnarterien und ihren Zusammenhang mit Apoplexie. Würzburg: F. E. Thein 1849

Peters, A.: The formation and structure of myelin sheaths in the central nervous system. J. Biophys. Biochem. Cytol. *8*, 431-446 (1960)

Peters, A.: The surface fine structure of the choroid plexus and ependymal lining of the rat lateral ventricle. J. Neurocytol. *3*, 99-108 (1974)

Peters, A., Palay, S. L., Webster, H. de F.: The finestructure of the nervous system: the cells and their processes. New York: Hoeber, Harper, and Row 1970

Peters, A., Palay, S., Webster, H. de F.: The fine structure of the nervous system. The neurons and supporting cells. Philadelphia, London, Toronto: W. B. Saunders 1976

Phillips, D. E.: An electron microscopic study of macroglia and microglia in the lateral funiculus of the developing spinal cord in the fetal monkey. Z. Zellforsch. *140*, 145-167 (1973)

Pick, A.: Rückenmarks-Erweichung, -Kompression; Myelitis; Rückenmarks-Abszeß. In: Handbuch der pathologischen Anatomie des Nervensystems. Flatau, E., Jacobsohn, L., Minor, L. (Hrsg.), Bd. 2, S. 846–879. Berlin: S. Karger 1904

Plenk, V. H.: Perizyten an Kapillaren des Zentralnervensystems. Anat. Anz. *66*, 369–377 (1929)

Plum, F., Siesjö, B. K.: Recent advances in CSF physiology. Anesthesiology *42*, 708–730 (1975)

Pollard, J. D., Fitzpatrick, L.: An ultrastructural comparison of peripheral nerve allografts and autografts. Acta Neuropathol. (Berl.) *23*, 152–165 (1973)

Pope, A.: Discussion. In: Biology of Neuroglia. Windle, W. F. (ed.), p. 225. Springfield/Ill.: Ch. C. Thomas Publ. 1958

Privat, A.: Sur l'origine des divers types de névroglie chez le rat. In: VIth Internat. Congr. Neuropath., pp. 447–448. Paris: Masson et Cie., Editeurs 1970

Privat, A.: Postnatal gliogenesis in the mammalian brain. Int. Rev. Cytol. *40*, 281–323 (1975)

Privat, A., Leblond, C. P.: The subependymal layer and neighboring region in the brain of the young rat. J. Comp. Neurol. *146*, 277–285 (1972)

Pruijs, W. M.: Über Mikroglia, ihre Herkunft, Funktion und ihr Verhältnis zu anderen Gliaelementen. Z. Gesamte Neurol. Psychiatr. *108*, 298–331 (1927)

Quincke, H.: Zur Physiologie der Zerebrospinalflüssigkeit. Du Bois Reymond's Arch. Anat. Phys., Phys. Abt., pp. 153–177, 1872

Raff, M. C.: Two distinct populations of peripheral lymphocytes in mice distinguishable by immunofluorescence. Immunology *19*, 637–650 (1970)

Raff, M. C., Wortis, H. H.: Thymus dependence of θ-bearing cells in the peripheral lymphoid tissues of mice. Immunology *18*, 931–942 (1970)

Rafferty, N. S., Gfeller, E.: Duration of nuclear labeling after intraperitoneal injection of tritiated thymidine into Rana Pipieus. Anat. Rec. *163*, 246 (1969)

Raisman, G.: Neuronal plasticity in the septal nuclei of the adult rat. Brain Res. *14*, 25–48 (1969)

Rapoport, S. I.: Blood-brain barrier in physiology and medicine. New York: Raven Press 1976

Rehm, O.: Die Cerebrospinalflüssigkeit. Physikalische, chemische und zytologische Eigenschaften und ihre klinische Verwertung. In: Histologische u. histopathologische Arbeiten. Nissl, F. (Hrsg.), Bd. 3, S. 201–296. Jena: G. Fischer 1910

Rehm, O.: Beiträge zur Kenntnis des Liquor cerebrospinalis. I. Zellformen. Dtsch. Z. Nervenheilkd. *117–119*, 517–532 (1931)

Rhodin, J. A. G.: Ultrastructure of mammalian venous capillaries, venules, and small collecting veins. J. Ultrastruct. Res. *25*, 452–500 (1968)

Ribbert, H.: Über multiple Sclerose des Gehirns und Rückenmarks. Virchows. Arch. [Pathol. Anat.] *90*, 243–260 (1882)

Rijssel, T., Van: Circulation of cerebrospinal fluid in carassius gibelio. Arch. Neurol. Psychiatr. (Chic.) *56*, 522–543 (1946)

Rio Hortega, P. del: Noticia de un nuevo y fácil método para la coloración de la neuroglia y del tejido conectivo. Trab. Lab. Invest. Biol. Univ. Madr. *15*, 367–368 (1917)

Rio Hortega, P. del: El tercer elemento de los centros nerviosos. I. La microglia en estado normal. II. Intervención de la microglia en los precesos patológicos. III. Naturaleza probable de la microglia. Bol. Soc. Esp. Biol. *9*, 69–120 (1919a)

Rio Hortega, P. del: Poder fagocitario y movilidad de la microglia. Bol. Soc. Exp. Biol. *9*, 154–166 (1919b)

Rio Hortega, P. del: La microglia y su transformación en células en bastoncito y en cuerpos gránuloadiposos. Trab. Lab. Invest. Biol. Univ. Madr. *18*, 37–82 (1920)

Rio Hortega, P. del: Estudios sobre la neuroglia –La glia de escasas radiaciones (oligodendroglia). Bol. Real. Soc. Exp. Hist. Nat. *21*, 64–92 (1921a)

Rio Hortega, P. del: El tercer elemento de los centros nerviosos: histogenesia y evolución normal; éxodo y distribución regional de la microglia. Mem. Real. Soc. Esp. Hist. Nat. *11*, 213–268 (1921b)

Rio Hortega, P. del: Histogénesis y evolución normal; éxodo y distribución regional de la microglia. Arch. Neurobiol. (Madr.) *2*, 215-255 (1921c)

Rio Hortega, P. del: Concepts histogénique, physiologique et physiopathologique de la microglia. Ann. Med. Psychol. (Paris) *88*, 347-349 (1930a)

Rio Hortega, P. del: Concepts histologenique, morphologique, physiologique et physiopathologique de la microglie. Rev. Neurol. (Paris) *37*, 956-987 (1930b)

Rio Hortega, P. del: Microglia. In: Cytology and cellular pathology of the nervous system. Penfield, W. (ed.), Vol. II, pp. 483-534. New York: Hafner Publ. Co. 1965, facsimile of 1932 edition

Rio Hortega, P. del: The microglia. Lancet *1939/I* (236), 1023-1026

Rio Hortega, P. del, Asua, F. J. de: Sobre la fagocitosis en los tumores y en otros procesos patologicos. Arch. Cardiol. Haematol. *2*, 161-220 (1921)

Rio Hortega, P. del, Penfield, W.: Cerebral cicatrix. The reaction of neuroglia and microglia to brain wounds. Bull. John Hopkins Hosp. *41*, 278-303 (1927)

Robain, O.: Gliogenese post-natale chez le lapin. J. Neurol. Sci. *11*, 445-461 (1970)

Robbins, D., Fahimi, H. D., Cotran, R. S.: Fine structural cytochemical localization of peroxidase activity in rat peritoneal cells. Mononuclear cells, eosinophils, and mast cells. J. Histochem. Cytochem. *19*, 571-575 (1971)

Robertson, W. F.: A textbook of pathology in relation to mental disease. Edinburgh: W. F. Clay 1900a

Robertson, W. F.: A microscopic demonstration of the normal and pathological histology of mesoglia cells. J. Med. Sci. *46*, 733-752 (1900b)

Robin, C.: Recherces sur quelques particularités de la structure des capillaires de l'Encéphale. J. Physiol. Hom. Animaux *2*, 537-548 (1859)

Robinson, N.: Enzyme response of traumatized tissue after intracortical injection into 5 day old rat brain. J. Neurol. Neurosurg. Psychiat. *35*, 865-872 (1972)

Roessmann, U., Friede, R. L.: Entry of labeled monocytic cells into the central nervous system. Acta Neuropathol. (Berl.) *10*, 359-362 (1968)

Romeis, B.: Mikroskopische Technik. München, Wien: R. Oldenbourg 1968

Ronai, P.: High resolution autoradiography with ^{51}Cr. Int. J. Appl. Radiat. Isot. *20*, 471-472 (1968)

Roos, B.: Makrophagen: Herkunft, Entwicklung und Funktion. In: Handbuch der allgemeinen Pathologie. Studer, A., Cottier, H. (Hrsg.), Bd. 7/3, S. 2-128. Berlin, Heidelberg, New York: Springer 1970

Rorke, L. B., Gilden, D. H., Wroblewska, Z., Santoli, D.: Human brain in tissue culture. IV. Morphological characteristics. J. Comp. Neurol. *161*, 329-340 (1975)

Rose, M., Rose, S.: Die Topographie der architektonischen Felder der Großhirnrinde am Kaninchenschädel. J. Psychol. Neurol. *45*, 264-276 (1933)

Rosen, W. C., Basom, C. R., Gunderson, L. L.: A technique for the light microscopy of tissues fixed for fine structure. Anat. Rec. *158*, 223-237 (1967)

Roser, B.: The distribution of intravenously injected peritoneal macrophages in the mouse. Aust. J. Exp. Biol. Med. Sci. *43*, 553-562 (1965)

Roser, B.: The distribution of intravenously injected Kupffer cells in the mouse. J. Reticuloendothel. Soc. *5*, 455-471 (1968)

Roser, B.: The migration of macrophages in vivo. In: Mononuclear phagocytes. Furth, R., Van (ed.), pp. 166-174. Oxford, Edinburgh: Blackwell Sci. Publ. 1970a

Roser, B.: The origins, kinetics, and fate of macrophage populations. J. Reticuloendothel. Soc. *8*, 139-161 (1970b)

Rotstadt, J.: Zur Cytologie der Cerebrospinalflüssigkeit. Z. Gesamte Neurol. Psychiatr. *31*, 228-274 (1916)

Rouget, M. C.: Memoire sur le développement de la structure et les propriétés physiologiques des capillaires sanguines et lymphatiques. Arch. Physiol. *5*, 603-663 (1873)

Rouget, M. C.: Note sur le devéloppement de la tunique contractile des vaissaux. C.R. Acad. Sci. (Paris) *79*, 559-568 (1874)

Rouget, M. C.: Sur la contractilite des capillaires sanguins. C.R. Acad. Sci. [D] (Paris) *88*, 916-918 (1879)
Roussy, G., Lhermitte, J., Oberling, C.: La nevroglie et les reactions pathologiques. Rev. Neurol. (Paris) *37/I*, 878-955 (1930)
Rubinstein, L. J., Klatzo, I., Miquel, J.: Histochemical observations on oxidative enzyme activity of glial cells in a local brain injury. J. Neuropathol. Exp. Neurol. *21*, 116-136 (1962)
Russell, D. S.: Intravital staining of microglia with trypan blue. Am. J. Pathol. *5*, 451-458 (1929)
Russell, G. V.: The compound granular corpuscle or gitter cell: A review, together with notes on the origin of this phagocyte. Tex. Rep. Biol. Med. *20*, 338-351 (1962)
Rydberg, E.: Cerebral injury in new-born children consequent on birth trauma; with an inquiry into the normal and pathological anatomy of the neuroglia. Acta Pathol. Microbiol. Scand. Suppl. *10*, 1-247 (1932)
Samorajski, T., Ordy, J. M., Zeman, W., Curtis, H. J.: Early and longterm effects of deuteron irradiation on cells in the cerebellum of adult mice. J. Cell. Biol. *38*, 213-220 (1968)
Sandberg-Wollheim, M., Turesson, I.: Lymphocyte subpopulations in the cerebrospinal fluid and peripheral blood in patients with multiple sclerosis. Scand. J. Immunol. *4*, 831-836 (1975)
Santha, K., von: Untersuchungen über die Entwicklung der Hortega'schen Mikroglia. Arch. Psychiatr. *96*, 36-67 (1932)
Santha, K., von, Juba, A.: Weitere Untersuchungen über die Entwicklung der Hortegaschen Mikroglia. Arch. Psychiatr. *98*, 598-613 (1933)
Santolaya, R. C., Echandia, E. L. R.: The surface of the choroid plexus cell under normal and experimental conditions. Z. Zellforsch. *92*, 43-51 (1968)
Sasaki, S.: Experimental studies on phagocytes in the brain. Folia Psychiatr. Neurol. Jap. *9*, 283-303 (1955)
Sato, M.: ^{3}H-thymidine autoradiographic studies on the origin of reaktive cells in the brain of mice infected with Japanese encephalitis virus (Japan.). Brain Nerve (Tokyo) *20*, 1239-1250 (1968)
Sayk, J.: Cytologie der Cerebrospinalflüssigkeit. Jena: VEB G. Fischer 1960
Sayk, J.: Histiozytäre und hämatogene Zellen und die Beziehungen zu Austausch- und Transportfunktionen im Liquorraum. In: Neue Forschungsergebnisse des Hirnstoffwechsels und der Entmarkungsenzephalomyelitis. Schmidt, R. M. (Hrsg.), S. 210-220. Halle/Saale: Wissenschaftl. Beitr. Martin-Luther-Universität 1974
Schaarschmidt, W., Lierse, W.: Ultrastrukturelle Reaktion der multipotenten Glia im Kleinhirn der Ratte nach Behandlung mit 6-Aminonikotinamid. Acta Anat. (Basel) *93*, 184-193 (1975)
Schaeffer, H. E., Käufer, C., Fischer, R.: Vergleichende fermentcytochemische Untersuchungen an Blut- und Knochenmarkzellen bei Laboratoriumstieren. Virchows Arch. [Zellpathol.] *4*, 310-334 (1970)
Schaltenbrand, G.: Plexus und Meningen. In: Handbuch der mikroskopischen Anatomie des Menschen. Bargmann, W. (Hrsg.), Bd. IV/2, S. 1-139. Berlin, Göttingen, Heidelberg: Springer 1955
Schaltenbrand, G., Bailley, P.: Die perivasculäre Piagliamembran des Gehirns. J. Psychol. Neurol. *35*, 199-278 (1928)
Schaly, G. A.: Over heet voorkommen van de Cellen van Rouget op den Wand van den Mensch. Inaug.-Diss. Groningen 1926
Scharrer, E.: Die Bildung von Meningocyten und der Abbau von Erythrocyten in der Paraphypophyse der Amphibien. Z. Zellforsch. *23*, 244-252 (1936)
Scheibel, M. E., Scheibel, A. B.: Neurons and Neuroglia. In: Biology of Neuroglia. Windle, W. F. (ed.), pp. 5-23. Springfield/Ill.: Ch. C. Thomas 1958
Scheid, W.: Untersuchungen über den Zerfall der Liquorzellen in vitro. Dtsch. Z. Nervenheilkd. *152*, 170-201 (1941)

Schlote, W.: Nervus opticus und experimentelles Trauma. Beitrag zur Zytologie und Zytopathologie eines zentralnervösen Markfasersystems. In: Monographien aus dem Gesamtgebiet der Neurologie und Psychiatrie. Müller, M., Spatz, H., Vogel, P. (Hrsg.), Heft 131. Berlin, Heidelberg, New York: Springer 1970

Schmaus, H.: Akute Myelitis. In: Ergebnisse der allgemeinen Pathologie und pathologischen Anatomie. Lubarsch, O., Ostertag, R. (Hrsg.), Bd. 9, S. 716-783. Wiesbaden: J. F. Bergmann 1904

Schmaus, H., Sacki, S.: Vorlesungen über die pathologische Anatomie des Rückenmarks. Wiesbaden: Bergmann 1901

Schmidt, R. M.: Der Liquor cerebrospinalis. Berlin: VEB Verlag Volk und Gesundheit 1968

Schmidt, R. M., Seifert, B.: Beitrag zur ultra-strukturellen Darstellung der Liquorzellen. Dtsch. Z. Nervenheilkd. *192*, 209-225 (1967)

Scholz, W.: Für die allgemeine Pathologie degenerativer Prozesse bedeutsame morphologische histochemische und strukturphysiologische Daten. In: Handbuch der speziellen pathologischen Anatomie und Histologie. Lubarsch, O., Henke, F., Rossle, Scholz, W. (eds), Vol. XIII/1. Nervensystem, pp. 42-265. Berlin, Göttingen, Heidelberg: Springer 1957

Schönenberg, H.: Untersuchungen über Vitalspeicherung in Liquorzellen sowie phasenkontrast- und fluoreszenzmikroskopische Beobachtungen über den Zerfall der Liquorzellen. Z. Kinderheilk. *72*, 157-180 (1952)

Schönenberg, H.: Der Liquor cerebrospinalis im Kindesalter. Stuttgart: G. Thieme 1960

Schotland, D. L., Cowen, D., Geller, L. M., Wolf, A.: A histochemical study of the effects of an antimetabolite 6-aminonicotinamide on the lumban spinal cord of the adult rat. J. Neuropathol. Exp. Neurol. *24*, 97-107 (1965)

Schultz, R. L., Pease, D. C.: Cicatrix formation in the rat cerebral cortex as revealed by electron microscopy. Am. J. Pathol. *35*, 1017-1041 (1959)

Schultz, R. L., Maynard, E. A., Pease, D. C.: Electron microscopy of neurons and neuroglia of cerebral cortex and corpus callosum. Am. J. Anat. *100*, 369-408 (1957)

Schultze, B., Hörning, N., Maurer, W.: Blut-Hirn-Schranke und Placentar-Schranke für ^{3}H-Thymidin und ^{3}H-Cytidin bei der Maus. (Untersuchungen mit Ganzkörper-Autoradiographie.) Z. Naturforsch. *27b*, 554-558 (1972)

Schupman, A.: Altersabhängiges Proliferationsverhalten ortsständiger Zellen am normalen und mechanisch geschädigten N. ischiadicus des Kaninchens. Autoradiographische Untersuchung. Inaug.-Diss. Tübingen 1976

Schwalbe, G.: Der Arachnoidalraum, ein Lymphraum und sein Zusammenhang mit dem Perichoroidalraum. Zentralbl. Med. Wiss. *7*, 465-467 (1869)

Schwalbe, G.: Lehrbuch der Neurologie. Erlangen: E. Besold 1881

Schwarze, E.-W.: Zytomorphologischer Vergleich der „kleinen und großen Rundzellen" des Liquor cerebrospinalis mit Lymphozyten des peripheren Blutes. Verh. Dtsch. Ges. Pathol. *57*, 262-268 (1973)

Schwarze, E. W.: The origin of (Kolmer's) epiplexus cells. A combined histomorphological and histochemical study. Histochemistry *44*, 103-104 (1975)

Seno, S., Fang, C. H., Himei, S., Hsueh, C. L., Nakashima, Y.: Hemopoietic recovery in bone marrow of lethally irradiated rats following parabiosis. Acta Haematol. (Basel) *55*, 321-331 (1976)

Shabo, A. L., Maxwell, D. S.: The morphology of the arachnoid villi: a light and electron microscopic study in the monkey. J. Neurosurg. *29*, 451-463 (1968a)

Shabo, A. L., Maxwell, D. S.: Electron microscopic observations on the fate of particulate matter in the cerebrospinal fluid. J. Neurosurg. *29*, 464-474 (1968b)

Shabo, A. L., Maxwell, D. S.: The subarachnoid space following the introduction of foreign protein: an electron microscopic study with peroxidase. J. Neuropathol. Exp. Neurol. *30*, 506-524 (1971)

Shands, J. W., Axelrod, B. J.: Mouse peritoneal macrophages: tritiated thymidine labeling and cell kinetics. J. Reticuloendothel. Soc. *21*, 69-76 (1977)

Sherwin, A. L., Richter, M., Cosgrove, J. B., Rose, B.: Studies of the blood cerebrospinal fluid barrier to antibodies and other proteins. Neurology (Minneap.) *13*, 113-119 (1963)

Shevach, E. M., Jaffe, E. S., Green, I.: Receptors for complement and immunoglobulin on human and animal lymphoid cells. Transplant. Rev. *16*, 3-28 (1973)

Shimizu, N.: Histochemical studies on the phosphatase of the nervous system. J. Comb. Neurol. *93*, 201-217 (1950)

Shimizu, N., Kumamoto, T.: Histochemical studies on the glycogen of the mammalian brain. Anat. Rec. *114*, 479-497 (1952)

Shimoda, A.: Elektronenmikroskopische Untersuchungen über den perivaskulären Aufbau des Gehirns unter Berücksichtigung der Veränderungen bei Hirnödem und Hirnschwellung. Dtsch. Z. Nervenheilkd. *183*, 78-98 (1961)

Shuttleworth, E. C., Allen, N.: Acid hydrolases in pia-arachnoid and ependyma of rat brain. Neurology (Minneap.) *16*, 979-985 (1966)

Sidman, R. L.: Autoradiographic methods and principles for study of the nervous system with thymidine-H^3. In: Contemporary research methods in neuroanatomy. Nauta, W. J. H., Ebesson, S. O. (eds.), pp. 252-273. New York, Heidelberg, Berlin: Springer 1970

Silver, M., Walker, A. E.: Histological pathology of the thermocoagulation of cerebral cortex. J. Neuropathol. Exp. Neurol. *6*, 311-322 (1947)

Simmonds, W. J.: The absorption of blood from the cerebrospinal fluid in animals. Aust. J. Exp. Biol. Med. Sci. *30*, 261-270 (1952)

Sjöstrand, J.: Proliferative changes in glial cells during nerve regeneration. Z. Zellforsch. *68*, 481-493 (1965)

Sjöstrand, J.: Studies on the glial cells in the hypoglossal nucleus of the rabbit during nerve regenration. Acta Physiol. Scand. *67*, Suppl. 270, 1-18 (1966a)

Sjöstrand, J.: Morphological changes in glial cells during nerve regeneration. Acta physiol. scand. *67*, Suppl. 270, 19-43 (1966b)

Sjöstrand, J.: Changes of nucleoside phosphatase activity in the hypoglossal nucleus during nerve regeneration. Acta Physiol. Scand. *67*, Suppl. 270, 219-228 (1966c)

Sjöstrand, J.: Neuroglial proliferation in the hypoglossal nucleus after nerve injury. Exp. Neurol. *30*, 178-189 (1971)

Skoff, R. P., Vaughn, J. E.: An autoradiographic study of cellular proliferation in degenerating rat optic nerve. J. Comp. Neurol. *141*, 133-156 (1971)

Skoff, R. P., Price, D. L., Stocks, A.: Electron microscopic autoradiographic studies of gliogenesis in rat optic nerve. II. Time of origin. J. Comp. Neurol. *169*, 313-323 (1976)

Smith, B., Rubinstein, L. J.: Histochemical observations on oxidase enzyme activity in reactive microglia and somatic macrophage. J. Pathol. Bacteriol. *83*, 572-575 (1962)

Smith, C. W., Walker, B. E.: Glial and lymphoid cell response to tumor implantation in mouse brain. Tex. Rep. Biol. Med. *25*, 585-600 (1967)

Smith, M. L., Adrian, E. K.: On the presence of mononuclear leukocytes in dorsal root ganglia following transsection of the sciatic nerve. Anat. Rec. *172*, 581-587 (1972)

Sörnäs, R.: Transformation of mononucleаr cells in cerebrospinal fluid. Acta Cytol. *15*, 545-552 (1971)

Sotelo, C., Palay, S. L.: The fine structure of the lateral vestibular nucleus in the rat. I. Neurons and neuroglial cells. J. Cell. Biol. *36*, 151-179 (1968)

Spector, W. G.: The macrophage in inflammation. Ser. Haematol. *3*, 132-144 (1970)

Spencer, P. S., Thomas, P. K.: Ultrastructural studies of the dyingback process. II. The sequestration and removal by Schwann cells and oligodendrocytes of organelles from normal and diseased axons. J. Neurocytol. *3*, 763-783 (1974)

Spielmeyer, W.: Histopathologie des Nervensystems. Berlin: Springer 1922

Spritzer, A. A., Watson, J. A., Auld, J. A., Guettnoff, M. A.: Pulmonary macrophage clearance. The hourly rates of transfer of pulmonary macrophages to the oropharynx of the rat. Arch. Environ. Health *17*, 726-734 (1968)

Starck, D.: Embryologie. Stuttgart: G. Thieme 1955

Stensaas, L. J.: Pericytes and perivascular microglial cells in the basal forebrain of the neonatal rabbit. Cell Tissue Res. *158*, 517-541 (1975)

Stensaas, L. J.: The ultrastructure of astrocytes, oligodendrocytes, and microglia in the optic nerve of urodele amphibians (A. punctatum, T. pyrrhogaster, T. viridescens). J. Neurocytol. *6*, 269-286 (1977)

Stensaas, L. J., Gilson, B. C.: Ependymal and subependymal cells of the caudato-pallial junction in the lateral ventricle of the neonatal rabbit. Z. Zellforsch. *132*, 297-322 (1972)

Stensaas, L. J., Horsley, W. W.: Production of lymphoid tissue in the rat brain by implants containing phytohemagglutinin. Acta Neuropathol. (Berl.) *31*, 71-84 (1975)

Stensaas, L. J., Reichert, W. H.: Round and amoeboid microglial cells in the neonatal rabbit brain. Z. Zellforsch. *119*, 147-163 (1971)

Stensaas, L. J., Stensaas, S. S.: Astrocytic neuroglial cells, oligodendrocytes and microgliacytes in the spinal cord of the toad. II. Electron microscopy. Z. Zellforsch. *86*, 184-213 (1968)

Stenwig, A. E.: The origin of brain macrophages in traumatic lesions, Wallerian degeneration, and retrograde degeneration. J. Neuropathol. Exp. Neurol. *31*, 696-704 (1972)

Stöcker, E., Pfeifer, U.: Autoradiographische Untersuchungen mit ^{3}H-Thymidin an der regenerierenden Rattenleber. Z. Zellforsch. *79*, 374-388 (1967)

Stroebe, H.: Experimentelle Untersuchungen über die degenerativen und reparatorischen Vorgänge bei der Heilung von Verletzungen des Rückenmarks, nebst Bemerkungen zur Histogenese der sekundären Degeneration im Rückenmark. Beitr. Pathol. Anat. *15*, 383-490 (1894)

Sumner, B. E. H.: The nature of the dividing cells around axotomized hypoglossal neurones. J. Neuropathol. Exp. Neurol. *33*, 507-518 (1974)

Szécsi, S.: Neue Beiträge zur Cytologie des Liquor cerebrospinalis: Über Art und Herkunft der Zellen. Z. Gesamte Neurol. Psychiatr. *6*, 537-588 (1911)

Takano, I.: Electron microscopic studies on retrograde chromatolysis in the hypoglossal nucleus and changes in the hypoglossal nerve following its severance and ligation. Okajimas Folia Anat. Jap. *40*, 1-69 (1964)

Takeuchi, S.: Contribution to the immunological function of the Hortega's cells by tissue culture (Japan.). Jap. Rinshobyoriketsuekishi *2*, 341-354 (1933)

Talanti, S.: Studies on the subcommissural organ of the bovine fetus. Anat. Rec. *134*, 473-489 (1959)

Tani, E., Evans, J. P.: Electron microscope studies of cerebral swelling. III. Alterations in the neuroglia and the blood vessels of the white matter. Acta Neuropathol. (Berl.) *4*, 624-639 (1965)

Tennyson, V. M., Pappas, G. D.: Electron microscopic studies of the developing telencephalic choroid plexus in normal and hydrocephalic rabbits. In: Disorders of the developing nervous system. Field, W. S., Desmond, M. M. (eds.), pp. 267-318. Springfield, Ill.: Ch. C. Thomas 1961

Tennyson, V. M., Pappas, G. D.: Fine structure of the developing telencephalic and myelencephalic choroid plexus in the rabbit. J. Comp. Neurol. *123*, 379-412 (1964)

Terry, L. C.: Discussion of the lecture of Feigin, 1969

Terry, L. C., Bray, G. M., Aguayo, A. J.: Schwann cell multiplication in developing rat unmyelinated nerves - a radioautographic study. Brain Res. *69*, 144-148 (1974)

Testa, M.: Le cellule di Gluge, le cellule à bastoncello di Nissl et la mesoglia. Folia Med. (Napoli) *14*, 725 (1928)

Thomas, H.: Licht- und elektronenmikroskopische Untersuchungen an den weichen Hirnhäuten und den Pacchioni'schen Granulationen des Menschen. Z. Mikrosk. Anat. Forsch. *75*, 270-327 (1966)

Tilney, F., Riley, H. A.: The form and functions of the central nervous system. New York: Paul B. Hoeber 1938

Torack, R. M.: Ultrastructure of capillaries reaction to brain tumors. Arch. Neurol. *5*, 416-428 (1961)
Torack, R. M., Barrnett, R. J.: Nucleoside phosphatase activity in membranous fine structures of neurones and glia. J. Histochem. Cytochem. *11*, 763-772 (1963)
Törö, I.: Histologische Untersuchungen über die Beziehungen zwischen reticuloendothelialem System und Histaminwirkung. Z. Mikrosk. Anat. Forsch. *52*, 552-571 (1942)
Torvik, A.: Phagocytosis of nerve cells during retrograde degeneration. An electron microscopic study. J. Neuropathol. Exp. Neurol. *31*, 132-146 (1972)
Torvik, A.: The relationship between microglia and brain macrophages. Experimental investigations. Acta Neuropathol. (Berl.) Suppl. *4*, 297-300 (1975)
Torvik, A., Skjörten, F.: Electron microscopic observations on nerve cell regeneration and degeneration after axon lesions. I. Changes in nerve cell cytoplasm. Acta Neuropathol. (Berl.) *17*, 248-264 (1971 a)
Torvik, A., Skjörten, F.: Electron microscopic observations on nerve cell regeneration and degeneration after axon lesions. II. Changes in the glial cell. Acta Neuropathol. (Berl.) *17*, 265-282 (1971 b)
Torvik, A., Söreide, A. J.: Nerve cell regeneration after axon lesions in new born rabbits. J. Neuropathol. Exp. Neurol. *31*, 683-695 (1972)
Treves, A. J., Feldman, M., Kaplan, H. S.: Primary cultures of human spleen macrophages in vitro. J. Immunol. Methods. *13*, 279-287 (1976)
Trumpy, J. H.: Transneuronal degeneration in the pontine nuclei of the cat. II. The glial proliferation. Ergeb. Anat. Entwicklungsgesch. *44*, 47-72 (1971)
Tschaschin, S.: Über die „ruhende Wanderzelle" und ihre Beziehungen zu den anderen Zellformen des Bindegewebes und zu den Lymphozyten. Folia Haematol. (Leipz.) *17*, 317-397 (1914)
Tsujiyama, Y.: Normal and pathological figures of neuroglia stained with Tsujiyama's method. In: Morphology of neuroglia. Nakai, J. (ed.), p. 165. Tokyo: Shoin 1963
Tsusaki, T., Yamasaki, Y., Tange, Y., Eriguchi, K., Eida, T.: Über die Lymphozyten im Plexus chorioideus partis lateralis ventriculi telencephali. Yokohama Med. Bull. *2*, 234-248 (1952)
Tyler, R. W. C., Everett, N. B.: A radioautographic study of hemopoietic repopulation using irradiated parabiotic rats. Blood *28*, 873-890 (1966)
Tyler, R. W. C., Everett, N. B.: Radioautographic study of cellular migration using parabiotic rats. Blood *39*, 249-266 (1972)
Usui, K.: The actions and absorption of subarachnoid blood. I. Experimental hydrocephalus. II. Absorption of intact red blood cells from the subarachnoid space into the blood. Nagoya J. Med. Sci. *31*, 1-23 (1968)
Vaughn, J. E.: Electron microscopic study of the vascular response to axonal degeneration in rat optic nerve. Anat. Rec. *151*, 428 (1965)
Vaughn, J. E.: An electron microscopic analysis of gliogenesis in rat optic nerves. Z. Zellforsch. *94*, 293-324 (1969)
Vaughn, J. E., Pease, D. C.: Electron microscopic studies of Wallerian degeneration in rat optic nerves. II. Astrocytes, oligodendrocytes and adventitial cells. J. Comp. Neurol. *140*, 207-266 (1970)
Vaughn, J. E., Peters, A.: A third neuroglia cell type. An electron microscopic study. J. Comp. Neurol. *133*, 269-288 (1968)
Vaughn, J. E., Skoff, R. P.: Neuroglia in experimentally altered central nervous system. Struct. Funct. Nerv. Tissue *5*, 39-72 (1972)
Vaughn, J. E., Hinds, P. L., Skoff, R. P.: Electron microscopic studies of Wallerian degeneration in rat optic nerves. I. The multipotential glia. J. Comp. Neurol. *140*, 175-206 (1970)
Vernon-Roberts, B.: Lymphocyte to macrophage transformation in the peritoneal cavity preceding the mobilization of peritoneal macrophages to inflamed areas. Nature (Lond.) *222*, 1286-1288 (1969a)

Vernon-Roberts, B.: The effects of steroid hormones on macrophage activity. Int. Rev. Cytol. *25*, 131-159 (1969b)
Vialli, M.: Istologia comparata e istofisiologia dei plessi corroidei nella serie dei vertebrati. Riv. Sper. Freniatr. *54*, 120-187, 351-411 (1930)
Vimtrup, B. S.: Beiträge zur Anatomie der Kapillaren: Über contractile Elemente in der Gefäßwand der Blutkapillaren. Z. Anat. Entwicklungsgesch. *65*, 150-182 (1922)
Vimtrup, B.: Beiträge zur Anatomie der Kapillaren. II. Weitere Untersuchungen über contractile Elemente in der Blutgefäßwand der Blutkapillaren. Z. Anat. *68*, 469-482 (1923)
Virchow, R.: Über das granulierte Aussehen der Wandungen der Gehirnventrikel. Allg. Z. Psychiatr. *3*, 242-250 (1846)
Virchow, R.: Über die Erweiterung kleiner Gefäße. Arch. Pathol. Anat. Physiol. Klin. Med. *3*, 427-462 (1851)
Virchow, R.: Über eine im Gehirn und Rückenmark des Menschen aufgefundene Substanz mit der chemischen Reaction der Cellulose. Arch. Pathol. Anat. Physiol. Klin. Med. *6*, 135-138 (1854)
Virchow, R.: Zur pathologischen Anatomie des Gehirns. Arch. Pathol. Anat. *38*, 129-142 (1867)
Visintini, F.: Sulla presenza di cellule ramificate simili alla microglia, nel cuore, nei muscoli volontari e nella vescia urinaria. Riv. Patol. Nerv. Ment. *37*, 36-47 (1931)
Vogel, F. S., Kemper, L.: Modification of Hortega's silver impregnation methods to assist in the identification of neuroglia with electron microscopy. In: Proc. 4th Internat. Congr. Neuropathology, München. Jacob, A. (ed.), Vol. II, pp. 66-71. Stuttgart: G. Thieme 1962
Volkman, A.: The origin and turnover of mononuclear cells in peritoneal exudates in rats. J. Exp. Med. *124*, 241-254 (1966)
Volkman, A.: Disparity in origin of mononuclear phagocyte populations. J. Reticuloendothel. Soc. *19*, 249-268 (1976)
Volkman, A., Gowans, J. L.: The production of macrophages in the rat. Br. J. Exp. Pathol. *46*, 50-61 (1965a)
Volkman, A., Gowans, J. L.: The origin of macrophages from bone marrow in the rat. Br. J. Exp. Pathol. *46*, 62-70 (1965b)
Wachstein, M., Meisel, E.: Histochemistry of hepatic phosphatases at a physiologic pH. With special reference to the demonstration of bile canaliculi. Am. J. Clin. Pathol. *27*, 13-23 (1957)
Waggener, J. D., Beggs, F.: The membranous coverings of neural tissues: An electron microscopy study. J. Neuropathol. Exp. Neurol. *26*, 412-426 (1967)
Wagner, H.-J., Pilgrim, Ch., Brandl, J.: Penetration and removal of horseradish peroxidase injected into the cerebrospinal fluid: Role of cerebral perivascular spaces, endothelium and microglia. Acta Neuropathol. (Berl.) *27*, 299-315 (1974)
Waksman, B. H.: Animal investigations in autosensitization: Nervous system. Ann. N.Y. Acad. Sci. *124*, 299-309 (1965)
Walker, B. E.: Infiltration and transformation of lymphoid cells in areas of spinal cord injury. Tex. Rep. Biol. Med. *21*, 615-630 (1963)
Walker, W. S.: Functional heterogeneity of macrophages in the induction and expression of acquired immunity. J. Reticuloendothel. Soc. *20*, 57-65 (1976)
Walsh, R. J., Brawer, J. R., Lin, P. S.: Supraependymal cells in the third ventricle of the neonatal rat. Anat. Rec. *190*, 257-270 (1978)
Warr, G. W., Sljivic, V. S.: Origin and stimulation of liver macrophages during stimulation of the mononuclear phagocyte system. Cell Tissue Kinet. *7*, 559-565 (1974)
Watanabe, M.: Histological changes of the arachnoid in various intracranial diseases, especially in optochiasmatic arachnoiditis (Japan.). J. Jap. Surg. *51*, 59-66 (1950)
Watson, W. E.: An autoradiographic study of the incorporation of nucleic acid precursors by neurons and glia during nerve regeneration. J. Physiol. (Lond.) *180*, 741-753 (1965)

Wechsler, W., Hager, H.: Elektronenmikroskopische Untersuchungen der Waller'schen Degeneration der peripheren Säugetiernerven. Beitr. Pathol. Anat. *126*, 352–380 (1962)

Weed, L. H.: Studies on cerebrospinals fluid: II. Theories of drainage of cerebrospinal fluid with analysis of the methods of investigation. J. Med. Res. *31*, 21–49 (1914a)

Weed, L. H.: Studies on cerebrospinal fluid. IV. The dural source of cerebrospinal fluid. J. Med. Res. *31*, 93–117 (1914b)

Weed, L. H.: The cells of the arachnoid. John Hopkins Hosp. Bull. *31*, 343–350 (1920)

Weed, L. H.: The absorption of cerebrospinal fluid into the venous system. Am. J. Anat. *31*, 191–221 (1923)

Weed, L. H.: The meninges, with special reference to the cell coverings of the leptomeninges. In: Cytology and cellular pathology of the nervous system. Penfield, W. (ed.), Vol. II, pp. 611–634. New York: Hafner Publ. Co. 1965, facsimile of 1932 edition

Weed, L. H.: Meninges und cerebrospinal fluid. J. Anat. *72*, 181–215 (1938)

Weigeldt, H.: Studien zu Phasiologie und Pathologie des Liquor cerebrospinalis. Jena: Gustav Fischer 1923

Weil, A., Davenport, H. A.: Staining of oligodendroglia and microglia in celloidin sections. Arch. Neurol. Psychiatr. (Chic.) *30*, 175–178 (1933)

Weiss, P., Wang, H., Taylor, A. C., Edds, M. V.: Proximo-distal fluid convection in the endoneurial spaces of peripheral nerves demonstrated by colored and radioactive (isotope) tracers. Am. J. Physiol. *143*, 521–540 (1945)

Wells, A. Q., Carmichael, E. A.: Microglia: an experimental study by means of tissue culture and vital staining. Brain *53*, 1–10 (1930)

Wendell-Smith, C. P., Blunt, M. J., Baldwin, F.: The ultrastructural characterization of microglial cell types. J. Comp. Neurol. *127*, 219–240 (1966a)

Wendell-Smith, C. P., Blunt, M. J., Baldwin, F.: The ultrastructural characterization of neuroglial cell types. J. Anat. *100*, 943 (1966b)

Wender, M., Sniatala, M.: Zur Feinstruktur der Liquorzellen. Wien. Z. Nervenheilkd. *27*, 38–44 (1969)

Wenzel, D., Felgenhauer, K.: The development of the blood-CSF barrier after birth. Neuropädiatrie *7*, 175–181 (1976)

Werdelin, O.: The origin, nature, and specificity of mononuclear cells in experimental autoimmune inflammations. Acta Pathol. Microbiol. Scand. [A] Suppl. *232*, 1–91 (1972)

Wernet, P., Kunkel, H. G.: Blockage of T lymphocyte receptors and the shedding phenomenon in connective tissue and other disorders. Fed. Proc. *32*, 975–983 (1973)

Westergaard, E., Brightman, M. W.: Transport of proteins across normal cerebral arterioles. J. Comp. Neurol. *152*, 17–44 (1973)

Westman, J.: The lateral cervical nucleus in the cat. III. An electron microscopic study after transsection of spinal afferents. Exp. Brain Res. *7*, 32–50 (1969)

Wetz, K., Crichton, R. R.: Ferritin. Struktur, Funktion und medizinische Aspekte. Blut *27*, 275–283 (1973)

Widal, J., Sicard, L., Ravaut, G.: Cytodiagnostic de la meningite tuberculeuse. C.R. Soc. Biol. (Paris) *52*, 838–843 (1900)

Widmann, J. J., Fahimi, H. D.: Proliferation of mononuclear phagocytes (Kupffer cells) and endothelial cells in regenerating rat liver. Am. J. Pathol. *80*, 349–360 (1975)

Wieczorek, V., Stahl, J., Bock, R.: Zum Vorkommen von Riesenzellen im Liquor cerebrospinalis. Dtsch. Z. Nervenheilkd. *192*, 246–264 (1967)

Williams, P. L., Hall, S. M.: Chronic Wallerian degeneration – an in vivo and ultrastructural study. J. Anat. *109*, 487–503 (1971)

Wislocki, G. B.: The cytology of the cerebrospinal pathway. In: Special Cytology. Cowdry, E. V. (ed.), Vol. II, pp. 1069–1107. New York: P. B. Hoeber 1928

Wislocki, G. B., Leduc, E. H.: Vital staining of the hematoencephalic barrier by silver nitrate and trypan blue, and cytological comparisons of the neurohypophysis, pineal body, area postrema, intercolumnar tubercle and supraobtic crest. J. Comp. Neurol. *96*, 371-398 (1952)

Wislocki, G. B., Leduc, E. H.: The cytology of the subcommissural organ, Reissner's fibers, periventricular glial cells and posterior collicular recess of the rat's brain. J. Comp. Neurol. *101*, 283-309 (1954)

Wolf, A., Kabat, E., Newman, W.: Histochemical studies on tissue enzymes. III. A study of the distribution of acid phosphatases with special reference to the nervous system. Am. J. Pathol. *19*, 423-440 (1943)

Wolff, J.: Beiträge zur Ultrastruktur der Kapillaren in der normalen Großhirnrinde. Z. Zellforsch. *60*, 409-431 (1963)

Wong-Riley, M. T. T.: Terminal degeneration and glial reactions in the lateral geniculate nucleus of the squirrel monkey after eye removal. J. Comp. Neurol. *144*, 61-92 (1972)

Woollam, D. H. M., Millen, J. W.: Perivascular spaces of the mammalian central nervous system. Biol. Rev. Cambr. Philos. Soc. *29*, 251-283 (1954)

Woollam, D. H. M., Millen, J. W.: The perivascular spaces of the mammallian central nervous system and their relation to the perineuronal and subarachnoid spaces. J. Anat. *89*, 193-200 (1955)

Woollard, H. H.: Vital staining of the leptomeninges. J. Anat. *58*, 89-100 (1924)

Wüllenweber, G.: Über die Funktion des Plexus chorioideus und die Entstehung des Hydrocephalus internus. Z. Neurol. *88*, 208-219 (1924)

Wustmann, O.: Bewegungsvorgänge im Liquorsystem. Klin. Wochenschr. *1*, 666-668 (1934)

Yanagihara, T., Goldstein, N. P., Svien, H. J., Bahn, R. C.: Foreign body reaction of the brain. Enzyme-histochemical study in dogs. Neurology *17*, 337-345 (1967)

Young, M. B.: Effect of bilateral nerve injury on the migration of labelled mononuclear cells to hypoglossal nuclei. J. Neuropathol. Exp. Neurol. *36*, 74-83 (1977)

Zimmermann, K. W.: Der feinere Bau der Blutkapillaren. Z. Anat. Entwicklungsgesch. *68*, 29-109 (1923)

Zinkernagel, R. M., Blanden, R. V.: Macrophage activation in mice lacking thymus-derived (T) cells. Experientia *31*, 591-592 (1975)

Subject Index

Schriftenreihe Neurologie

Neurology Series

Herausgeber:
H. J. Bauer, H. Gänshirt, P. Vogel

Die Bezieher des Archiv für Psychiatrie und Nervenkrankheiten, der Zeitschrift für Neurologie/Journal of Neurology und des Zentralblatt für die gesamte Neurologie und Psychiatrie erhalten die Schriftenreihe zu einem um 10 Prozent ermäßigten Vorzugspreis

Band 1: **W. Kahle:** Die Entwicklung der menschlichen Großhirnhemisphäre
1969. 55 Abbildungen.
VII, 116 Seiten
ISBN 3-540-04703-4

Band 2: **A. Prill:** Die neurologische Symptomatologie der akuten und chronischen Niereninsuffizienz. Befunde zur pathogenetischen Wertigkeit von Stoffwechsel-, Elektrolyt- und Wasserhaushaltsstörungen sowie zur Pathologie der Blut/Hirn-Schrankenfunktion.
1969. 49 Abbildungen.
VIII, 177 Seiten
ISBN 3-540-04704-2

Band 3: **K. Kunze:** Das Sauerstoffdruckfeld im normalen und pathologisch veränderten Muskel. Untersuchungen mit einer neuen Methode zur quantitativen Erfassung der Hypoxie in situ.
1969. 67 Abbildungen.
VIII, 118 Seiten
ISBN 3-540-04705-0

Band 4: **H. Pilz:** Die Lipide des normalen und pathologischen Liquor cerebrospinalis
1970. 4 Abbildungen, 23 Tabellen.
VIII, 123 Seiten
ISBN 3-540-05007-8

Band 5: **F. Rabe:** Die Kombination hysterischer und epileptischer Anfälle. Das Problem der „Hysteroepilepsie" in neuer Sicht. Mit einem Geleitwort von E. Bay.
1970. VII, 112 Seiten
ISBN 3-540-05008-6

Band 6: **J. Ulrich:** Die cerebralen Entmarkungskrankheiten im Kindesalter. Diffuse Hirnsklerosen. Mit einem Geleitwort von F. Lüthy
1971. 35 Abbildungen, 1 Farbtafel.
XV, 202 Seiten
ISBN 3-540-05244-5

Band 7: **K.H. Puff:** Die klinische Elekromyographie in der Differentialdiagnose von Neuro- und Myopathien. Eine Bilanz.
1971. 12 Abbildungen.
VIII, 84 Seiten
ISBN 3-540-05527-4

Band 8: **K. Piscol:** Die Blutversorgung des Rückenmarkes und ihre klinische Relevanz.
1972. 37 Abbildungen, 3 Tabellen.
VI, 91 Seiten
ISBN 3-540-05740-4

Band 9: **M. Wiesendanger:** Pathophysiology of Muscle Tone.
1972. 4 figures. VI, 46 pages
ISBN 3-540-05761-7

Band 10: **H. Spiess:** Schädigungen am peripheren Nervensystem durch ionisierende Strahlen. Mit ausführlicher englischer Zusammenfassung.
1972. 35 Abbildungen.
VIII, 71 Seiten
ISBN 3-540-05763-3

Band 11: **B. Neundörfer:** Differentialtypologie der Polyneuritiden und Polyneuropathien
1973. 18 Abbildungen. X, 205 Seiten
ISBN 3-540-06062-6

Band 12: **H. Lange-Cosack, G. Tepfer:** Das Hirntrauma im Kindes- und Jugendalter. Klinische und hirnelektrische Längsschnittuntersuchungen an 240 Kindern und Jugendlichen mit frischen Schädelhirntraumen. Unter Mitarbeit von H.-J. Schlesener. Mit einem Geleitwort von W. Tönnis
1973. 45 Abbildungen in 83 Teilfiguren. XIII, 212 Seiten
ISBN 3-540-06262-9

Band 13: **S. Kunze:** Die zentrale Ventrikulographie mit wasserlöslichen, resorbierbaren Kontrastmitteln.
1974. 24 Abbildungen. VI, 77 Seiten
ISBN 3-540-06782-5

Band 14: **E. Sluga:** Polyneuropathien. Typen und Differenzierung Ergebnisse bioptischer Untersuchungen.
1974. 20 Abbildungen, 5 Schemata.
X, 155 Seiten
ISBN 3-540-06945-3

Band 15: **H. F. Herrschaft:** Die regionale Gehirndurchblutung. Meßmethoden. Regulation, Veränderung bei den cerebralen Durchblutungsstörungen und pharmakologische Beeinflußbarkeit.
1975. 25 Abbildungen, 34 Tabellen.
X, 239 Seiten
ISBN 3-540-07363-9

Band 16: **R. Heene:** Experimental Myopathies and Muscular Dystrophy. Studies in the Formal Pathogenesis of the Myopathy of 2, 4-Dichlorophenoxyacetate.
1975. 17 figures. VI, 97 pages
ISBN 3-540-07376-0

Band 17: **T. Tsuboi, W. Christian:** Epilepsy. A Clinical, Electroencephalographic and Statistical Study of 466 Patients.
1976. 11 figures, 45 tables.
VII, 171 pages
ISBN 3-540-07735-9

Band 18: **E. Esslen:** The Acute Facial Palsies. Investigations on the Localization and Pathogenesis of Meato-Labyrinthine Facial Palsies. With a foreword by U. Fisch
1977. 127 figures, 22 tables.
X, 164 pages
ISBN 3-540-08018-X

Band 19: **J. Jörg:** Die elktrosensible Diagnostik in der Neurologie Mit einem Geleitwort von E. Bay
1977. 33 Abbildungen, 5 Tabellen.
VIII, 126 Seiten
ISBN 3-540-08236-0

Band 20: **S. Poser:** Multiple Sclerosis
1978. With 28 figures.
VIII, 93 pages
ISBN 3-540-08644-7

Springer-Verlag
Berlin
Heidelberg
New York